Research Methods in Neurochemistry

Edited by
Neville Marks

New York State Research Institute for Neurochemistry and Drug Addiction
Ward's Island, New York, New York

and

Richard Rodnight

Department of Biochemistry
Institute of Psychiatry
University of London
London, Great Britain

Volume 1

Ⴔ PLENUM PRESS • NEW YORK-LONDON • 1972

Library of Congress Catalog Card Number 76-183563
ISBN 0-306-36001-2

© 1972 Plenum Press, New York
A Division of Plenum Publishing Corporation
227 West 17th Street, New York, N. Y. 10011

United Kingdom edition published by Plenum Press, London
A Division of Plenum Publishing Company, Ltd.
Davis House (4th Floor), 8 Scrubs Lane, Harlesden, London, NW10 6SE, England

Printed in the United States of America

Contributors to This Volume

ALAN A. BOULTON   Psychiatric Research Unit, University Hospital, Saskatoon, Saskatchewan, Canada

STEPHEN R. COHEN   New York State Research Institute for Neurochemistry and Drug Addiction, Ward's Island, New York

CARL W. COTMAN   Department of Psychobiology, University of California at Irvine

ALAN N. DAVISON   M.R.C. Membrane Biology Group, Department of Biochemistry, Charing Cross Hospital Medical School, London

JOSEPH D. FENSTERMACHER   Office of the Associate Scientific Director for Experimental Therapeutics, National Institutes of Health, National Cancer Institute, Bethesda, Maryland

M. GOLDSTEIN   Department of Psychiatry, Neurochemistry Laboratories, New York University Medical Center, New York

LLOYD A. HORROCKS   Department of Physiological Chemistry, The Ohio State University, Columbus, Ohio

PATRICIA V. JOHNSTON   Children's Research Center and the Burnsides Research Laboratory, University of Illinois at Urbana-Champaign

JOHN R. MAJER   Department of Chemistry, University of Birmingham, Edgbaston, Birmingham, England

RENÉE K. MARGOLIS   Department of Pharmacology, State University of New York, Downstate Medical Center, Brooklyn

RICHARD U. MARGOLIS   Department of Pharmacology, New York University School of Medicine, New York

BRUCE S. MCEWEN   The Rockefeller University, New York

WILLIAM T. NORTON   The Saul R. Korey Department of Neurology, Albert Einstein College of Medicine, New York

SHIRLEY E. PODUSLO   The Saul R. Korey Department of Neurology, Albert Einstein College of Medicine, New York

SIDNEY ROBERTS   Department of Biological Chemistry, School of Medicine, and the Brain Research Institute, University of California Center for the Health Sciences, Los Angeles

BETTY I. ROOTS   Department of Zoology, University of Toronto

SOLOMON H. SNYDER   Department of Pharmacology and Experimental Therapeutics and Department of Psychiatry, The Johns Hopkins University School of Medicine, Baltimore, Maryland

MARTHA SPOHN   M.R.C. Membrane Biology Group, Department of Biochemistry, Charing Cross Hospital Medical School, London

GRACE Y. SUN   Laboratory of Neurochemistry, Cleveland Psychiatric Institute, Cleveland, Ohio

KENNETH M. TAYLOR   Department of Pharmacology and Experimental Therapeutics and Department of Psychiatry, The Johns Hopkins University School of Medicine, Baltimore, Maryland

L. S. WOLFE   Department of Neurology and Neurosurgery, McGill University, and Donner Laboratory of Experimental Neurochemistry, Montreal Neurogical Institute, Montreal, Canada

RICHARD E. ZIGMOND   The Rockefeller University, New York

CLAIRE E. ZOMZELY-NEURATH   Roche Institute of Molecular Biology, Nutley, New Jersey

Introduction

On picking up this first volume of a new series of books the reader may ask the two questions: (a) why research methods? and (b) why in neurochemistry? The answers to these questions are easy—they more than justify the volumes to come and show the strong need for their existence.

It is customary to think of methods as a necessary but unexciting means to an end—to relegate advances in methodology to a minor role in the creative, original portion of advances in science. This is not the case; the pace-setting function of methodology is well illustrated in most areas of neurobiology. To formulate our questions to Nature (which is the essence of experimental design), methodology is needed; to get answers to our questions we have to devise yet new methods. The chapters of the present volume fully illustrate how the development of a new method can cut a new path— how it can open new fields, just as the microscope founded histology. Heterogeneity of structures presents a formidable challenge for methodology in the nervous system, yet methods for separating the structures are essential if we ever want to decipher the enigma of functional contribution of the elements to the whole. The problem is not only physical separation—clearly methods are essential to study complex structures *in situ*. Once we separate a structure, more new methods are needed to analyze and to identify its elements. Much as we have tried over many years (and are still engaged in trying), with Dr. Marks, to devise methods for measuring protein turnover and for measuring protein breakdown in the living brain, a good method that would open this important area to study still eludes us (no wonder therefore that Dr. Marks became one of the concerned editors).

No method is the final one, nor can any one be best for all purposes; in addition to developing new, more specific, sensitive, and rapid procedures, we often have to dust off old-established ones from our shelves and modify them to a particular new purpose. The need for these adaptations as well as the development of new methods makes us look forward to a number of volumes in addition to this very well executed initial one, and to welcome them — in spite of the ever-increasing burden of the information explosion.

I should close with the second question: why neurochemistry? Surely, few readers of this book have to be convinced of the importance of the nervous system. Some say that just because the brain is at the top end of the human anatomy it does not prove that that's the important end. They might be right; undoubtedly many functions of the nervous system — memory, emotion, learning — generate a great deal of trouble for us. But among its possible properties is creativity, which needs to function optimally if we want to create ... new research methods in neurochemistry.

ABEL LAJTHA

New York, June 1972

Preface

The present volume is the first of a series which aims to provide investigators in the neurosciences with detailed descriptions of experimental procedures for the biochemical study of the nervous system. We hope that the tremendous growth in neurochemistry as a branch of biochemistry with its own specialized methodology is sufficient justification for its aim. Sound methods form the basis of advances in any experimental subject and this is especially true in this relatively new and expanding field. Neurochemistry embraces many specialities, with the consequences that descriptions of techniques are often minimal and scattered among a wide variety of literature sources.

The arrangement and selection of chapters for the present volume has been dictated largely by the tradition of subdivision already established in biochemistry. Thus chapters on subcellular fractionation and specific molecular constituents have been grouped separately from those concerned with studies on intact tissues or animals. A separate section has been accorded to biogenic amines because of their central importance and the unique roles that they play in nerve function. In so complex an organ as the brain special importance is assigned to ultrastructural studies, which are grouped together with the section on subcellular components. A major objective of the present series is to present within each chapter sufficient detail for ongoing experiments without the need for the investigator to have extensive recourse to the literature. As such it is aimed primarily at the skilled research worker, although we hope it will also facilitate teaching programs and assist research students embarking on their chosen careers. Authors have been urged to stress methods that can be employed with available equipment rather than describe procedures requiring expensive instruments outside the range of most laboratories. We anticipate that one advantage of a continuing series will be to add refinements to established methods, or provide new approaches to old problems when deemed appropriate or justified by new developments. However, the series is not intended to replace older texts where well proven methods still have their rightful place and have yet to be superseded by newer procedures. It is our sincere hope that this collection of modern methods may make a lasting and valuable contribution to the advancement of neurochemical knowledge and ultimately to the amelioration of diseases afflicting the nervous system.

Finally we wish to acknowledge the assistance and encouragement of Plenum Press and above all the many contributors who have made this volume possible. Suggestions for areas to be covered or improvements for future volumes are most welcome.

RICHARD RODNIGHT, *London*
NEVILLE MARKS, *New York*

May 1972

Contents

Chapter 3

**Separation of Myelin Fragments from the Central
    Nervous System**

   Martha Spohn and Alan N. Davison

Chapter 4

**Principles for the Optimization of Centrifugation Conditions
    for Fractionation of Brain Tissue**

   Carl W. Cotman

Chapter 5

Brain Ribosomes

Claire E. Zomzely-Neurath and Sidney Roberts

Chapter 6

Isolation of Brain Cell Nuclei

Bruce S. McEwen and Richard E. Zigmond

Section II. PROPERTIES OF INTACT NEURAL TISSUES

Chapter 7

Ventriculocisternal Perfusion as a Technique for Studying Transport and Metabolism within the Brain
Joseph D. Fenstermacher

Chapter 8

The Estimation of Extracellular Space of Brain Tissue *in Vitro*
Stephen R. Cohen

Section III. COMPONENTS OF NEURAL TISSUES

Chapter 9

Ethanolamine Plasmalogens

Lloyd A. Horrocks and Grace Y. Sun

Chapter 10

Methods for Separation and Determination of Gangliosides

L. S. Wolfe

Section IV. BIOLOGICALLY ACTIVE AMINES

Chapter 12

Assay of Biogenic Amines and Their Deaminating Enzymes in Animal Tissues

Solomon H. Snyder and Kenneth M. Taylor

Chapter 13

Enzymes Involved in the Catalysis of Catecholamine Biosynthesis

M. Goldstein

Chapter 14

**Detection and Quantitative Analysis of Some Noncatecholic Primary
Aromatic Amines**

Alan A. Boulton and John R. Majer

Research Methods in Neurochemistry

Volume 1

Section I
ULTRASTRUCTURE AND FRAGMENTATION OF NEURAL TISSUES

Chapter 1

Nervous System Cell Preparations: Microdissection and Micromanipulation

Betty I. Roots and Patricia V. Johnston

Department of Zoology, University of Toronto
Toronto, Canada
and
Children's Research Center and the Burnsides
Research Laboratory, University of Illinois at
Urbana-Champaign, Illinois

I. INTRODUCTION: A BRIEF HISTORY

A classic approach to the elucidation of any complex structure, whether it be a living organism or an inanimate body, is to separate the component parts and study them in isolation. The degree of structural complexity of nervous systems and the consequent difficulty in interpreting gross observations, both morphological and functional, has stimulated numerous attempts to isolate individual units. More than 100 years ago Deiters (1865) published drawings of neurons which he had dissected from parts of the nervous system. The most striking drawings are those of cells he dissected from the anterior horn of spinal cord. In more recent years cells prepared by hand dissection have been the subject of many studies, the most prominent being those of Lowry (1952, 1953, 1956), Giacobini (1956, 1959, 1962, 1964), and Hydén (1959, 1960, 1964). Chemical and biochemical studies of single cells are limited by the sensitivity of the analytical methods available and ways have been sought to obtain cells in greater number and by less laborious techniques than hand dissection.

The first attempt at bulk separation of neurons and glia was made by McIlwain (1954) who, by using enzymes to break up the tissue, succeeded

3

in preparing a cell suspension but did not separate the component cell types. Chu (1954) made histological observations on cells from the anterior horn of human spinal cord, preparing his cell suspension by homogenizing the tissue with small glass beads. Korey (1957) prepared a suspension of glia from white matter by homogenizing small pieces of tissue in a Waring blendor in which the blades had been dulled and flattened. The suspension was then filtered through a siliconized silk grid and returned to the blendor. This cycle was repeated several times and the final suspension was passed through a finer silk grid. As the primary means of preparing cell suspensions, Roots and Johnston (1964) passed the tissue through a graded series of sieves, a procedure which has been adopted by several subsequent workers. Recently Norton and Poduslo (1969, 1970) combined enzymic digestion and sieving as a means of tissue disintegration.

The methods developed for the isolation of individual cell types fall into two categories, micromanipulation by which relatively small numbers of cells are prepared, and macroscale methods involving various centrifuge techniques. Centrifugation on a discontinuous gradient was introduced by Korey (1957), who also used a relatively homogeneous nervous tissue as starting material, namely white matter, a precedent followed more recently by Fewster, Scheibel, and Mead (1967). Rose (1965) applied centrifugation, also on discontinuous gradients, to the separation of cell fractions from suspensions prepared from the highly heterogeneous mammalian cortex, by passing the tissue through sieves. Most of the methods developed in the following years involve variation in the media used, the speed of centrifugation, and the combination of techniques. For example, Satake and Abe (1966) and Freysz et al. (1967) used organic solvents during preparation of the fractions; Bocci (1966) used low-speed centrifugation as opposed to the high speeds used by Rose; Satake et al. (1968) combined centrifugation with separation by sieving, and Norton and Poduslo (1969, 1970) combined enzyme digestion with separation by centrifugation. The use of zonal cen-

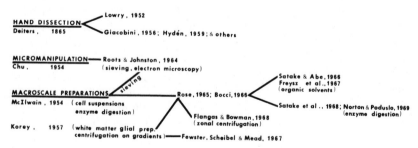

Fig. 1. The historical development of procedures for the isolation of neuronal and glial perikarya. (Modified from Johnston and Roots, 1970.)

trifugation was introduced by Flangas and Bowman (1968). These developments and the relationships between them are illustrated in Fig. 1.

Microdissection and micromanipulation techniques have the important advantage of providing cell preparations having a high degree of purity. These methods are of special interest to investigators who wish to study discrete functional units. They are, for example, invaluable to workers interested in the effects of the application of drugs, neurotransmitters, etc., to specific nuclei; to those conducting morphological and ultrastructural studies on pathological states affecting small areas of the brain; and to workers attempting to relate learning experiences to chemical changes in small groups of cells. Such micromethods are the subject of this chapter.

II. PREPARATION BY MICRODISSECTION

A. Freeze-Dried Tissue

Nerve cell perikarya were first isolated for neurochemical studies by Lowry who developed a technique for dissecting single cell bodies from freeze-dried sections of tissue (Lowry, 1952, 1953, 1956).

Small pieces of tissue, not more than a few millimeters in any dimension, are frozen by placing them on a piece of hardened filter paper and plunging them into liquid nitrogen or isopentane cooled to a slush with liquid nitrogen. The tissue is then allowed to warm up to -20 to $-10\,°C$ in a cold room maintained at this temperature before attaching it to the block-holder for sectioning. At no time must the temperature rise above $-10\,°C$ or ice-crystal artefacts may develop.

A piece of $\frac{5}{8}$-inch alloy metal rod with a cross-grooved end makes a convenient block-holder. The block of tissue is attached to the holder with a paste of mashed brain in the following way. A good blob of paste is applied to the holder which is then chilled to just above freezing. The frozen tissue block is pushed into the paste and the whole is immediately plunged into a beaker of cold petroleum ether which is maintained at a low temperature by a bath of petroleum ether and Dry Ice. Success in mounting depends upon the relative temperatures of the block and the paste. The block should freeze the paste, not be melted by it.

When the block and holder are cooled, sections are cut with a microtome in a cryostat. The cutting temperature is critical. If it is too high the section will be compressed and if it is too low the section will fragment. The optimal temperature for cutting usually lies between -15 and $-20\,°C$. Sections are cut singly with a slow, steady motion. They are kept flat by holding a small camel's hair brush against the cutting face of the block as the section is cut. The brush is moved slightly faster than the block. The thickness of the section is determined by the size of the cell bodies in the tissue. For rabbit dorsal root ganglion and anterior horn 25 μm is suitable.

As they are cut, sections are transferred to a holder with a pointed wooden or plastic stick or fine forceps tipped with paper or thin flexible plastic. Holders are made from aluminum blocks in which holes 7 μm in diameter have been drilled, clipped between two 3 × 1 inch glass slides. Details of a section holder are shown in Fig. 2. As soon as a holder is filled, the cover is replaced to prevent evaporation of water from the sections at the temperature of the cryostat. One to four section holders are placed in

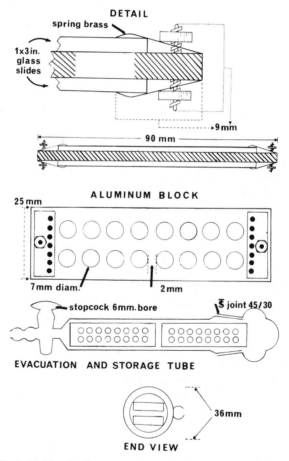

Fig. 2. Holder for frozen sections and glass evacuation tube for drying frozen sections. (Redrawn from Lowry, 1953.)

a special drying tube (see Fig. 2) which is then transferred to a small constant temperature box at -30 to $-40\,°C$. The tube and its contents are allowed to reach this lower temperature and then a vacuum of 0.1 Torr or less is applied to dry the sections. A liquid nitrogen or Dry Ice trap is used to condense the water removed. At no time must the temperature be allowed to rise above $-10\,°C$. After 1–6 hr, depending on the number of sections, they are dry and the tube may be removed from the cold box, but vacuum is maintained until room temperature is reached.

Individual cell bodies may be dissected from freeze-dried sections prepared in this way by freehand teasing out with fine needles under a magnification of about $\times 90$. Lowry *et al.* (1956) used needles ground to a blade-shaped point, but fine steel needles or entomological pins of no special shape mounted in glass handles may be used with equal success. It is desirable for the experimenter to wear a mask during these operations to prevent blowing the section away. A dust shield will prevent contamination from the air.

Sections are transferred with "hair points," which are short pieces of hair mounted in a glass holder, and held down during dissection by hair loops. The preparation of hair points and loops is described in Section V.

It is recommended that experimenters wishing to use this technique begin by working with dorsal root ganglion as the cell bodies are easy to see in the freeze-dried sections. From this tissue the investigator may proceed to other parts of the nervous system for which experience is required to recognize the cell bodies.

B. Fresh Tissue

1. Neuronal Perikarya

The dissection of nerve cell bodies from fresh tissue was pioneered by Giacobini (1956) and Hydén (1959). Giacobini worked with spinal and sympathetic ganglion cells and anterior horn cells of spinal cord. Hydén used mammalian brain. Since they are encapsulated, the cells of spinal and sympathetic ganglia can readily be located. With mammalian brain the most difficult part of the technique is identifying the cell body. However, this difficulty may be overcome relatively easily if the problem is approached in the following way.

At first as large an animal as possible should be used. Pig, sheep, and ox brains (which can be obtained fresh from local abattoirs) are preferable, but rabbit brains are also suitable for use during the period when the investigator is gaining experience. Furthermore, the investigator is well advised to begin by using nuclei containing large cells such as the lateral vestibular nucleus or red nucleus before proceeding to the cells of his choice. The size difference between comparable cells of different species may be illustrated by the following example. Deiters' neurons from the lateral vestibular nucleus of ox brain are approximately 200 μm long and 100 μm wide (see Fig. 5) whereas those from rabbit brain are 70 × 70 μm and from rat brain 40 μm in diameter. The advantages of starting with large cells are obvious.

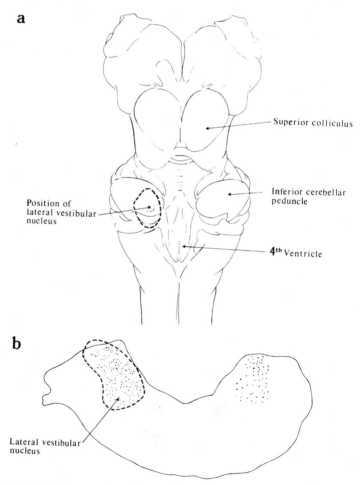

Fig. 3. (a) Brainstem of ox. The position of the lateral vestibular nucleus is outlined. (b) A section through the medulla showing the position of the lateral vestibular nucleus.

A slice is taken through the desired locus; in the case of the lateral vestibular nucleus this passes through the medulla at the level of the inferior cerebellar peduncles (Fig. 3). A piece of tissue containing the cells wanted for study is excised and placed on a glass slide. The uppermost surface of the piece should be observed very carefully at a suitable magnification under a stereomicroscope and differences in texture and color noted. (For ox brain a magnification of × 20 is adequate; for rabbit brain × 30 should be used; and for rat brain × 40.) Then a solution of methylene blue in an isotonic Ringer's solution (1 part in 10,000) should be applied while the surface is kept under observation. The dye is taken up preferentially by the neurons and their position may be related to the textural and color differences previously noted. (The position of the nucleus in the slice may also be verified by staining with methylene blue.) Perikarya with processes of varying lengths may now readily be dissected out by gentle teasing with a pair of fine needles.

This procedure should be repeated using progressively less stain until the neurons can be recognized and dissected out without its use. The dissection is then carried out in a drop of Ringer's solution. Advantage may be taken of the yellow lipofuscin pigment which is present in the neurons of adult animals. Illumination can be adjusted in such a way that the pigment can be seen, thus facilitating identification of neuronal somata. A piece of aluminum foil placed under the slide to reflect the light is often useful. Once the technique has been mastered on large cells, the investigator should have little difficulty in proceeding to smaller cells. The only difference is that higher magnifications must be used.

Giacobini (1956) used micromanipulators during dissection but in our experience and that of others, this is not essential. Some investigators (Hydén, 1959) use 0.25 M sucrose solution rather than a Ringer solution for the dissection medium.

2. Glia and Neuropil

With the exception of spinal ganglion cells, neurons in the vertebrate nervous system are surrounded by a complexity of cells and cell processes termed the neuropil. Components are oligodendrocytes, astrocytes, dendrites, and synaptic endings. Opinions differ as to the relative proportions of these components in the neuropil immediately surrounding individual nerve cell bodies. Some authors (Hamberger, 1964; Hydén, and Pigon, 1960) claim that oligodendrocytes predominate with not more than 10% astrocytes and a negligible quantity of dendrites and nerve endings. Clumps of tissue dissected from around neuronal somata are therefore regarded as oligodendrocytes by these authors. Others (Epstein and O'Connor, 1965) have a different view of the heterogeneity of such clumps of tissue and term them neuropil. Whatever views the investigator may hold on this matter, the technique for preparing these clumps is the same.

A piece of fresh nervous tissue is removed as described in the previous section and placed in a drop of medium on a slide. Single nerve cell bodies with adhering neuropil/glia may then be lifted out of the tissue with a stainless steel microspatula. Alternatively, they may be removed directly from the cut surfaces of the original brain slice. The neuropil/glia may then be dissected off by gentle manipulation with fine needles. It sticks together easily and can be formed into a spheroid clump.

The capsular cells of spinal and sympathetic ganglia provide a more homogeneous population of glial cells, and these have been studied by Giacobini (1956, 1959). These cells also may be separated from the neurons with fine needles.

III. PREPARATION OF NEURONAL PERIKARYA BY MICROMANIPULATION USING CELL SUSPENSIONS

The outstanding advantage of the method (Roots and Johnston, 1964) to be described below is that considerable numbers of neuronal perikarya can be obtained free from extraneous matter. If particular brain nuclei are selected as the starting material, a relatively homogeneous collection of cells can be obtained.

Although this method may be applied to any part of the nervous system, when the ratio of neuronal perikarya to other matter in the starting material is high more cells can be obtained in unit time.

The nucleus or other area from which perikarya are to be prepared is excised from fresh brain. As for hand dissection, it is recommended that in the first instance a large animal be used; also preferable is a nucleus containing large cells, e.g., the lateral vestibular nucleus. Furthermore, nuclei from six brains should be pooled. After the initial experience both the amount of material and the size of the animal may be reduced.

The dimensions in the description below are for the lateral vestibular nucleus of ox; sizes for other material are given later.

The excised tissue is placed in cold (4 °C) medium. In the first instance the investigator should use 0.25 M sucrose since the cells are more easily seen in this medium. When no difficulty is experienced in recognizing cells, then the transition may be made to other media. The choice of media is, of course, dictated by the needs of the individual investigator. In general, however, maintenance of the integrity of the cell (the retention of surface structures and the reduction of the effects of anoxia on cellular organelles) will be of concern to most workers. A number of media constituents and factors are now known to assist in the maintenance of cellular integrity. These appear to act largely by decreasing the effects of shear stresses during preparation of the suspension. They include the use of gangliosides in media, a medium of low pH (Johnston and Roots, 1970) and the use of albumin (Satake *et al*, 1968). The medium used by Norton and Poduslo (1970) which includes albumen and calf serum also seems to be successful in maintaining the integrity of both neurons and glia. A detailed account of this medium is given in Chapter 2 of this book.

The tissue is then placed on a nylon sieve (5–6 cm in diameter) with apertures of 300–350 μm square which is attached to a Büchner flask which is packed in crushed ice. A sieve may be made simply and conveniently from a wide-necked polyethylene bottle with a polyethylene screw cap. The bottom of the bottle is cut away, leaving a section approximately 3 inches deep attached to the neck. The center of the cap is cut away, leaving only a narrow rim. Pieces of monofilament nylon cloth with apertures of appropriate size are fitted by placing them over the neck of the bottle and screwing the modified cap into place.

The tissue is forced through the sieve by applying firm pressure above with a glass pestle with a flat surface and suction below from a high-vacuum pump. Fresh medium is added to the material as required and the underside of the sieve is cleared from time to time. The resulting coarse suspension is then sucked through a finer monofilament nylon cloth (apertures 108–110 μm square) into a flask packed in ice while a continuous jet of medium is applied from a wash bottle. The fine suspension produced is allowed to settle for 10 min at 4 °C.

A sample of 10–20 ml is then withdrawn from the bottom of the flask. A few drops of this suspension are transferred to a cavity slide and observed at a magnification of × 20 with a stereomicroscope fitted with a cold stage. While microscopes with fitted cold stages are available commercially, an investigator who does not have one at his disposal may construct a substitute very readily. A metal cylinder of a suitable height for the microscope is filled with brine, which is then frozen by placing in a deep freeze at −20 °C or below. Several layers of filter paper are placed on the lid until the fluid in a cavity slide maintains a temperature of about 4 °C. With an insulating jacket of expanded polystyrene, such a stage can be used over a period of 2–3 hr depending upon the ambient temperature.

Neuronal perikarya can be seen suspended in the medium. The angle of incidence of the light is critical and should be adjusted for optimal visibility of cell somata. The accumulations of yellow lipofuscin pigment in neurons from adult animals are valuable aids to recognition. Either an efficient heat filter (a vessel of water is excellent for this purpose) should be placed between the light source and the object, or light should be conducted along a Plexiglas, Perspex, or Lucite rod $\frac{3}{4}$ to 1 in. in diameter and about 12 in. long.

Neuronal perikarya are transferred from the suspension by means of a nylon loop to another cavity slide containing fresh medium. The loop is brought up under the cell which may then be lifted out of the fluid. The loop is then turned over (i.e., through 180°) so that the cell is on the underside and lowered into the fresh medium until the cell just touches the bottom of the slide. The cells adhere slightly to the glass so that the loop may be withdrawn, leaving the cell in the cavity slide. A "jacket" of filter paper on the collecting slide helps to combat condensation. The microscope should also be fitted with a plastic shield to prevent contamination by air-borne particles (Fig. 4). By this method an experienced worker can collect 70 or more cells per minute. A small collection of perikarya is shown in Fig. 5 together with one perikaryon shown at higher magnification. When a collection slide is filled, the medium may be withdrawn by means of a fine pipette operated by mouth suction (any particles of extraneous matter may also be

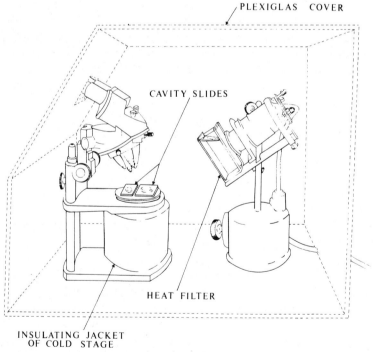

Fig. 4. An illustration of the microscope and accessories used in the microdissection and micromanipulation of perikarya.

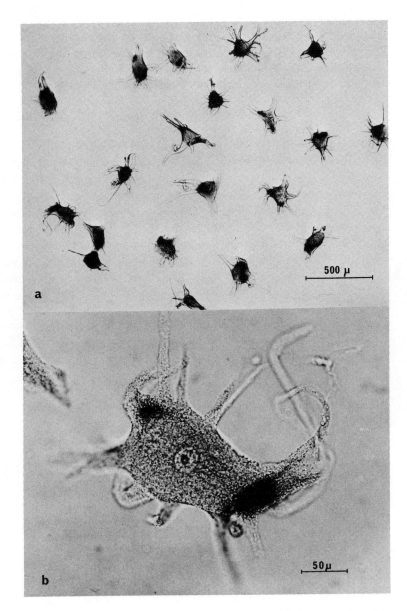

Fig. 5. (a) A small collection of neuronal perikarya. (b) A neuronal perikaryon isolated from the lateral vestibular nucleus of ox brain. (From Roots and Johnston, 1964.)

removed in this way), and the perikarya frozen rapidly and stored at
− 20° C or below for subsequent analysis.

Glial perikarya may be recognized also in the suspension and may
be collected in the same way using a smaller nylon loop. Sieves with apertures
of 300 μm square and 74 μm square are used for rabbit lateral vestibular
nucleus. For rat cortical cells sieves with apertures of 130 μm and 40 μm
should be used.

IV. HANDLING NEURONAL AND GLIAL PERIKARYA
FOR ELECTRON MICROSCOPY AND ADJUNCT TECHNIQUES

Preparation for electron microscopy of isolated cells may readily be
carried out in polyethylene planchets 2 cm in diameter such as are used for
counting radioactive material (Johnston and Roots, 1965). Cells adhere
sufficiently well to the polyethylene to enable solutions to be changed by
decanting or withdrawal by pipette. Moreover, embedding media do not
adhere to the planchet and the final block is readily popped out. Transfer
is made to the planchet by means of a nylon loop in the way described
in the previous section.

Embedded cells can be cut out individually with a single-edged razor
blade if the blocks are warmed slightly. This is most easily achieved by

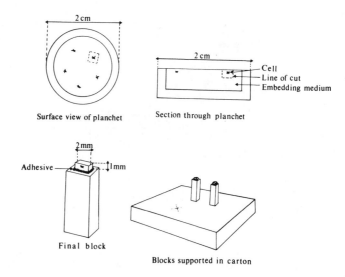

Fig. 6. An illustration of the method of preparing single perikarya for
electron microscopy.

means of a closed metal box filled with hot, but not boiling, water. The block is placed on filter paper on the surface of the box and cutting is done under a stereomicroscope. The small blocks each containing one cell are then stuck onto previously prepared blank blocks by means of epoxy adhesive. These blocks may be conveniently supported in light cardboard cartons, during the curing of the adhesive (Fig. 6).

Nylon loops can be used for supporting cells for special needs.

V. PREPARATION OF INSTRUMENTS USED IN THE TECHNIQUES

   a. Nylon and Hair Loops. Glass tubing 8 mm in diameter is pulled to form a Pasteur-type pipette. The end is bent to form a hook by means of which the pipette is suspended. The region of taper is then heated cautiously with a microburner until the pipette falls under its own weight, thus pulling a very fine tube (Fig. 7). The finest end of the tube is broken off at the point where the internal diameter is little more than twice the diameter of the thread to be inserted. A short length of the chosen thread is then inserted to form a

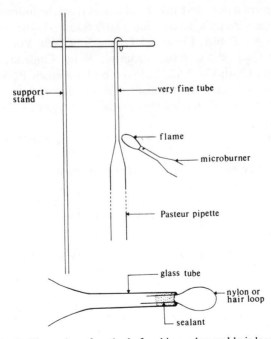

Fig. 7. Illustration of method of making nylon and hair loops.

loop and sealed in by touching a drop of Japan gold size or Plexiglas, Perspex, or Lucite dissolved in chloroform on a glass rod to the end so that the tip becomes filled by capillarity. Japan gold size is the most satisfactory sealant as it does not contaminate media.

For most purposes, loops made from 12- and 15- denier nylon thread are the most satisfactory. A 12-denier thread gives a loop of 150–200 μm in diameter.* Loops of 60 μm in diameter can be made from 9-denier thread. Loops made from finer thread are not sufficiently rigid to be useful.

b. Hair Points. These are made by sealing short lengths of hair (or nylon thread) into glass holders in the way described above. The degree of stiffness and resilience is determined by the thickness of the hair (or thread) and by the length of the piece used.

c. Microburner. A simple microburner suitable for the preparation of glass holders can be made from a Pyrex glass Pasteur-type pipette. The pipette is attached to the gas supply by rubber tubing and the size of the flame is controlled by a hosecock screw clamp.

APPENDIX: SOURCES OF MATERIALS

Monofilament nylon cloth may be obtained from the following suppliers: General Biological Supply House Inc., 8200 South Hoyne Ave., Chicago, Ill. 60620, U.S.A.; Tobler, Ernst and Traber, Inc., New York, N.Y. 10007, U.S.A.; P.K. Dutt & Co. Ltd., Bromley, Kent, England; or Nippon-Nakano Bolting Cloth Co. Ltd., Tokyo Yofuku-Kaikan Building, No. 13, Hachiman-Cho, Ichigaya, Shinjukuku, Tokyo, Japan.

For nylon thread manufacturers in the investigator's country should be approached.

Stainless steel thread may be obtained from A.B. Kanthal, Hallstahammar, Sweden.

Gold size may be obtained from artists' suppliers.

ACKNOWLEDGMENTS

We thank Dr. O.H. Lowry, Williams and Wilkins Co. and Academic Press, Inc. for permission to reproduce illustrations.

---

* The diameter of the loop is determined by the thickness and resilience of the thread. Hair forms the largest loops, although good loops may be made from the fine hair of newborn babies, a material which has long been used by embryologists for manipulation of small cells.

Dr. Johnston is supported by Grant HD 03598 from the National Institutes of Health.

We are indebted to Miss I.R. Nosyk for the drawings and to Mr. Stuart Waterman for photographic assistance.

REFERENCES

Bocci, V. (1966) *Nature (Lond.)* **212**, 826.

Chu, L.-W. (1954) *J. Comp. Neurol.* **100**, 381.

Deiters, O. (1865) *Untersuchungen über Gehirn und Rückenmark des Menschen und der Säugethiere*, Schultz, Braunschweig.

Epstein, M. H., and O'Connor, J. S. (1965) *J. Neurochem.* **12**, 389.

Fewster, M. E., Scheibel, A. B., and Mead, J. F. (1967) *Brain Res.* **6**, 401.

Flangas, A. L., and Bowman, R. E. (1968) *Science* **161**, 1025.

Freysz, L., Bieth, R., Judes, C., Jacob, M., and Sensenbrenner, M. (1967) *J. Physiol. Paris* **59**, 239.

Giacobini, E. (1956) *Acta Physiol. Scand.* **36**, 276.

Giacobini, E. (1959) *Acta Physiol. Scand.* **45** (Suppl. 156), 1.

Giacobini, E. (1962) *J. Neurochem.* **9**, 169.

Giacobini, E. (1964) in *Morphological and Biochemical Correlates of Neural Activity* (M. M. Cohen and R. S. Snider, eds.), Harper and Row, New York, p. 15.

Hamberger, A. (1964) *Bol. Inst. Estud. Méd. Biol. Méx.* **22**, 129.

Hydén, H. (1959) *Nature (Lond.)*, **184**, 433.

Hydén, H., and Egyhazi, E. (1964) *Proc. Nat. Acad. Sci. U.S.* **52**, 1030.

Hydén, H., and Pigon, A. (1960) *J. Neurochem.* **6**, 57.

Johnston, P. V., and Roots, B. I. (1965) *Nature (Lond.)* **205**, 778.

Johnston, P. V., and Roots, B. I. (1970) *Int. Rev. Cytol.* **29**, 265.

Korey, S. R. (1957) in *Metabolism of the Nervous System*, (D. Richter, ed.), Pergamon Press, London, p. 87.

Lowry, O. H. (1952) *Science,* **116**, 526.

Lowry, O. H. (1953) *J. Histochem. Cytochem.* **1**, 420.

Lowry, O. H., Roberts, N. R., and Chang, M.-L. W. (1956) *J. Biol. Chem.* **222**, 97.

McIlwain, H. (1954) *Proc. Univ. Otago Med. Sch.* **32**, 17.

Norton, W. T., and Poduslo, S. E. (1969) *Fed. Proc.* **28**, 734.

Norton, W. T., and Poduslo, S. E. (1970) *Science* **167**, 1144.

Roots, B. I., and Johnston, P. V. (1964) *J. Ultrastruct. Res.* **10**, 350.

Rose, S. P. R. (1965) *Nature (Lond.)* **206**, 621.

Satake, M., and Abe, S. (1966) *J. Biochem. Tokyo* **59**, 72.

Satake, M., Hasegawa, S., Abe, S., and Tanaka, R. (1968) *Brain Res.* **11**, 246.

Chapter 2

The Bulk Separation of Neuroglia and Neuron Perikarya

Shirley E. Poduslo and William T. Norton

The Saul R. Korey Department of Neurology
Albert Einstein College of Medicine
New York, New York

I. INTRODUCTION

Morphological studies of the central nervous system reveal an incredibly complex meshwork of neuronal and glial somata, axons, dendrites and glial processes, myelin and capillaries. It is apparent that biochemical studies of this tissue reflect the sum of the individual properties of each separate cell type. Yet we know that neurons, astrocytes, oligodendroglia, microglia, and the other cells composing the brain have quite different functions and quite different biochemical properties. Even specialized regions of a single cell, for example, the dendritic tree, neuron perikaryon and axon, have their own particular ultrastructure, function, and complement of subcellular organelles; and therefore most probably have a unique composition and chemistry. Over the years many efforts have been made to resolve this complex tissue and determine the contribution made by each separate component to the biochemistry of the brain. It is beyond the scope of this chapter to discuss all the approaches, but they include microscopical histochemistry, quantitative histochemistry of different cortical layers and brain regions, microchemistry of hand-dissected cells, macrochemistry of grossly separated areas, studies of tumors, tissue culture of pure cell lines, and subcellular fractionation of constituents known to arise from a particular cell such as synaptosomes, myelin, and neuronal and glial nuclei.

    The recent development of techniques for the bulk separation of neurons and glia affords the most promising approach to the determination of their individual properties. Cell suspensions are routinely prepared for tissue culture from many organs, usually with immature or embryonic tissue where intercellular adhesion is not a major problem. Moreover, separation of such suspensions is usually not required. The complexity of the nervous system, with its intertwined processes and minimal extracellular space, presumably inhibited even the attempt to extend these methods to brain. Credit for the first serious effort to prepare a cell suspension and CNS cells in bulk must be given to Korey and co-workers (Korey, 1957; Korey *et al.*, 1958). They isolated a glial-rich fraction from white matter by first sieving a mince through nylon mesh and then separating the suspension on a density gradient. The fraction obtained was not well characterized and by today's standards was undoubtedly crude. However, the basic techniques employed by them have been adapted by most subsequent investigators.

It wasn't until 10 years after Korey's work that Rose (1967) demonstrated the apparent feasibility of the bulk isolation of neuron and glia-rich fractions. In the interim, however, Roots and Johnston (1964) and Johnston and Roots (1965) had shown that neuronal perikarya could be obtained intact, with parts of processes still attached, after brain tissue had been disrupted by simple mechanical sieving (see Chapter 1). These encouraging findings have stimulated other investigators to devise various methods for preparing cell suspensions and separating the component cells. These methods have been reviewed recently (Rose, 1968; Rose, 1969; Johnston and Roots, 1970) and there have been a number of developments since.

It is necessary first to prepare a suspension of cells by some means which disrupts the intercellular adhesion without disrupting the cells. Following the lead of Korey (1957), Roots and Johnston (1964), and Rose (1967), most investigators have used direct mechanical means without pretreatment. In these techniques the tissue is gently forced through fine meshes of nylon and steel. Others have pretreated the tissue to loosen the intercellular adhesion before sieving. Hemminki (Hemminki *et al.*, 1970; Hemminki, 1970) incubates with a mixture of hyaluronidase and collagenase, and Rappaport (1966) has used tetraphenyl boron, a K^+ complexing agent. However, neither of these workers has attempted to separate cells from the suspension. A quite different approach has been utilized by Satake and Abe (1966) who immerse brain in a mixture of acetone, glycerol, and water which presumably partially "fixes" and hardens the cells. This technique has also been used and extended by Freysz *et al.* (1968, 1969).

The techniques for separating a tissue suspension from cortex to produce both neuronal and glial fractions are obviously of greater applicability than those which attempt the isolation of only one cell type. All of these separation methods involve centrifugation on a density gradient containing Ficoll or sucrose or both. When cortical tissue is used, it is a general finding that neuronal perikarya, largely shorn of processes, are obtained with much less difficulty and in higher purity than neuroglia. Rose and his colleagues have devised (Rose, 1967) and subsequently improved (Rose and Sinha, 1969; Rose and Sinha, 1970) methods for isolating neuron-enriched and glia-enriched fractions, but now conservatively call their glial-enriched fraction neuropil. Hamberger and co-workers (Blomstrand and Hamberger, 1969; Blomstrand and Hamberger, 1970; Hamberger *et al.,* 1970) obtain both types of cells by a modification of the Rose technique; Flangas and Bowman (1968) claim to obtain a glial-rich as well as a neuron fraction utilizing the zonal centrifuge for separation; and Freysz *et al.* (1968, 1969) also obtain both neurons and glia. Recently Sellinger and co-workers Sellinger *et al.,* 1971; Johnson and Sellinger, 1971) have also designed a method for obtaining both types of cells.

If only glia, and especially oligodendroglia, are desired, then white matter is a more logical starting material. Aside from the early work of Korey previously mentioned, the only published work on the isolation of glia exclusively is that of Fewster *et al.* (1967), Fewster and Mead (1968), and Takahashi *et al.* (1970). They both use modifications of Rose's technique with bovine brain white matter as a source.

A third category of techniques includes those apparently suitable only for the isolation of neurons. These include the methods of Satake and Abe (1966) and Bocci (1966). McKhann *et al.* (1969) have isolated neurons from fresh and frozen human brain using the method of Varon and Raiborn (1969) developed for embryonic chick ganglia. The second method of Satake *et al.* (1968) which uses disruption in buffered salt plus Ficoll solutions, a medium favored by many investigators, is designed to selectively isolate large multipolar neurons from brain stem by collecting them on a sieve through which only small cells can pass.

The method of Roots and Johnston (1964), which is also designed for the isolation of large neurons, is not properly a bulk separation technique. The details of this technique, together with the description of methods for obtaining cells by hand dissection, are described in detail in Chapter 1.

In this chapter we describe in detail methods we have developed for isolating nervous system cells (Norton and Poduslo, 1970; Norton and Poduslo, 1971). Tissue suspensions are prepared by sieving after the minced tissue has been treated with trypsin. Cells are isolated from the suspension by density gradient centrifugation. These methods have the advantage of permitting the isolation in high yield of both neuronal perikarya and as-trocytes from rat brain and oligodendroglia from white matter. Thus all three major cell types of the central nervous system can be obtained. In addition, these methods are apparently widely applicable for use with different CNS regions and different species.

II. THE ISOLATION OF NEURONAL PERIKARYA AND ASTROCYTES FROM RAT BRAIN

Reagents

Hexose-albumin-phosphate (HAP) medium: 10 m*M* KH$_2$PO$_4$–NaOH buffer (pH 6.0) containing 5% glucose, 5% fructose, and 1% bovine serum albumin (Cohn fraction V, Sigma Chemical Co.).*

Trypsinization Medium: HAP medium containing 1% trypsin (2X crystallized, salt-free, ex beef pancreas, Nutritional Biochemicals Corp.).

Density gradient solutions: 0.9 *M* sucrose, 1.35 *M* sucrose, 1.55 *M* sucrose, and 2.0 *M* sucrose, all made up in HAP medium.

Buffered calf serum: A mixture of 9 : 1 (v/v) calf serum and phosphate buffer, pH 6.0.

All solutions are prepared fresh the day of the preparation and chilled before use. The trypsin is dissolved in the medium just before the tissue is added. The pH of the density gradient solutions are checked and brought to pH 6.0 by the addition of 0.4 *M* NaOH as necessary.

Special Apparatus

Nylon bolting cloth, 100–150 mesh. Bolting cloth is made of both silk and synthetic fibers and is used in flour manufacture. The nylon cloth is the most satisfactory. In the US it may be purchased from Tobler, Ernst and Traber, 420 Saw Mill River Rd., Elmsford, N.Y.

Stainless steel screen, 200 mesh. This is an ASTM standard sieve having openings of 74 μ. The usual stock item in laboratory supply houses is brass, but it may be obtained in steel on special order.

Method

Rats in the age range of 10–30 days give the most satisfactory preparations, although older animals can also be used. They are decapitated without anesthesia, the brains removed rapidly, trimmed of cerebellum and stem, weighed, and placed in a beaker of ice-cold HAP medium. From 1 to 6 brains can be processed at a time using the rotor specified, but up to 24 brains can be processed per day. Once the procedure is started it must be carried through without interruption. The tissue is placed on a polyethylene plate and chopped with a sharp blade into a fine mince. The minced brain is added to the trypsinization medium (10 ml/g of tissue) and shaken under oxygen for 90 min at 37 °C.

After incubation, the flask is cooled in ice and 0.2 volume of ice-cold buffered calf serum is added. All subsequent steps are performed at 0–4 °C.

---

* Note that the buffer concentration is in error in Norton and Poduslo (1970).

The mixture is centrifuged at 140 g for 5 min to precipitate the bulk of tissue. The supernatant is discarded and the softened tissue is washed twice by resuspending it in medium and centrifuging as before. This treatment with calf serum and washing is to remove trypsin. Calf serum can be eliminated if the incubated tissue is thoroughly washed with medium. The small pieces of tissue are again suspended in the HAP medium and filtered with vacuum through the nylon bolting cloth. This is accomplished by stretching the bolting cloth over a porcelain Hirsch or Buchner funnel and saturating it with medium; the tissue suspension is transferred to the cloth and gently stroked through the mesh with a blunt rounded glass rod while vacuum is applied. Medium is added to the tissue during this process to keep the cloth and tissue wet. To complete the disruption, the resultant suspension is then passed three times through the 200-mesh stainless steel screen. This sieving is also accomplished with the aid of a vacuum, the screen being placed on top of a funnel as before. This final suspension is adjusted with HAP medium to a volume of 10–20 ml per gram of brain for the density gradient centrifugation. At this stage it consists of free-floating cells, capillaries, erythrocytes, processes, myelin, little if any undissociated tissue, and small particulate matter. Neuronal perikarya can easily be distinguished in the phase microscopy, but glial cells are difficult to pick out against the background of other material.

We have separated the cells by centrifugation in a number of systems in which discontinuous density gradients of sucrose or Ficoll, or both, are used. The technique given here appears to be the most satisfactory. Discontinuous gradients are prepared in the 39-ml tubes of the Spinco SW-27 rotor. The gradient consists of (from the bottom up): 5 ml of 2.0 M sucrose in HAP (density 1.286 g/ml), 5 ml of 1.55 M sucrose in HAP (density 1.227 g/ml), 5 ml of 1.35 M sucrose in HAP (density 1.204 g/ml), and 14 ml of 0.9 M sucrose in HAP (density 1.154 g/ml). The cell suspension is layered on these gradients, 10 ml per tube, and the tubes are centrifuged at 3300 g for 10 min. Four layers are formed which are removed with a Pasteur pipette. Very little pellet is seen. Layer A, which consists of the 0.9 M sucrose–suspension interface and the supernatant above it, contains myelin, cell processes, and very small subcellular particles; layer B (on 1.35 M sucrose) is the crude glial layer; layer C (on 1.55 M sucrose) contains a mixed population of neurons, astrocytes, oligodendroglia and capillaries; and layer D (on 2.0 M sucrose) is the neuronal fraction.

The neuronal fraction (layer D) is used without further purification. The crude glial layer (B) is less pure and is carried through a second centrifugation step. This fraction from two tubes (equivalent to 2 g of brain tissue) is diluted slowly with HAP medium to 25 ml and layered onto a discontinuous gradient of 5 ml of 0.9 M sucrose in HAP over 5 ml of 1.4 M

sucrose in HAP. These tubes are centrifuged at 3300 g, but for 20 min this time. The purified glial cells collect at the interface between 1.4 M and 0.9 M sucrose. Any contaminating myelin will layer on the 0.9 M sucrose.

Both cell fractions can be concentrated without breaking the cells by first gradually diluting the suspensions at least 5-fold with HAP and then centrifuging them for 10 min at 630 g. Before centrifugation, a portion of the suspension can be taken for counting. If the counting cannot be done soon, the cells may be preserved by the addition of formalin, and refrigerated and counted when convenient. We generally use a phase hemacytometer without staining the cells.

III. THE ISOLATION OF OLIGODENDROGLIA FROM BOVINE WHITE MATTER

Reagents

Trypsinization medium: HAP medium as described above, containing 0.1 % trypsin.

Density gradient solutions: 0.9 M sucrose, 1.4 M sucrose, and 1.55 M sucrose, all made up in HAP.

All solutions are prepared fresh each day, adjusted to pH 6.0 if necessary, and cooled.

Method

Calf brains are removed from the animal at the slaughterhouse within 15 min after death. They are immediately placed in plastic bags, packed in ice, and taken to the laboratory. The isolation is started within 2–3 hr after the animal is slaughtered. Approximately 30–40 g of white matter dissected free of gray matter is obtained from the corpus callosum and centrum semiovale of one brain. This is minced as fine as possible with a very sharp blade. The tissue is incubated with shaking in the trypsinization medium (0.1 % trypsin in HAP) for 90 min at 37 °C. For 30–40 g of white matter 100 ml of medium is used. The softened tissue is then washed free of trypsin as previously described. The washed tissue pellet is suspended in 0.9 M sucrose in HAP (rather than in HAP alone) and screened as before through the nylon mesh and then at least three times through the 200-mesh stainless steel screen. All undissociated tissue must be thoroughly disrupted. These filtration steps require somewhat more vigorous conditions than used for rat brain. The tissue is tougher and a higher vacuum and prolonged stroking with the glass rod is needed. The suspension is then adjusted to 200 ml per 30–40 g of original tissue with 0.9 M sucrose in HAP.

Isolation of the oligodendroglia is achieved by centrifugation on a density gradient, but one of different composition from that used for neurons and astrocytes. The Spinco SW-25.2 rotor is used which has 60-ml tubes. A discontinuous gradient is prepared which consists of (from the bottom up): 8 ml of 1.55 M sucrose in HAP, 8 ml of 1.4 M sucrose in HAP, and 8 ml of 0.9 M sucrose in HAP; on this is layered 35 ml of the cell suspension. The tubes are centrifuged at 3300 g for 10 min.

A thick semipaste of myelin floats to the top of tube and can be removed with a relatively wide-tipped Pasteur pipette. The reddish colored layer at the interface of 0.9 M sucrose and 1.4 M sucrose contains red blood cells, capillaries, and oligodendroglia. The main oligodendroglial layer is at the interface of 1.55 M sucrose and 1.4 M sucrose and extends down into the 1.55 M sucrose layer. Any neurons which may arise from adventitious gray matter are found in the pellet. The oligodendroglial layer does not require any further purification. It can be concentrated by gradually diluting it with HAP and centrifuging at 630 g for 10 min.

This method has been scaled up to process 200 g of white matter per day. The tissue suspension is prepared as above and adjusted to 1000 ml per 200 g of white matter. Gradients are prepared in 650-ml polycarbonate bottles and the HB-4 rotor of the Sorvall RC-3 centrifuge is used. The suspension (250 ml) is layered over a gradient consisting of 100 ml of 0.9 M sucrose, 150 ml of 1.4 M sucrose, and 100 ml of 1.55 M sucrose, all prepared in HAP as before. The bottles are centrifuged at 3500 rev/min (3400 g) for 20 min. Everything below the reddish layer on 1.4 M sucrose is taken as the oligodendroglial layer. The pooled fractions from four bottles can be diluted slowly to 2 liters with HAP and concentrated by centrifuging at 1500 rev/min for 12 min in the HB-4 rotor.

IV. MISCELLANEOUS APPLICATIONS AND MODIFICATIONS

The full 90-min incubation in trypsin is essential if both astrocytes and neurons are desired from rat brain. However, neurons alone may be obtained, with many processes still attached, after only 30 min of incubation in the trypsinization medium.

The oligodendroglial isolation method has so far been applied only to bovine white matter. There is, however, no reason to expect it to behave differently with white matter of any other mammal. The method for isolating neurons and astrocytes has been used successfully with mouse, dog, and cat brain, without modification. Other species and different CNS regions have been processed successfully, but in some cases minor changes in the method may be required to adapt it for the particular goal. For example, the following modifications were made for the isolation of large motor neurons from rabbit cord. The cord was split lengthwise, the gray matter scraped out, minced, and trypsinized with 0.5 % trypsin in HAP for 30 min. The tissue was washed as usual, taken up in 0.9 M sucrose in HAP, screened through the nylon bolting cloth and then through a 100-mesh steel screen, rather than a 200-mesh screen. These large neurons have different sedimentation rates than the rat cortical neurons. Preliminary experiments using a simple gradient consisting of 1.75 M sucrose in HAP as the bottom layer, overlaid with 1.4 M sucrose in HAP, 0.9 M sucrose in HAP and the suspension, indicate neurons collect on the 1.75 M sucrose layer after centrifugation at 3300 g for 10 min. This fraction is still contaminated with oligodendroglia and capillary fragments, but the neurons have retained much larger portions of their processes than the rat neurons prepared by method A. They closely resemble photographs of large neurons prepared by hand dissection.

Preliminary experiments show that neurons may be obtained from human brain, either fresh or frozen. Cells from frozen human brain are apparently not as well preserved as those from fresh tissue. They also require a different gradient since they collect on less dense sucrose solutions than the rat neurons. A pellet of free nuclei is also found below 2.0 M sucrose when suspensions of frozen brain are centrifuged. Thus, while the method is applicable to a wide variety of CNS tissues, it is important not to use it uncritically. Modifications in the amount of trypsin, time of trypsinization, and composition of the gradient are the important variables to adjust so that optimum results can be achieved.

V. GENERAL COMMENTS

A rather large number of approaches to cell separation were tried before this technique was devised. The problem is a two-part one: first a cell suspension must be made and then the suspension must be fractionated. The number of parameters involved in each of these steps is formidable. Very many attempts were made to perfect a direct mechanical disruption of tissue. In our hands it appeared that while suspensions of neuronal perikarya could be obtained, intact glial cells were infrequently seen. The use of hydrolytic enzymes to liberate cells from a tissue matrix is, of course, well established (see Chapter 1). Crude pancreatin or purified trypsin presumably act on the intercellular glycoproteins, reducing cell-to-cell adhesion, without appreciable damage to cell membranes if their action is limited. It was believed that such an approach could produce satisfactory suspensions, even though other investigators had reported that enzymic digestion did not prove satisfactory with nervous tissue (Rose, 1967; Johnston and Roots,

1970). In initial experiments we evaluated crude pancreatin, trypsin, hyaluronidase, neuraminidase, pronase, papain, and various mixtures of these. Only trypsin or mixtures containing trypsin seemed promising.

Of course, the composition of the medium and pH are equally important variables, and trypsin used in a variety of balanced salt solutions at pH 7–7.5 was completely ineffective. The present HAP medium was arrived at on purely empirical grounds through a series of trial-and-error experiments. In particular, it might seem contradictory to include albumin in the medium with trypsin, and this may be the reason that the relatively high levels of trypsin and long incubation periods are required. However, the added protein apparently has a protective action on the cell membranes. It is interesting that other methods include a high molecular weight material such as Ficoll, polyvinylpyrollidone, or ganglioside in their media for cell stabilization.

The selection of gradient composition and centrifugation conditions present equally difficult problems. Most investigators use Ficoll density gradients to maintain nearly isotonic conditions. Sucrose is less difficult to remove preparatory to analysis but does perhaps make the design of a gradient and choice of forces and times more difficult. The main reason for this is the rather peculiar behavior of osmometers when centrifuged on gradients of increasing tonicity. Thus the conditions given in the methods are not equilibrium conditions, but rather represent a compromise rate-zonal separation. If the gradients are centrifuged at higher g forces and longer times, the separation is not improved, cells migrate to regions of higher density, and quite different distributions of cells and particulates are found.

There are a few practical points to stress if one is to perform the method successfully. The tissue must be finely minced, both to enable the trypsin to penetrate and to aid the screening process, since larger pieces are more difficult to sieve. Thus the degree of myelination is important; the more myelin in the tissue, the more difficult it is to mince thoroughly and to disrupt completely. Therefore, heavily myelinated tissue should be passed through the steel screen at least three times and the suspension checked by phase microscopy to make sure no undisrupted tissue clumps remain. Also, a large quantity of myelinated processes tend to form a mat which can trap cells during the centrifugation. This can be minimized by either using more dilute suspensions or by suspending the cells in 0.9 M sucrose in HAP as done in method B rather than in HAP alone. When the suspension in the denser medium is placed on a gradient, the myelin floats up rather than sedimenting to the first gradient interface.

Occasionally with method A, neurons are obtained but astrocytes are very sparse or fragmented. As previously mentioned, longer trypsinization is required to free the extensive intertwined astrocytic processes. However, these cells also appear to be more fragile and sensitive to minor changes in technique than the neurons; thus a failure to obtain astrocytes can be a result of many factors: insufficient trypsin, too short incubation, incomplete or too severe sieving, too high temperatures, improper pH, etc. It is important to check the pH of the final solutions and adjust if necessary. We have also on occasion received batches of trypsin which do not dissolve completely but have a fine amorphous precipitate suspended in the medium. Although our evidence is not secure, we have recently suspected that poor yields of astrocytes may be obtained when such trypsin preparations are used. The necessity of monitoring each preparation by phase microscopy cannot be overemphasized. Slight variations in the procedure can have large effects and the only rapid check on the success of the procedure is microscopic examination.

All three types of cells are very sensitive to changes in the medium when they are taken off the very hypertonic gradient. If they are diluted too rapidly with HAP, or if an attempt is made to transfer them to saline or balanced salt media, they will invariably fragment. It is probable such transfers can be accomplished if done gradually enough.

VI. CELL PROPERTIES

The separate cell types are readily distinguishable from each other when examined by phase microscopy (see Fig. 1). The neurons are large cells having soma diameters ranging from 10 to 40 μ. They retain stumps of axons and dendrites, have abundant cytoplasm and large round nuclei with a single, prominent nucleolus (Fig. 1A). The astrocytes are largely intact, with highly ramified processes, small nuclei, and little perinuclear cytoplasm. The processes vary in length from 20 to 80 μ (Figs. 1B and 1C). The oligodendroglia are small round cells 8–15 μ in diameter with an occasional short process. At low or medium magnification it is difficult to distinguish some of these elements from free nuclei or erythrocytes (Fig. 1D). However, at 1000 × magnification under oil or in stained sections, the oligodendroglial fraction was found to consist of cells having a rim of cytoplasm surrounding a small round nucleus.

Electron micrographs of these three cell types showed they retained most of their characteristic features as seen *in situ* (Raine *et al.*, 1971). The triple-layered plasma membrane and nuclear envelope was preserved and the former showed only minor interruptions. Neurons contained abundant Nissl substance and their processes contained 240 Å microtubules. Astroglia contained finely granular areas in the cytoplasm, probably representing altered filaments. Occasionally intact groups of 100 Å filaments

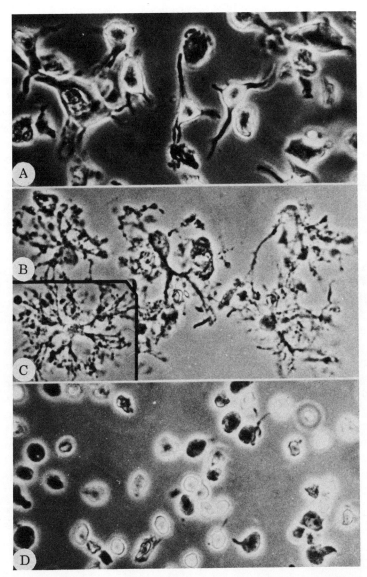

Fig. 1. A–D are all phase contrast photomicrographs at the same magnification, ×740. (A) Rat brain neuron fraction. Many cells have portions of processes attached. Note absence of small debris. (B) Rat brain astroglial fraction. Processes are extensive, branched, and of irregular diameters. (C) A single typical rat brain astroglial cell with symmetrically arranged, highly branched processes. (D) Bovine white matter oligodendroglial fraction. Only a few cells have a short process. Nuclei are not generally discernible at this magnification. Note the absence of astroglia and small debris. (Reproduced from Raine *et al.*, 1971.)

were seen. The oligodendroglia were characterized by a narrow rim of dense cytoplasm, rich in ribosomes and mitochondria. The characteristic microtubules were always seen. The short processes were loops of myelin either attached to or closely associated with the cell membrane.

The purity of the neurons and oligodendroglia is judged to be about 90% by light microscopy, and this high degree of purity is confirmed by electron microscope observations. The astrocyte fraction is less pure and is judged to have a particle purity of at least 50% astrocytes. However, when the DNA values of the astrocyte fraction are compared to the neuronal fraction, a cell purity of 66% can be calculated which, since the astrocytes are larger than the contaminating cells, represents a weight purity of 84% (Norton and Poduslo, 1971).

The total recovery of DNA in neurons plus astrocytes is 11% of the DNA in the rat brain sample. We calculate that this represents a recovery of 15–20% for neurons and about 3.5% for glia. However, since the term "glia" includes astrocytes, oligodendrocytes, and microglia, the recovery of astrocytes alone may be twice that figure. The recovery of oligodendroglia is also of the order of 10% of the total cells in the white matter sample.

The yield and chemical composition of these three cell types is compared in Table I. On an individual cell basis the astrocytes are heavier than neurons and much heavier than the oligodendrocytes. All of these weights are consistent with the microscopic dimensions of the cells and the fact that the astrocytes retain elaborate processes. Neurons and astrocytes have similar DNA/RNA ratios, but neurons have a higher percentage of RNA, as expected from their abundant Nissl substance. The oligodendroglia have a much higher DNA/RNA ratio than the other two cells, owing to the low volume of cytoplasm, but the percentage of RNA is actually rather high. The astrocytes have the highest lipid content, and the lipid composition of astrocytes and neurons is very similar (Norton and Poduslo, 1971), both

Table I.   Properties of Isolated Cells

	Rat		Bovine
	Neurons	Astrocytes	oligodendroglia
Yield, cells/g tissue	17×10^6	3.5×10^6	11.4×10^6
Weight, pg/cell	178	590	25–50
DNA, pg/cell	8.2	11.2	5.5
DNA/RNA ratio	0.34	0.38	2.9
Gangliosides, % dry wt.	0.23	0.60	0.25
Lipid, % dry wt.	24.1	38.9	29.5
Cholesterol, % lipid	10.6	14.0	14.1
Galactolipid, % lipid	2.1	1.8	9.9
Phospholipid, % lipid	72.3	70.9	62.2

having little cerebroside or sulfatide. The oligodendroglia, however, have appreciable amounts of these two galactolipids, as would be expected since they are the myelin-generating cells. The ganglioside concentrations are surprising since they are believed to be primarily neuronal constituents. We feel they are probably constituents of all plasma membranes in the nervous system, and are therefore higher in astrocytes because of the very high surface/volume ratio of these isolated cells. All of these ganglioside figures are quite low, and none of these data should be taken as an argument against the major concentration of gangliosides being in the dendritic tree which is lost from the neuron on isolation.

It is difficult to compare the methods presented here with the other methods currently in use. Obviously this field of bulk separation of neurons and glia is still relatively new and not enough data have been accumulated to show whether any one technique is clearly superior to another. One of the major criticisms leveled against our techniques is the possibility that trypsin has a deleterious effect on cell proteins and enzyme systems. It is not possible to answer these criticisms in detail; however, it should be borne in mind that the trypsin is acting on the intact tissue, not on separated cells. Evidence that the cells have maintained their integrity is the following: (1) they respire linearly for up to 2 hr, (2) the plasma membrane and intracellular organelles are remarkably well preserved, (3) astrocytes contain appreciable amounts of the very soluble glial-specific protein, S-100, and (4) the cells exclude trypan blue. It is probable that at the present time no one method will satisfy the many requirements of all investigators. Major questions to be asked about all techniques are how closely the properties of isolated cells correspond to those of brain cells in living tissue and whether they are representative samples of the total *in vivo* population. What the method described here offers is the ability to produce clean fractions of the three major cell types of the CNS, in the highest yield and with the highest degree of preservation so far reported.

ACKNOWLEDGMENT

The work described in this chapter was supported by U.S.P.H.S. grants NS-02476 and NS-03356 and grant 584-B-2 from the National Multiple Sclerosis Society.

REFERENCES

Blomstrand, C., and Hamberger, A. (1969) *J. Neurochem.* **16**, 1401.
Blomstrand, C., and Hamberger, A. (1970) *J. Neurochem.* **17**, 1187.

Bocci, V. (1966) *Nature* **212**, 826.
Fewster, M. E., Scheibel, A. B., and Mead, J. F. (1967) *Brain Res.* **6**, 401.
Fewster, M. E., and Mead, J. F. (1968) *J. Neurochem.* **15**, 1041.
Flangas, A. L., and Bowman, R. E. (1968) *Science* **161**, 1025.
Freysz, L., Bieth, R., Judes, C., Sensenbrenner, M., Jacob, M., and Mandel, P. (1968) *J. Neurochem.* **15**, 307.
Freysz, L., Bieth, R., and Mandel, P. (1969) *J. Neurochem.* **16**, 1417.
Hamberger, A., Blomstrand, C., and Lehninger, A. L. (1970) *J. Cell Biol.* **45**, 221.
Hemminki, K. (1970) *Febs Letters* **9**, 290.
Hemminki, K., Huttunen, M. O., and Jarnefelt, J. (1970) *Brain Res.* **23**, 23.
Johnson, D. E., and Sellinger, O. Z. (1971) *J. Neurochem.* **18**, 1445.
Johnston, P. V., and Roots, B. I. (1965) *Nature* **205**, 778.
Johnston, P. V., and Roots, B. I. (1970) *Int. Rev. Cytol.* **29**, 265.
Korey, S. R. (1957) in *Metabolism of the Nervous System* (D. Richter, ed.), Pergamon Press, New York, p. 87.
Korey, S. R., Orchen, M., and Brotz, M. (1958) *J. Neuropath. Exp. Neurol.* **17**, 430.
McKhann, G. M., Ho, W., Raiborn, C., and Varon, S. (1969) *Arch. Neurol.* **20**, 542.
Norton, W. T., and Poduslo, S. E. (1970) *Science* **167**, 1144.
Norton, W. T., and Poduslo, S. E. (1971) *J. Lipid Res.* **12**, 84.
Raine, C. S., Poduslo, S. E., and Norton, W. T. (1971) *Brain Res.* **27**, 11.
Rappaport, C. (1966) *Proc. Soc. Exp. Biol. Med.* **121**, 1016.
Roots, B. I., and Johnston, P. V. (1964) *J. Ultrastruct. Res.* **10**, 350.
Rose, S. P. R. (1967) *Biochem. J.* **102**, 33.
Rose, S. P. R. (1968) in *Applied Neurochemistry* (A. N. Davison and J. Dobbing, ed.), F. A. Davis Co., Philadelphia, p. 332.
Rose, S. P. R. (1969) in *Handbook of Neurochemistry* (A. Lajtha, ed.), Vol. 2, Plenum Press, New York, p. 183.
Rose, S. P. R., and Sinha, A. K. (1969) *J. Neurochem.* **16**, 1319.
Rose, S. P. R., and Sinha, A. K. (1970) *Life Sci.* pt. II, **9**, 907.
Satake, M., and Abe, S. (1966) *J. Biochem. (Tokyo)* **59**, 72.
Satake, M., Hasegawa, S., Abe, S., and Tanaka, R. (1968) *Brain Res.* **11**, 246.
Sellinger, O. Z., Azcurra, J. M., Johnson, D. E., Ohlsson, W. G., and Lodin, Z. (1971) *New Biology* **230**, 253.
Takahashi, Y., Hsu, S., and Honma, S. (1970) *Brain Res.* **23**, 284.
Varon, S., and Raiborn, C. W. (1969) *Brain Res.* **12**, 180.

Chapter 3

Separation of Myelin Fragments from the Central Nervous System

Martha Spohn and Alan N. Davison*

M.R.C. Membrane Biology Group
Department of Biochemistry
Charing Cross Hospital Medical School
London, England

I. INTRODUCTION

Myelin consists of compact multilamellae of low density (approx. 1.103). The membrane contains cholesterol, phospholipids, and characteristically cerebroside; only small amounts of ganglioside are found. About 25% of the myelin is protein, mainly proteolipid protein, but a unique basic protein with encephalitogenic properties is also present. The composition of most vertebrate myelin is similar but there are differences in the composition of central and peripheral nerve myelin. Myelin isolated from developing brain has a different composition from that in the adult and it is possible to separate two fractions from "early" myelin (Banik and Davison, 1969; Agrawal *et al.*, 1970). Present methods for the isolation of myelin depend on differential and density gradient centrifugation of nervous tissue homogenates. Several methods are available; choice should be made according to the purpose of the work. Thus the method of Autilio *et al.* (1964) leads to a highly purified preparation, but myelin and possibly soluble components may be lost during the course of the isolation. The method described here is suitable for isolation of myelin from vertebrate central nervous tissue and leads to myelin fractions which may be further purified by repeated washing if required.

* Present address: Institute of Neurology, Queen Square, LONDON, WCIN 3BG.

II. RECOMMENDED PROCEDURE

Animals may be lightly anesthetized before decapitation. The dissected brains should be washed free of blood by rinsing the tissue in ice cold 0.32 M sucrose, followed by careful blotting on wet filter paper. The tissue is weighed in precooled beakers, the whole operation being carried out as quickly as possible to avoid a rise in temperature. Sucrose should be of reagent-grade purity and solutions should be of neutral pH. It is convenient to prepare 1.2 M sucrose and use this as stock solution for further dilutions. The stock sucrose solution can be kept at $-10\,°C$ for up to 2 weeks (see Table I). More dilute solutions should be freshly prepared.

A. Step 1

Disruption of Tissue

The weighed tissue may be disrupted in 0.32 M sucrose to give a 10% (w/v) suspension. Various forms of homogenizers have been used by different

Table I. Properties of Aqueous Sucrose Solutions

Molarity at 20°C[a]	Concentration g/liter at 20°C	Relative proportions (Parts by volume) 1.2 M	H₂O	Vol. of 1.2 M sucrose (ml)	Density at 20°C[b]
0.1	34.2	1	11	83.3	1.013
0.2	68.5	1	5	166.7	1.027
0.25	85.6	5	19	208.3	1.033
0.3	102.7	1	3	250.0	1.040
0.32	109.5	4	11	266:7	1.043
0.4	136.9	1	2	333.3	1.054
0.5	171.2	5	7	416.7	1.067
0.6	205.4	1	1	500.0	1.081
0.7	239.6	7	5	583.3	1.094
0.8	273.8	2	1	666.7	1.107
0.85	291.0	17	7	708.3	1.114
0.9	308.1	3	1	750.0	1.121
1.0	342.3	5	1	833.3	1.134
1.1	376.5	11	1	916.7	1.147
1.2	410.8	1	0	1000.0	1.160
1.3	445.0				1.173
1.4	479.2				1.187
1.5	513.5				1.200
1.6	547.7				1.213
1.7	581.9				1.223
1.8	616.1				1.238
1.9	650.4				1.251
2.0	686.4				1.264

[a] Molecular weight sucrose 342.3. [b] Source: C. De Duve *et al.* (1959).

investigators (Gregson, 1965). The one most commonly employed for nervous tissue is a Potter-Elvehjem type fitted with a Teflon pestle and driven by an electric motor. Pestle clearance of 0.125–0.2 mm diameter, and speeds of 1000–2000 rev/min give good disruption. The recommended procedure is homogenization for 1.5–2 min, the pestle being moved three times up and down the tube. The tube must be kept in ice during this operation. The original volume of 0.32 M sucrose used for homogenization may conveniently be four to five times the weight of tissue and the final concentration of the homogenate adjusted to approximately 100 mg of original tissue per milliliter.

B. Step 2a and 2b

Removal of Nuclei and Cell Debris

A 10% (w/v) tissue homogenate in 0.32 M sucrose when centrifuged at 10^3 g for 10 min sediments nuclei, cell debris, broken capillaries, and blood cells, leaving the bulk of myelin together with synaptosomes and mitochondria in the supernatant. Up to 20% of myelin may sediment with the nuclear pellet, and in order to recover some of this myelin the pellet may be resuspended in 0.32 M sucrose and the suspension recentrifuged (step 2b). Even then, some myelin sediments with the pellet.

When higher yields of myelin are required, the speed may be reduced to as little as 800 g for 10 min with the risk of a lower degree of purity of the final myelin fraction (Rose, 1962).

C. Step 3

Separation of Crude Mitochondrial Pellet

Myelin together with synaptosomes and mitochondria is sedimented by centrifugation of the supernatant from step 2 at 1.35×10^4 g for 15 min to give a crude mitochondrial pellet (pellet 2).

D. Step 4

Separation of Myelin

Myelin can be separated from the remaining constituents of the crude mitochondrial pellet by many variations of density gradient centrifugation. These methods take advantage of the large vesicle size and low density of myelin. Myelin is less dense than 0.8 M sucrose and will therefore float over a solution of this concentration, thus separating from the other components of the tissue suspension which are sedimented through denser sucrose solutions.

The recommended procedure involves upward floatation of myelin from a suspension in 0.8 M sucrose. Pellet 2 is suspended in a small volume of 0.32 M sucrose and the concentrated suspension mixed with an equal volume of 1.2 M sucrose. The mixture should be diluted with 0.8 M sucrose to give a concentration of approximately 100 mg of original tissue per milliliter. Aliquots of this solution should be layered over half their volume of 1.2 M sucrose, and covered with a small layer (about 0.2 of their volume) of 0.3 M sucrose. The relative volumes will depend on the size of the available rotors and tubes. Centrifugation at 5.3 $\times$ $10^4 g$ (5–5.4 $\times$ 10^4) for 1 hr gives a good separation of myelin at the 0.8 M – 0.32 M sucrose interface.

E. Step 5

Purification of Myelin by Osmotic Shock

It has been generally observed that "myelin" thus isolated consists mainly of myelin lamellae contaminated with axonal material in the form of fragments of distorted myelinated axons (Gray and Whittaker, 1962; Laatsch et al., 1962; Adams et al., 1963; De Robertis et al., 1963). Myelin can be obtained in a much purer form by subjecting the above crude fraction to an osmotic shock by suspending it in water, followed by centrifugation (Laatsch et al., 1962; Davison et al., 1962; Autilio et al., 1964) at 1.2 $\times$ $10^4 g$ for 10 min to form a pellet consisting of almost pure, vesicularized myelin.

F. Steps 6 and 7

Further Purification of Myelin

When a very high degree of purity of myelin is essential, the above fraction may be resuspended in 0.32 M sucrose and layered over 0.85 M sucrose, followed by centrifugation at 7.5 $\times$ $10^4 g$ for 30 min. The resulting myelin (interface) may be suspended in ice-cold water (as in step 5) and recentrifuged at 7.5 $\times$ $10^4 g$ for 15 min (Suzuki et al., 1967). This allows the complete recovery of myelin as a pellet. At this stage some sucrose is still contaminating the pellet, and in order to remove it the washing process can be repeated exhaustively. The disadvantages of extensive purification of the fraction are numerous. The yield of myelin falls with the rise of the number of steps involved, owing to unavoidable losses on manipulation, and most important of all is the risk of isolating an artificial product not completely representative of myelin in situ.

III. ALTERNATIVE METHODS FOR THE ISOLATION
OF MYELIN

All of the methods for the isolation of myelin are based on the fact that the lipid-rich myelin vesicles formed on homogenization of nervous tissue in isotonic solutions have the lowest density of any membrane fraction. Sucrose is normally used for the initial homogenization of the tissue. The original method of Laatsch *et al.* (1962) involves upward flotation of myelin from a tissue homogenate in 0.88 *M* sucrose. The myelin is purified by osmotic shock followed by reflotation. In a modified method of Autilio *et al.* (1964), Suzuki *et al.* (1967) homogenized the tissue in 0.32 *M* sucrose and layered the homogenate over 0.85 *M* sucrose; the myelin was subjected to osmotic shock and sedimented by centrifugation. The process of "layering" and "water washing" was repeated several times. Davison and co-workers (Adams *et al.,* 1963; and Cuzner *et al.,* 1965), used a technique of layering a suspension of the mitochondrial fraction of the brain over 0.8 *M* sucrose followed by purification of the myelin interface by water shock treatment. De Robertis and co-workers (De Robertis *et al.,* 1963) separated myelin from many other subcellular structures of brain tissue by layering crude mitochondrial suspensions in 0.32 *M* sucrose over a continuous sucrose gradient, the density of the sucrose ranging from 1.4 *M* at the bottom of the tube to 0.8 *M* sucrose at the top. All the methods described above are variations of sucrose density gradient centrifugation of tissue homogenates or of the crude mitochondrial fraction. The speeds and times of centrifugation vary from investigator to investigator as do the necessary solutes added to the basic sucrose medium (e.g., buffers, EDTA, $CaCl_2$, $MgCl_2$), etc. For details the reader is referred to the original publications.

As an alternative to sucrose Kornguth *et al.* (1967) and Thompson *et al.* (1967) used centrifugation in a density gradient of cesium chloride for fractionation of subcellular elements of nervous tissue. However, in CsCl myelin layers out at a mean density of 1.11 gm/ml (0.85 *M* CsCl) as opposed to 1.08 gm/ml (0.65 *M*) in sucrose. The reason for the difference in density of myelin in the two media remains unexplained.

Kurokawa *et al.* (1965) separated myelin from a crude mitochondrial suspension in 0.32 *M* sucrose by layering over a Ficoll gradient. In order to isolate myelin in larger amounts, Murdock and co-workers (Murdock *et al.,* 1969) have recently developed a zonal centrifugation method using a Beckman preparative ultracentrifuge. Basically this is an adaptation of a sucrose density gradient procedure used by them in a previous study (Lowden *et al.,* 1966). Shapiro and his colleagues (Shapiro *et al.,* 1970) have described a similar method.

Peripheral nerve myelin has been isolated from beef intradural spinal roots by O'Brien *et al.* (1967) and from monkey brachial plexus by Horrocks (1967). A special problem is presented by the presence of collagen in peripheral nerve samples, which makes homogenization difficult and isolation of myelin questionable (see Adams *et al.,* 1968).

IV. CRITERIA FOR PURITY

It is advisable to check all fractionations by electron microscopy by fixing in glutaraldehyde and staining with OsO_4. Sections should be taken from all areas of the block; axoplasmic debris and mitochondria should be minimal (see Figs. 1 and 2). Electron microscopic examination may be especially useful in checking that the myelin constituents responsible for staining of the intraperiod line are not removed during the purification procedure. Gel electrophoresis will show the presence of the characteristic bands of basic encephalitogenic protein typical for the myelin of each species (Mehl and Halaris, 1970) and estimation of this protein in separated myelin gives a very accurate assessment of the myelin content (Gaitonde and Martenson, 1970). Table II shows the composition of purified rat myelin; similar details for other species are available (e.g., Smith, 1967; Davison, 1970; Norton, 1971). Purity of the myelin can also be assessed by chemical and enzymic criteria. Thus 95–99% of isolated myelin when free of sucrose is soluble in chloroform–methanol (2:1, v/v) solution (Kies *et al.,* 1965;

Table II.   Proteins and Lipid Composition of Purified Myelin
Isolated from Adult Rat Brain[a]

Constituent	Amount in purified myelin units/g wet wt. of brain	Approx. % of whole brain values
Dry weight[b]	45.5 mg	
Total protein	7.0 ± 0.7 mg (9)	8
Total nucleic acids	0.01 mg	0.4
Total lipid NANA[c]	66.5 μg	10
Cholesterol	13.4 ± 1.6 μg (5)	24
Cerebroside	5.4 ± 0.7 μm (2)	45
Lipid phosphorus	12.3 ± 1.2 μm (7)	17
Ethanolamine phospholipid	6.7 (2)	24
Phosphatidyl choline	5.0 (2)	13
Sphingomyelin[d]	2.7 (2)	25

[a] Analyses are from our own laboratory for purified myelin as isolated in step 5 (above) except for the dry weight which was from Suzuki *et al.* (1967) who found 27% protein in their sample. Equal amounts of basic and proteolipid protein are present (Mehl and Halaris, 1970) together with a small amount of a third type of protein (Wolfgram, 1966).
[b] Myelin probably contains about 40% water (Norton, 1971).
[c] N-Acetylneuraminic acid.
[d] High values may be due to lysophosphatidyl ethanolamine and other minor phospholipids.

STEP 1.　　　　TISSUE–(weighed)
　　　　　　　　　Homogenize in 0.32 M sucrose solution.
　　　　　　　TISSUE HOMOGENATE 10% w/v (wet weight in sucrose solution)
STEP 2a.　　　　Centrifuge at 10^3 g for 10 min.

　　　　　　NUCLEAR PELLET　　　　　　　　　　　SUPERNATANT 1
STEP 2b.　　　　Resuspend in the original vol
　　　　　　　　of 0.32 M sucrose solution　　　　　　　Combine
　　　　　　　　centrifuge as in Step 2a.

　　　　　　NUCLEI + CELL DEBRIS　　　　　　SUPERNATANT 2
　　　　　　(Pellet 1)
STEP 3.　　　　　　　　Centrifuge at 1.35×10^4 g
　　　　　　　　　　　　for 15 min.

　　　　　　CRUDE MITOCHONDRIA　　　　　SUPERNATANT
　　　　　　(Pellet 2)　　　　　　　　　(Microsomes + Supernatant)
　　　　　　　　Resuspend in 0.32 M sucrose (small volume). Mix with an equal volume
　　　　　　　　of 1.2 M sucrose. Dilute with 0.8 M sucrose.
　　　　　　CRUDE MITOCHONDRIAL SUSPENSION (approx. 10 ml/g original
　　　　　　tissue)
　　　　　　　　Layer over half the volume of 1.2 M sucrose.
　　　　　　　　Centrifuge at 5.3×10^4 g for 1 hr.
STEP 4.

　　　　　　CRUDE MYELIN　　　NERVE ENDINGS　　MITOCHONDRIA
　　　　　　Interface between　　Interface between　Pellet
　　　　　　0.32 M and 0.8 M　　0.8 M and 1.2 M
　　　　　　sucrose　　　　　　　sucrose
　　　　　　　　Remove the interface and measure the volume of the suspenson.
　　　　　　　　Mix with 10 times its volume of ice cold water. Allow to stand
　　　　　　　　for at least 20 min at 0-4°C. Centrifuge at 1.2×10^4 g for 10 min.
STEP 5.

　　　　　　PURIFIED MYELIN PELLET
STEP 6.　　　　Suspend the pellet in 0.32 M sucrose (approx. 10 ml/g original
　　　　　　　　tissue) Layer aliquots of the suspension over equal volumes of 0.85
　　　　　　　　M sucrose. Centrifuge at 7.5×10^4 g for 30 min.
　　　　　　PURIFIED MYELIN AT THE INTERFACE
　　　　　　　　Resuspend at 10 times its volume of water. Centrifuge at 7.5×10^4 g
　　　　　　　　for 15 min.
STEP 7.

　　　　　　PURIFIED MYELIN (PELLET)

Fig. 1. Scheme for the isolation of myelin. All apparatus and solutions should be pre-cooled to 0–4°C, and all operations carried out at this low temperature. Density gradient centrifugations should be carried out in swing-out rotors.

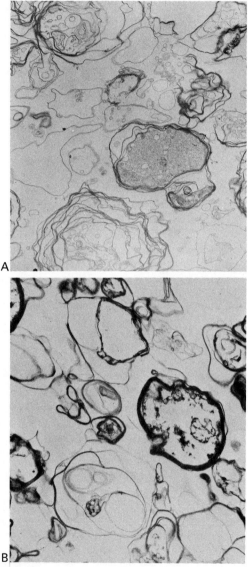

Fig. 2. Electron micrographs of (A) unwashed crude rat myelin. Myelin prepared from adult rat brain in 0.32 M sucrose was rapidly fixed by glutaraldehyde, postfixed in Millonig's osmium fixative. The section was stained by lead and uranyl acetates. The picture shows some intact axoplasm with free mitochondria; small vesicles possibly derived from swollen organelse are present. Other myelin whorls of varying degrees of compactness arer elatively free of contamination. × 21,000. (B) Washed purified myelin prepared by the above method. × 31,000. (Courtesy of Dr. N. A. Gregson, Guy's Hospital Medical School, London S.E.1.) (Reduced for reproduction 65%.)

Table III. Enzyme Activity of Rat Brain Myelin

	Purified myelin[a]	Other fractions	
Enzymee	Specific activity	Typical localization	Specific activity
Succinate dehydrogenase (E.C. 1.3.99.1)	0.15 (3)	Mitochondria	11.90
Na$^+$ +K$^+$, Mg^{2+} Activated ATPase (E.C. 3.6.1.3)	3.7 (3)	Microsomes Nerve ending particles	33.8 29.7
Acetylcholinesterase (E.C. 3.1.1.7)	2.2 (2)	Microsomes Nerve ending particles	10.6 8.9
5′-Nucleotidase (E.C. 3.1 3.5)	0.65 (2)	Microsomes Supernatant	1.87 1.09
Leucine aminopeptidase (E.C. 3.4.1.1)	0.33 (3)	Microsomes Nerve ending particles	0.41 0.20
2′,3′-Cyclic nucleotide 3′-phosphohydrolase	202 (3)	Microsomes Nerve ending particles	53.05 11.60

[a] Results show specific enzyme activities (μmoles of substrate utilized/hr/mg protein) from Banik and Davison (1969) for adult rat brain myelin. Number of separate analyses are shown in parentheses.

Autilio *et al.,* 1964), and relatively little nucleic acid (less than 0.5 of that in the whole tissue) and lipid NANA (less than 100 μg/100 mg dry myelin) should be present. Myelin contains about 70–80 % of its dry weight as lipid; almost all the remainder is protein. Myelin is especially rich in the galactolipid cerebroside and sulfatide (see Table II) and the ratio of cholesterol–phospholipid–galactolipid provides a good index of myelin purity, for other membranes tend to contain relatively more phospholipid and much less galactolipid than myelin.

Assay of enzyme activity gives a useful means of monitoring the purity of isolated myelin fractions (Table III, Adams *et al.,* 1963). Only traces of succinate dehydrogenase activity should be detectable and other enzymes (e.g., adenosinetriphosphatase) should have activities similar to that shown in Table III. Specific activity of 2′,3′-cyclic nucleotide 3′-phosphohydrolase gives a measure of overall purity of the fraction.

V. YIELD OF MYELIN

The amount of myelin obtainable depends on the method used and is generally related to the purity of the final product. Thus, based on cerebroside estimations, Cuzner and Davison (1968) found 50 % of the total brain

cerebroside lipid in myelin whereas Suzuki *et al.* (1968) recovered only
28.4% of whole brain glycolipids in rat myelin (see Table II). In practice,
various amounts of myelin are found to contaminate many subcellular
fractions and for quantitative recovery it is necessary to relayer and centrifuge each subcellular fraction.

Norton and Autilio (1966) have calculated that myelin accounts for
50% of the white matter dry weight in the ox but only 25% of the wet weight.
From earlier analyses Norton (1971) estimates that a 100-g sample of bovine
centrum ovale white matter has 78 g water and of the 28 g solids, 11 g is
protein, 15.4 g lipid, and 1.7 g salts, gangliosides, and other water-soluble
molecules. Of the 28 g solids, 3.9 g is myelin protein and 10.4 g myelin
lipid. These figures give a useful minimal estimate of the myelin content of
bovine white matter.

It will be clear from this account that the method best adopted will
depend on the purpose of the investigation. The technique described here
appears to us to have the most general application.

REFERENCES

Adams, C. W. M., Abdulla, Y. H., Turner, D. R., and Bayliss, O. B. (1968) *Nature
    (London)* **220**, 171.
Adams, C. W. M., Davison, A. N., and Gregson, N. A. (1963) *J. Neurochem.* **10**, 383.
Agrawal, H. C., Banik, N. L., Bone, A. H., Davison, A. N., Mitchell, R. F., and Spohn, M.
    (1970) *Biochem. J.* **120**, 635.
Autilio, L., A., Norton, W. T., and Terry, R. D. (1964) *J. Neurochem.* **11**, 17.
Banik, N. L., and Davison, A. N. (1969) *Biochem. J.* **115**, 1051.
Cuzner, M. L., and Davison, A. N. (1968) *Biochem. J.* **106**, 29.
Cuzner, M. L., Davison, A. N., and Gregson, N. A. (1965) *J. Neurochem.* **12**, 469.
Davison, A. N. (1970) in *Myelination* (A. N. Davison and A. Peters, eds.), C. C Thomas,
    Springfield, Ill., p. 80.
Davison, A. N., Gregson, N. A., and Williams, P. L. (1962) *J. Physiol. Lond.* **161**, 41.
deDuve, C., Berthet, J., and Beaufay, H. (1959) *Progr. Biophys. Biophys, Chem.* **9**, 325.
DeRobertis, E., DeIraldi, A. P., Arnaiz, G. R. L., and Salganicoff, L. (1962) *J. Neurochem.*
    9, 23.
DeRobertis, E., Arnaiz, G. R. L., Salganicoff, L., DeIraldi, A. P., and Zieher, L. M. (1963)
    J. Neurochem. **10**, 225.
Gaitonde, M. K., and Martenson, R. E. (1970) *J. Neurochem.* **17**, 551.
Gray, E. G., and Whittaker, V. P. (1962) *J. Anat. Lond.* **96**, 79.
Gregson, N. A. (1965) in *Neurochemistry* (C. W. M. Adams, ed.), Elsevier, Amsterdam,
    p. 207.
Horrocks, L. A. (1967) *J. Lipid Res.* **8**, 569.
Kies, M. W., Thompson, E. B., and Alvord, E. C. (1965) *Ann. N. Y. Acad. Sci.* **122**, 148.
Kornguth, S. E., Walberg Anderson, J., Scott, G., Kubinski, H. (1967) *Exp. Cell Res.* **45**,
    656.
Kurokawa, M., Sakamoto, T., and Kato, M. (1965) *Biochem. J.* **97**, 833.
Laatsch, R. H., Kies, M. W., Gordon, S., Alvord, E. C., Jr. (1962) *J. Exp. Med.* **115**, 777.
Lowden, J. A., Moscarello, M. A., and Morecki, R. (1966) *Can. J. Biochem.* **44**, 567.
Mehl, E., and Halaris, A. (1950) *J. Neurochem.* **17**, 659.

Murdock, D. D., Katona, E., and Moscarello, M. A. (1969) *Can. J. Biochem.* **47,** 818.
Norton, W. T. (1971) in *The Cellular and Molecular Basis of Neurologic Disease* (E. S. Goldensohn and S. M. Appel, eds.), Lea & Febiger, Philadelphia (in press).
Norton, W. T., and Autilio, L. A. (1966) *J. Neurochem.* **13,** 4.
O'Brien, J. S., Sampson, E. L., and Stern, M. B. (1967) *J. Neurochem.* **14,** 357.
Rose, S. P. R. (1962) *Biochem. J.* **83,** 614.
Shapiro, R., Binkley, F., and Windram, I. J. (1970) *Proc. Soc. Exp. Biol. Med.* **133,** 239.
Smith, M. E. (1967) *Adv. Lipid Res.* **5,** 241.
Suzuki, K., Poduslo, S. E., and Norton, W. T. (1967) *Biochem. Biophys. Acta* **144,** 375.
Suzuki, K., Poduslo, J. F., and Poduslo, S. E. (1968) *Biochem. Biophys. Acta* **152.** 576.
Thompson, E. J., Goodwin, H., and Cummings, J. N. (1967) *Nature (London)* **215,** 168.
Wolfgram, F. (1966) *J. Neurochem.* **13,** 461.

Chapter 4

Principles for the Optimization of Centrifugation Conditions for Fractionation of Brain Tissue

Carl W. Cotman

Department of Psychobiology
University of California at Irvine
Irvine, California

I. INTRODUCTION

Classes of subcellular particles separate by centrifugation procedures because of significant differences in their sedimentation rates and buoyant densities. Most centrifugation procedures devised for brain make use of differences in both sedimentation rate and buoyant density. Preliminary enrichment by rate is achieved by differential centrifugation, usually in angle rotors, followed by separation by buoyant density on density gradients in zonal or conventional rotors. Particles separate by differential centrifugation because they differ in size, density, and shape. Particles separate on density gradients because they differ in buoyant density (isopycnic centrifugation) or because prior to isopycnic banding their sedimentation rates differ (rate zonal centrifugation).

II. FACTORS AFFECTING SUBCELLULAR SEPARATIONS

A. Properties of Subcellular Particles

Two major factors affect the manner in which subcellular particles separate: the properties of the particles and those of the centrifugation technique. Currently one of the central limitations in preparing highly purified subcellular fractions from brain is the close similarity in particle density and sedimentation rate. In order to evaluate how to improve separations and overcome these intrinsic limitations, we analyze the physical properties of a particle that determine its buoyant density and sedimentation rate. These theoretical factors can provide guidelines for understanding, developing, and modifying separation procedures. In a subsequent section (Section IV) we describe certain of the critical factors of the separation technique which allow for maximum resolution.

1. Sedimentation Properties of Brain Subcellular Particles and Particular Problems Encountered in Fractionating Brain Tissue

Brain contains an abundance of subcellular structures, the buoyant densities and sedimentation rates of which are clustered quite closely together. This clustering makes it difficult to find conditions to achieve entirely satisfactory separation. The success of a separation depends on effectively utilizing those differences which exist.

The separation of brain subcellular particles by rate sedimentation has been examined by Cotman *et al.* (1970) and Kuhar *et al.* (1970, 1971) who have noted that populations of subcellular particles differ in sedimentation rate. Overlap, rather than complete separation, however, is the general situation. Rate sedimentation analysis as a technique for exploring function particularly as a property of structure size and for enrichment prior to isopycnic banding has been studied in detail to a very limited extent. Additional well-defined experiments would be profitable. Two technical considerations should be pointed out regarding rate sedimentation analysis in brain. It is well known that membranes shear into vesicles of a size determined by the shear conditions. Since rate separations in most cases are based on size, the homogenization technique dramatically influences the resulting rate separation. Ideally, the shear conditions optimal for preserving a class of subcellular structures should not reduce other structures to a similar size. Also, the separations obtained by differential centrifugation in most tissues are sharpened by recycling or washing the fractions. In brain, recycling is not as satisfactory since fragile structures such as synaptosomes become damaged by resuspension and recentrifugation, leading to a decrease rather than increase of the appropriate structure. Methods to stabilize these structures have not been studied. In subsequent sections (II,3; II,4; V) the basis of rate separations is described and the techniques appropriate for optimizing separations by rate are analyzed.

In Table I we have compiled from the literature a summary of the isopycnic banding densities of various brain subcellular particles. Particle density depends to a degree on the age of the animal, the species, previous treatment of the particle and the type of density gradient employed, in addition to technical considerations such as the sensitivity and fidelity of the assay method. While the isopycnic densities are not as yet precisely determined, it is evident that the densities of most brain particles overlap those of other particles. By isopycnic centrifugation on sucrose density gradients, glial and neuronal membranes, mitochondria, synaptosomes, lysosomes, and a portion of the microsome fraction all band close together. Since this is the case, a complete separation is not possible on the basis of density alone. However, most subcellular particles differ from each other enough so that partial separation is possible by isopycnic centrifugation, particularly when preceded by careful preliminary differential centrifugation. The separation of synaptosomes and mitochondria provides an illustration. In rat brain, synaptosomes are isopycnic at approximately 36% sucrose (w/w) while most nonsynaptosomal mitochondria sediment through 36% sucrose. By taking the leading edge of the synaptosomes and the trailing edge of the mitochondria, relatively pure fractions can be obtained.

2. Theoretical Parameters Determining Particle Density

In view of the critical nature of particle density in brain subcellular fractionations, it is important to analyze and evaluate the factors determining the density of a subcellular particle. The density of a subcellular particle is determined by the composite density of its components. This can vary, depending on the nature of the gradient and the exact state of the particle. The simplest practical case is that of a hydrated particle freely permeable to the gradient medium. In this case the density is equal to the density of its nondiffusible components (soluble and insoluble) plus the contribution from hydration. Membrane vesicles in hypertonic sucrose fall into this category. As a first approximation synaptosomes may be considered as membrane vesicles so that when they are equilibrated in hypertonic sucrose they, too, may be described by this model. Mitochondria are more complex. The thrust of a rather extensive literature is that mitochondria contain a space inaccessible to sucrose as well as a sucrose-accessible space (Bentzel and Solomon, 1967; deDuve, 1965; Gamble and Garlid, 1970). In these cases, when the gradient is not free to equilibrate with the total interior volume of the particle, the buoyant density will be a composite of the mass and volume contributions of its hydrated membrane and its solvent components (deDuve et al., 1959; Wallach, 1967). The mass of a given particle (μ) can be considered in terms of its components so that $\mu_p = \mu_m + \mu_s + \mu_h$ where μ_p is the mass of the particle, μ_m the mass of its membranes and nondiffusible solids, μ_s the mass of the solvents within the particle, and μ_h the mass of hydration layers of the particle. Then, since $\mu_i = \varrho_i V_i$

$$\varrho_p = \frac{\varrho_m V_m + \varrho_s V_s + \varrho_h V_h}{V_p} \qquad (1)$$

where ϱ_p is the effective density of the particle, V_p its total volume including the hydration layer, and $\varrho_m V_m$ the density and volume of its membranes and nondiffusible solids, $\varrho_s V_s$ the density and volume of its solvents, and $\varrho_h V_h$ the density and volume of its hydration layers. Measurements on mitochondria have yielded quantitative data on these different values and show excellent agreement between computed and measured isopycnic densities (Bentzel and Solomon, 1967; Loeb and Kimberg, 1970).

Thus substantial differences in the contribution of the solvent compartment and hydration can permit the isopycnic separation of particles having the same mass. Two particles inseparable on certain gradients become resolvable if conditions can be found where one or more of the factors making up the density are different. For example, synaptosomes do not completely separate from free mitochondria in sucrose gradients. In Ficoll-sucrose gradients, however, the separation is improved because synaptosomes show a larger decrease in density in these gradients than do mitochondria (Table I). The lighter buoyant density of synaptosomes on Ficoll-sucrose gradients compared to sucrose is in all probability due to the contribution of this solvent compartment to their buoyant density. Mitochondria are not affected. Since Ficoll is a macromolecule, having an estimated molecular weight of 400,000, it exerts a negligible osmotic pressure at the concentrations used for brain separations. Thus the solvent compartment remains under isotonic conditions during the separation and the aqueous components of the solvent compartment are not lost due to hypertonic conditions. These then contribute an additional buoyant force so that the net buoyant density is less in Ficoll gradients than in sucrose gradients where these components are lost. The additional buoyant force is more pronounced for synaptosomes than mitochondria.

As is evident from Eq. (1), the relative contribution of each component to the overall density is proportional to the volume of the component. The larger the vesicle, the greater and more significant the contribution of the solvent compartment to the effective density of the particle since the volume increases with the cube of the radius. Thus, large particles such as synaptosomes or large membrane fragments are more dependent on the medium than are small particles such as synaptic vesicles, microsomes, or perhaps small mitochondria.

Clearly, environmental factors that affect V_s and V_h can influence particle density. Wallach and co-workers (Wallach, 1967) have made the important observation that changes in pH or divalent ion concentration can selectively alter the isopycnic density of different particles on gradients where the solute is impermeable. These ionic effects possibly result from differences in the fixed charge of the vesicle (i.e., on the inner surface of the membrane and on the nondiffusible molecules within the vesicle). The osmotic activity of the solutes tends to shrink the vesicle while the fixed charges within the vesicle cause diffusible ions to accumulate within the vesicle lumen by a Donnan equilibrium and expand the vesicle (Steck *et al.,* 1970a). The volume of the vesicle fluid thus follows a Donnan-osmotic equilibrium across its membrane which will be reflected in the isopycnic density of the vesicle. These principles for altering particle density in impermeable gradients are effectively used for the separation of plasma membranes from microsomes (Wallach and Kamat, 1964; Graham *et al.,* 1968), but they have not yet been applied to brain.

A variety of techniques have been described which alter particle density in sucrose gradients. Most of these increase particle density by adsorbtion of a substance such as an antibody or by accumulation of a dense substance within the particle. Boone and co-workers (1969) and Roizman and Spear (1971) have used antibodies to plasma membranes to achieve an increase in the density of plasma membrane fractions homologous to their antibody. The limitation of such antibody techniques for a routine procedure is the relatively large quantity of specific antibody required. A more appropriate technique for most routine applications makes use of the formation of a heavy residue resulting as a product of specific enzyme-driven reactions. Microsomes from liver, for example, contain the enzyme glucose-6-phosphatase which hydrolyzes glucose-6-phosphate. Leskes and Siekevitz (1969) found that the released phosphate could be precipitated within the microsomal compartment by the presence of lead ions and the enclosed precipitate shifted the isopycnic density of these microsomes to a higher value. Similarly, mitochondria can be shifted to a higher density. Succinic dehydrogenase activity with iodonitrotetrazolium violet as electron acceptor catalyzes the formation of a dense formazan within the interior of the mitochondrion and the entrapped dense formazan causes the mitochondria to increase their density (Davis and Bloom, 1970). Mitochondria also become more dense after the accumulation of insoluble calcium phosphate salts during respiration-driven cation transport (Greenawalt *et al.,* 1964). It is apparent that most procedures such as histochemical reactions which lead to the formation of a dense impermeable product within a subcellular compartment should be suitable for selectively altering the density of the particle catalyzing the reaction.

The technique of altering particle density has provided a means to

Table I. Summary of Isopycnic Banding Densities of Various Brain Subcellular Particles

Particle	Gradient	Density (g/ml)	Source	Method of determination	Reference
Mitochondria whole brain	Sucrose	1.141–1.192	Rabbit Guinea pig Rat	Cytochrome oxidase Succinic dehydrogenase	Cotman, 1968 Hamberger et al., 1970 Whittaker, 1968
	Ficoll–0.32 M sucrose	1.116	Rat	Cytochrome oxidase	Cotman, 1968 Autilio et al., 1968
Neuronal (soma)	Sucrose	1.171–1.219	Neuron enriched fraction from rabbit brain	Cytochrome oxidase	Hamberger et al., 1970
Glial	Sucrose	1.156–1.187	Rat cultured glial cells (C6)	Cytochrome oxidase	Cotman et al., 1971a
	Sucrose	1.156–1.192	Glial enriched fraction from rabbit brain	Cytochrome oxidase	Hamberger et al., 1970
Synaptosomes	Sucrose	1.141–1.182	Rat	Morphology, enzymes	Cotman, 1968
	Sucrose	1.14–1.17	Guinea pig	Morphology, ACh	Whittaker, 1968
	Ficoll–sucrose	1.063–1.090	Rat	Morphology, various enzymes	Autilio et al., 1968
Synaptic plasma membrane	Sucrose	1.120–1.161	Rat	Morphology, enzymes	Cotman et al., 1968
	Sucrose	1.130–1.157	Rat	Morphology, enzymes	Rodriguez de Lores Arnaiz et al., 1967
	CsCl	1.150	Rat	Morphology, Na-K ATPase	Cotman, 1968
Synaptic vesicles	Sucrose	1.08	Rat		Cotman, 1968
	Sucrose	1.056[a]	Guinea pig	Morphology	Whittaker et al., 1964
	CsCl–sucrose	1.15	Rat		Cotman, 1968

Table I (*Continued*)

Particle	Gradient	Density (g/ml)	Source	Method of determination	Reference
Glial membranes	Sucrose	1.121–1.167	Rat cultured glial cells (C6)	Morphology, enzymes	Cotman *et al.*, 1970
Myelin	Sucrose	1.10	Bovine	Morphology, lipid analysis	Autilio *et al.*, 1964
	Ficoll-sucrose	1.04–1.07	Rat	Morphology	Cotman, 1968
	CsCl	1.04			
Lysosomes	Sucrose	1.15–1.19	Rat	Enzymes, morphology	Koenig *et al.*, 1964

a Not quite isopycnic.

isolate various subcellular structures otherwise not resolvable by rate sedimentation and isopycnic density and has allowed for progress on the study of their function. Lysosomes in liver, for example, isopycnically band with mitochondria, but they will accumulate the low-density detergent WR. 1339 after intravenous injection and as a result shift their density from 1.21 to 1.12 g/ml (de Duve, 1965). In this way it became possible to resolve lysosomes from liver mitochondria. The application of techniques to modify particle density in brain is a particularly appropriate means to overcome the intrinsic similarities in particle density and lead to improvements in fraction purity. Other techniques which lead to a change in particle density have been described (Heine and Schnaitman, 1971; Steck *et al.*, 1970b; Pollak and Munn, 1970; Thines-Sempoux *et al.*, 1969; Emmelot and Vaz Dias, 1970; Wattiaux-DeConinck and Wattiaux, 1969).

3. Theoretical Parameters Determining Sedimentation Rate

Particles not separable by isopycnic banding often separate by rate sedimentation. Microsomes and mitochondria, which have very similar isopycnic densities, separate easily by rate sedimentation. The quantity expressing the rate of migration for a particular particle in a centrifugation field is the sedimentation coefficient. It is the velocity of a particle in a centrifugation field of unity. Clearly, subcellular particles with the same sedimentation coefficient will not separate by rate sedimentation.

The properties of a particle that determine the sedimentation coefficient are given by the Svedberg equation, a general form of which can be written as

$$S = \frac{V_p (\varrho_p - \varrho_m)}{f_0} \tag{2}$$

where S is the sedimentation coefficient, V_p the volume, and ϱ_p the density of the particle; ϱ_m is the density of the media and f_0 is the frictional coefficient for a spherical particle (deDuve *et al.*, 1959; Schackman, 1959). This equation is derived from the relationship of the force on the particle exerted by the centrifugation field counterbalanced by the frictional force on the particle. The force on the particle is equal to $M\omega^2 x$, where M is the mass of the particle, ω the angular velocity, and x the distance between the particle and the center of the rotor. Since the particle displaces a volume of medium V of density ϱ_m, the effective mass of the particle is $(\varrho - V_m)$. Thus the driving force on the particle is $\omega^2 x(\varrho - V\varrho_m)$. This force is counterbalanced by the frictional force on the particle $f dx/dt$. Equating the two forces to describe the motion of the particle and substituting the density and volume of the particle for its mass gives

$$S = \frac{dx/dt}{\omega^2 t} = \frac{V_p(\varrho_p - \varrho_m)}{f_0} \tag{3}$$

The quantity $(dx/dt)/\omega^2 t$ is the sedimentation coefficient S, the sedimentation rate in a unit centrifugation field. It is measured in seconds or Svedberg units, $1S = 10^{-13}$ sec. The frictional coefficient f_0 for a spherical particle can be written according to Stokes' law as, $f_0 = 6\pi\eta r_0$, where η is the viscosity of the medium in poises and r_0 is the radius of the sphere in centimeters. Thus for a spherical particle Eq. (2) is written

$$S = \frac{2r_0^2(\varrho_p - \varrho_m)}{9\eta} \tag{4}$$

Equation (4) indicates that size and density both are important in determining the rate of sedimentation of a particle. The major factor determining differences in sedimentation rate is particle size. This is in accordance with the empirical findings obtained by analytical differential centrifugation (Section V). However, density also plays a part, so that a small particle with a large density can have the same sedimentation rate as a large particle with a small density. Equation (4) quantitates the nature of this counterbalancing relationship for a spherical particle. It does not, however, predict what effect particle shape will have on S. To apply this equation to nonspherical particles the frictional ratio or shape factor is introduced. The frictional ratio (θ) is the ratio of the frictional coefficient of the particle to that of a spherical particle of equal volume. For prolate ellipsoids with radii r_1/r_2 equal to 1, θ is also 1; for $r_1/r_2 = 3$, θ is 1.105, for $r_1/r_2 = 6$, θ is 1.277 (deDuve et al., 1959). Radius r_1 represents the half axis of revolution and r_2 the equatorial radius of the ellipsoid. This shape factor is introduced into the denominator of Eq. (4). Increases in θ as the sphere becomes more ellipsoid will tend to slow down particles. Particles sedimenting in density gradients can have increasing, decreasing, or constant sedimentation coefficients, depending on how the radius, density, and frictional ratio are affected by the gradient. For subcellular particles this must be determined experimentally.

Factors which modify the size, shape, and density of a particle will alter its sedimentation rate. If this modification is selective for one particle, its separation properties will change relative to other particles so that further resolution will be achieved. Methods to alter particle density as discussed in the previous section will alter sedimentation rate as well. However, the major factor determining $S_{20,w}$ is particle size because the sedimentation coefficient is proportional to radius squared [Eq. (4)] so that factors changing size will be most effective in altering sedimentation rate. Controlled sonication or selective aggregation are two means of achieving selective size alterations. For example, rough endoplasmic reticulum can be resolved from other microsomal membranes by introducing cesium ions. This treatment selectively aggregates the rough endoplasmic reticular fraction so that it sediments more rapidly than other microsomal components (Dallner and Ernster, 1968).

4. Application of Theory to Experimental Design

The purpose of developing quantitative relationships between the factors determining particle density and sedimentation coefficient is to provide a basis for approaching brain separation in a theoretical as well as an empirical manner. From this basis a protocol for determining the appropriate means of separation may be developed. Various alternatives may be tested sequentially. Are the particles separable by isopycnic banding on sucrose gradients? If differences in density are not sufficient for a satisfactory separation, are the particles separable by rate either because of differences in their size or shape or because of differential density changes during rate sedimentation in density gradients? Since these procedures are based on the physical properties of the particles, if a separation does not result on the basis of these properties, further experiments will only verify the similarity in these properties. In this type of situation a separation will not result. Either another separation technique must be found or a means must be devised to independently alter one or more of the centrifugation properties of the particles. Significant increases in resolution are usually not obtained by repeating many times a procedure based only on sedimentation rate or only on density when the properties of the particles do not change during the procedure. Particles are organized according to their sedimentation coefficients or their banding densities and no further separation results.

A critical factor in the design of separation procedures is the selection of a gradient to provide adequate resolution of the particle populations. The degree of resolution necessary is dependent on the centrifugation technique. Usually the particle populations should be resolved by two or more fractions.

In general, the gradient selected should have enough capacity so that the sedimenting zones are stable. In multicomponent systems a series of zones leaves the starting zone with little separation between them. As the zones sediment, they spread out in the gradient. The greatest capacity is therefore required through and immediately below the starting zone. The gradient should be steep and convex in this region (Anderson, 1966). However, if the gradient rises too steeply just under the sample zone, particles will overload the initial region and form a kind of barrier which prevents each particle from acting independently of the others and leads to nonideal sedimentation and trapping of other particles. Particularly when a particle is isopycnic at the initial region of the gradient, a barrier is easily formed. Very shallow gradients, on the other hand, have low capacity and without some increase in density cannot support the sedimentation of the zones. A gradient therefore should have a sufficient increase in density to maintain stability. Theoretical approaches for capacity and boundary stability have been developed and tested for one-particle systems (Berman, 1966; Spragg and Rankin, 1967; Brakke, 1964), but not for multicomponent systems with sedimentation coefficients and densities in the range of subcellular particles.

As discussed, the sedimentation behavior of a particle is determined by its sedimentation coefficient and its density. Hence two-particle separation problems can be reduced to four separate cases: (1) $S_1 > S_2$, $\varrho_1 = \varrho_2$; (2) $S_1 = S_2$, $\varrho_1 > \varrho_2$; (3) $S_1 > S_2$, $\varrho_1 > \varrho_2$; (4) $S_1 > S_2$, $\varrho_1 < \varrho_2$. In each section below we will discuss the principles for selecting a gradient most appropriate for each case. The problem in gradient design then is to determine the particular case most closely corresponding to the experimental situation.

We need to determine the resolution that will be achieved between two particles characterized by sedimentation coefficients S_1 and S_2 and densities ϱ_1 and ϱ_2 in different gradients. Resolution is defined as the distance between the two particles as percent of the gradient path. To determine resolution we use a computer program and calculate the position of each particle at a particular value of total applied force. The separation between the two particles as percent of gradient path (resolution) is expressed as a function of the migration distance of the faster particle in the gradient. In this way we observe the migration of the fastest particle in each gradient and the distance that the slower particle is behind the faster. Maximum resolution of the two particles is achieved when separation as percent of the gradient path is largest.

Case 1: $S_1 > S_2$, $\varrho_1 = \varrho_2$. Resolution in this case can be achieved only by differences in sedimentation rates; separation by isopycnic banding will not resolve the particles since their densities are equivalent.

Maximum resolution for this case is achieved in a homogeneous sucrose medium. For example, in 10% sucrose the particle with the larger $S_{20,w}$ reaches the end of the gradient path while the second particle is 47% of the gradient path behind the first (Fig. 1). Interestingly, resolution for this case is independent of the sucrose concentration. In both 25% and 10% sucrose the maximum separation between the two particles is 47% of the gradient path.

As illustrated in Fig. 1, increasing the slope of the gradient is accompanied by a loss of resolution. Any increase in gradient slope from 10% sucrose results in a decrease in the separation. In a linear 10–40% sucrose gradient, maximum resolution is only 14% of the gradient path. In this situation

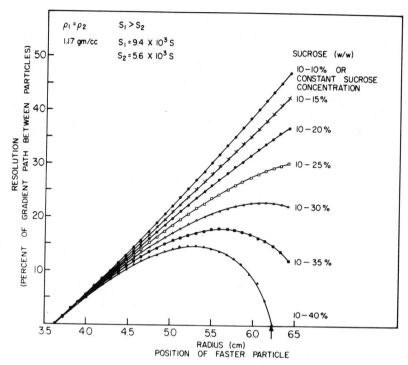

Fig. 1. A comparison of the separation of two particles for case 1 where $S_1 = 9.4 \times 10^3\ S$, $S_2 = 5.6 \times 10^3\ S$, $\varrho_1 = \varrho_2 = 1.17$ g/ml on 10% sucrose or various gradients. The separation between two particles (as percent of the gradient path between particles) is shown as a function of the position of the faster particle in the gradient. Thus, as the faster particle sediments into the gradient, the slower particle follows behind by a distance given as percent of the gradient path. Most of the $S_{20,w}$ values and densities are within the range of those found of various brain subcellular particles (Sections II and IV and Table I). The gradients were designed for a B XIV zonal rotor. The gradient ends at rotor volume (6.4 cm). The calculations were carried out on an Olivetti computer based on the method of Bishop (1966) and Halsall and Schumaker (1969) as described in the Appendix or by a similar program on a PDP computer. (From Cotman, Doyle and Banker, 1972a. Doyle, Banker, and Cotman, 1972). (See also Figs 2–6).

resolution reaches a maximum when the faster particle is midway into the gradient and then resolution returns to zero when both particles reach 38% sucrose, the isopycnic point of the particles. Thus it is critical in this type of gradient to determine the required total applied force to achieve maximum resolution because there is no separation at isopycnic banding.

Resolution depends not only on gradient slope but also on the initial sucrose concentration. For example, in gradients with a 10% change in sucrose concentration starting at 10% sucrose (10–20% sucrose) and 25%

sucrose (25–35% sucrose), resolution is 37% and 24%, respectively. The generalization that can be made is as follows: the farther away the particle density is from the initial sucrose density and the shallower the gradient slope, the better the separation.

The value of the density of the particles also influences the resulting separation, except in homogeneous sucrose media. In gradients, resolution depends on how close the sucrose density approaches the isopycnic banding density of the particles. This can be illustrated by the following example. For particles with $S_{20,w}$ values of 5.6 and 9.4 × 10^3 S and with a density such that the particles band at 23% sucrose, maximal resolution in 10–15% sucrose is 39%, while in 10–25% it is only 19%. For particles with the same $S_{20,w}$'s but which band at 38% sucrose, the separation in the 10–23% gradient is only 33% compared to 43% in the 10–15% gradient. Thus the further the particles' density is from that of the gradient, the better the separation.

The exact value of the $S_{20,w}$ for each particle influences the separation in all sucrose media and gradients. Resolution is determined by the ratio of the sedimentation coefficients, not by their absolute difference. We programmed the computer to vary the $S_{20,w}$ values of two particles. S_1/S_2 ratios that were the same, regardless of the absolute $S_{20,w}$ values, produced identical resolution in terms of percent gradient path. Increasing the ratio of sedimentation coefficients increases resolution as illustrated in Fig. 2. When S_1/S_2 is small, resolution is small. Resolution increases rapidly, then more gradually as the ratio approaches larger values. In 10% sucrose the separation increases from 21% to 57% as S_1/S_2 increases from 1.2 to 2.0 and from 87% to 90% as S_1/S_2 increases from 6.0 to 8.0. Steepening the slope of the gradient does not change resolution very significantly if the ratio of S_1/S_2 is very large. If S_1/S_2 is small, as is the case for most subcellular particles of interest, increases in gradient slope are accompanied by decreases in separation from homogeneous sucrose media. The effect of gradient slope on resolution at different values of S_1/S_2 is illustrated in Table II.

The general conclusion for this case is that maximum resolution is achieved in homogeneous sucrose media and is independent of this media as long as the media is less dense than that of the particles. The effect of increasing gradient slope depends on the values of the density of the particles and the ratio of S_1/S_2. Resolution is not markedly dependent on gradient slope if the density of the particles is significantly greater than the initial or final density of the sucrose in the gradient or if the ratio of sedimentation coefficients is very large.

Case 2: $S_1 = S_2, \varrho_1 > \varrho_2$. Particles that differ in density alone separate most effectively by isopycnic banding. Maximum resolution is simply limited by the length of the gradient because the lighter particle can be retained at

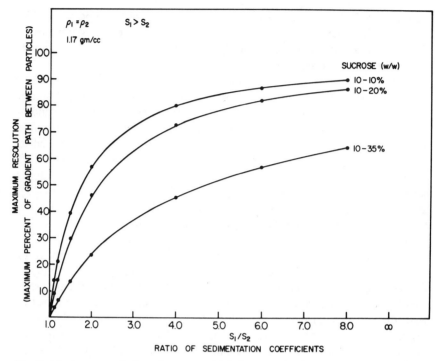

Fig. 2. Maximum resolution of two particles for case 1 where $\varrho_1 = \varrho_2 = 1.17$ g/ml on different gradients as the ratio of sedimentation coefficients (S_1/S_2) is varied (see explanation in Fig.1).

the sample zone while the heavier particle sediments to the end of the gradient.

Particles that differ in density alone can also be separated by rate in gradients. The best separations are achieved with conditions very similar to those for isopycnic banding. Maximum separation occurs in a homogeneous sucrose medium where the sucrose density is close to that of the lighter particle. The relevant question for this case is to determine the extent to which separations are affected by altering gradient properties.

Resolution in homogeneous media is rapidly lost when the density of the medium decreases from that of the lighter particle. Maximum resolution for particle of a density 1.14 and 1.17 g/ml in a 30% sucrose medium is 78% of the gradient path, whereas for a 25% medium resolution it is 44% and for a 10% medium it is only 7%. (Fig. 3). Thus the farther the density of the medium is from that of the lighter particle, the poorer the separation. It is

Table II.   Decrease in Resolution in 10–20% or 10–35% Sucrose
(w/w) Gradients Compared to 10% Sucrose[a]

Gradient	S_1/S_2	Percent decrease
10–20%	1.2	30
	1.5	24
	2.0	18
	4.0	9
10–35%	1.2	68
	1.5	64
	2.0	58
	4.0	43

[a] Decreases in resolution are given as percent change from 10% sucrose for each value of S_1/S_2. Gradients do not decrease resolution as markedly at large values of S_1/S_2 as at smaller ratios of S_1/S_2.

particularly interesting that there is very little separation in 10% sucrose for particles in case 2 when resolution for particles in case 1 is excellent.

The relationship between the densities of the two particles that determines the separation in homogeneous sucrose can be derived. Resolution depends on the interaction between particle densities and the sucrose medium. This relationship can be expressed as

$$\frac{(\varrho_1 - \varrho_m)}{(\varrho_1 - \varrho_m)} \times \frac{(\varrho_2 - \varrho_{20,w})}{(\varrho_1 - \varrho_{20,w})} \tag{5}$$

The relation is essentially one of a ratio of density differences. As long as this relationship remains constant, maximum resolution stays the same (Table III). Resolution improves with increases in the ratio of density differences. When the ratio is small, improvements occur quite rapidly and then as the ratio becomes large the increases are not as pronounced. In a homogeneous medium of 20% sucrose, maximal resolution increases from zero to 57% as the ratio of density differences increases from 1.0 to 2.0. When the ratio increases from 3.0–4.0, maximal resolution increases from 73–80%.

Resolution by rate for this case is independent of variations in $S_{20,w}$. As long as the ratio of S_1/S_2 equals one in either homogeneous media or density gradients, resolution remains the same.

In sucrose gradients the separation depends on the gradient slope and the initial or final sucrose concentration. If the final sucrose concentration is held constant and the gradient slope changed, resolution is lost compared to a homogeneous media of 30% sucrose. As shown in Fig.3, resolution is 78% in 30% sucrose, whereas in a 25–30% sucrose gradient resolution is 42%. Resolution in a 20–30% gradient is 26% and in a 10–30% gradient it is 14%. The separation in these gradients is nearly identical to that in a homo-

Table III.   Relationship Between Ratio of Density Differences and
Resolution for Different Particle Densities[a]

Particle densities (g/ml)		Density difference (g/ml)	Ratio of density difference	Resolution (%)
ϱ_1	ϱ_2			
$\varrho_m = 1.0842\ (20\%-20\%\ \text{sucrose})$				
1.098	1.098	0.0000	1.0	0
1.098	1.1013	0.0033	1.2	21
1.098	1.1066	0.0086	1.5	40
1.098	1.1169	0.0189	2.0	57
1.098	1.1446	0.0466	3.0	73
1.098	1.1892	0.0912	4.0	80
$\varrho_m = 1.0406\ (10\%-10\%\ \text{sucrose})$				
1.098	1.1351	0.0371	1.2	21
1.098	1.3071	0.2091	1.5	40

[a] Resolution is not dependent on the difference in densities of two particles, but on their ratio of density differences.

geneous media of the concentration of the initial sucrose. In 25% sucrose resolution is 43% compared to 44% in a 25–30% gradient. In 20% sucrose it is 25.5% compared to 26% in a 20–30% gradient; and in 10% it is 7% compared to 14% in a 10–30% gradient. These comparisons are illustrated in Fig. 3. Thus, decreasing the slope from homogeneous media by lowering the initial sucrose concentration when the homogeneous media is close to the isopycnic banding point of the lighter particle is accompanied by a large loss in the separation of the two particles. In gradients the best separation by rate is obtained in very shallow gradients in which the density of the initial and final portion of the gradient is close to the isopycnic banding density of the lighter particle. Resolution is relatively poor in very steep gradients (e.g., 10–30% sucrose) or in homogeneous media such as 10% sucrose where differences between the density of the media and particles is large.

Clearly, for this case the most separation is found at isopycnic banding. A number of practical considerations are of importance. In selecting a gradient for this case consideration should be given to the experimental purpose and the resolution of the instrument. For the separation of only two particles, the maximum resolution is obtained by using a medium of a density equal to that of the lightest particle so that this particle is stopped at the sample zone while the heavier particle sediments completely to the bottom of the tube or rotor. Continuous gradients inclusive of the density of the particles are most useful when (1) there are other populations of particles with densities heavier than ϱ_2 or lighter than ϱ_1; and (2) a precise determination of the density range of the population and shape of the distribution is required. Step gradients created by introducing a discontinuity or step in the density are useful for (1) grouping a population into a small volume and (2)

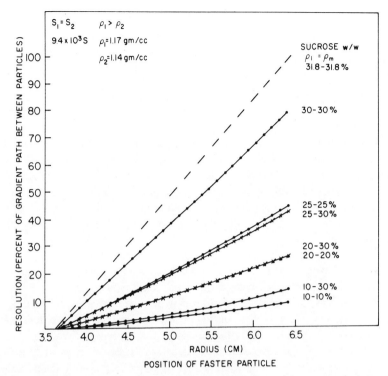

Fig. 3. Comparison of the separation of two particles for case 2 where $S_1 = S_2 = 9.4 \times 10^3\ S$ and $\varrho_1 = 1.17$ g/cm³ and $\varrho_2 = 1.14$ g/cm³ on various sucrose gradients (see explanation in Fig. 1).

for increasing the resolution between two populations by providing a plateau of constant density between two particles. Once the particles are separated by more than the resolution of the instruments, the separation is not further improved by further spreading of the gradient unless the zone is overloaded. A simple way to determine if the zone is overloaded is to recycle the band. It should come out as a symmetrical peak confined to its initial banding density.

There is sometimes a question as to how critical it is to achieve complete equilibrium of the particles in isopycnic banding. Essentially the complete separation is reached prior to isopycnic banding. The particles achieve full separation at relatively short times and sediment essentially in parallel as they asymptotically approach their isopycnic banding densities. This permits the selection of shorter centrifugation times and illustrates that complete isopycnic banding is not always critical for particle separations of $S_1 = S_2$. Somewhat the same considerations apply in steep gradients in case 3 when particles differ in both sedimentation coefficient and density (see Fig. 5, 10–40% gradient). It should be emphasized that these considerations apply only to ideal particles since it is well known that particularly during prolonged equilibration, interactions with the gradient lead to increased particle densities which may be selective for one particular class.

Case 3: $S_1 > S_2$, $\varrho_1 > \varrho_2$. The complex cases in which the particles differ in both S and density can be considered as a combination of the first two cases. In this case the larger particle is heavier and the smaller particle is lighter. Rate separation is better than in cases 1 or 2 because both density and $S_{20,w}$ are working for the separation. Maximum resolution occurs when the particles can reach their isopycnic points encompassing the entire gradient path, that is, one traveling to the end of the gradient and one remaining at the beginning. When either density or S differences are large relative to the other property, the rate separation will in fact approximate that for either case 1 or case 2.

The homogeneous sucrose medium which gives best resolution is one in which the density of the lighter particle approaches that of the medium. This was also optimal for case 2 when particles differed in density alone. Differences in $S_{20,w}$ improve resolution in homogeneous media especially when the density of the eighter particle is farther away from the density of the media. For example, when the density of the lighter particle (ϱ_2) is such that it bands at 31.8% sucrose and the density of the heavier particle (ϱ_1) is 1.17 so that it bands at 38%, sucrose and $S_1/S_2 = 9.4/5.6 = 1.7$, resolution in 30% sucrose is 89% of the path. If, however, the same two particles are assigned equal sedimentation coefficients and $S_1/S_2 = 1$ (case 2), resolution is reduced to 79%. In 20% sucrose, resolution for particles differing in both density and sedimentation coefficient is 60%, in contrast to 25.5% resolution when they differ in density alone. It is apparent that differences in sedimentation coefficient contribute positively to the separation in case 3.

In homogeneous media the exact relationship that determines resolution is the ratio of sedimentation coefficients (S_1/S_2) times the ratio of the density differences [Eq. (5)]. Equal resolution is produced as long as the product of the ratios is equal. When the ratio of density differences is 1.5 and S_1/S_2 is 1.2, resolution is 51%. Likewise, when the ratio of density differences is 1.2 and S_1/S_2 is 1.5, resolution is 51%. If the product of the ratios is 6.0, whether it is formed by 1.5×4.0 or by 2.0×3.0, resolution is 87% of the path. Therefore, it is simple to determine resolution in flat gradients for any set of particles in this case.

In density gradients the relation between resolution and sedimentation coefficient cannot be established as it can for homogeneous sucrose media, since the term expressing the density differences varies with changes in sucrose density. Resolution is most suitably analyzed by selecting particle densities of interest to subcellular separations ($\varrho_1 = 1.17$, $\varrho_2 = 1.14$ g/ml) and varying S_1/S_2 for particular gradients. Resolution is lost as the initial sucrose density decreases away from the density of the lighter particle. In 25–30% sucrose resolution is 50% when S_1/S_2 is 1.2. In 20–30% sucrose resolution for these particles is 35% of the gradient path. In 10–30% sucrose it is only 19%. When S_1/S_2 is large, there is a more gradual loss of resolution as the initial sucrose density decreases away from the isopycnic density of the lighter particle. The resolution in 25–30% sucrose when S_1/S_2 is 8.0 is 92%; in 20–30% sucrose it is 88%; in 10–30% sucrose, 79%. Thus separation is dependent on the initial concentration of the gradient as it relates to the ratio S_1/S_2 and particle densities.

We can evaluate resolution in gradients for sedimentation coefficients derived from subcellular particles from brain. Synaptosomes defined by the sedimentation of choline acetyltransferase have an apparent $S_{20,w}$ of about 5.6×10^3 and a density of 1.14 g/ml while mitochondria have an apparent $S_{20,w}$ of about 9.6×10^3 S and a density of 1.17 g/ml. The $S_{20,w}$ values describe the sedimentation of a hypothetical particle which sediments at the mean of the choline acetyltransferase population (50% point) and thus do not describe the entire population, only the mean. S_1/S_2 is 1.7 for these particles. In 10% sucrose these particles would be resolved by 52% of the gradient path while in a 10–25% sucrose gradient resolution is 38%. Since the ratio of sedimentation coefficients is relatively small, resolution is better in a 25–30% sucrose gradient in which the initial region of the gradient approaches the density of the lighter particle. In this gradient the particles separate by 64% of the gradient path. Resolution in a commonly used gradient for the separation of brain subcellular particles, such as 10–40% sucrose, is reduced by comparison to all above examples. The separation is only 21% of the gradient path.

It is of interest to compare the rate separations achieved for particles with $S_{20,w}$ values of 5.6 and 9.6×10^3 S and density values of 1.14 and 1.17 g/ml to the separations which would be realized if density values were equal, but $S_{20,w}$ 5.6 and 9.6×10^3 S (case 1), or if $S_{20,w}$ values were equal and densities 1.14 and 1.17 g/ml (case 2). In this way we can demonstrate the relative contributions of ϱ and $S_{20,w}$ to the rate separation of these particles. The comparison of particles with different $S_{20,w}$ and densities to those in which the densities are considered equal is illustrated in Fig 4. In 10% sucrose there is little difference in resolution and it is clear that sedimentation coefficients are primarily responsible for resolution in this medium. In 10–25% sucrose or 10–40% sucrose, density differences have a more beneficial effect on resolution. In Fig. 5 resolution for these particles in case 3 is compared to resolution when the sedimentation coefficients are considered equal. Resolution in 30% sucrose is mainly due to density differences and is rapidly

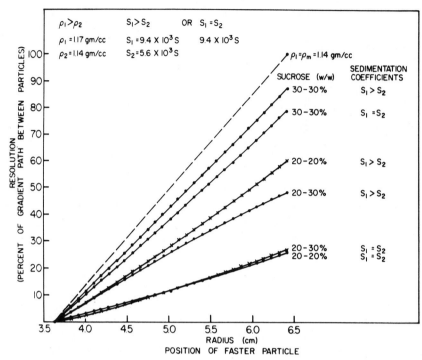

Fig. 4. The separation of two particles for case 3 ($S_1 > S_2$, $\varrho_1 > \varrho_2$) on various gradients compared to the separation of two particles for case 1 ($S_1 > S_2$, $\varrho_1 = \varrho_2$). Sedimentation coefficients and densities used are given in the figure (see explanation in Fig. 1).

lost in less dense homogeneous media or shallow gradients. It is evident that the major determinate of resolution is the sedimentation coefficient for these particles in 10% sucrose; in 30% sucrose it is the densities, but both the sedimentation coefficient and density interact to aid the separation in case 3, particularly on gradients between the extremes.

In summary, resolution can be achieved by density differences, $S_{20,w}$ differences, or both. Optimal gradients for separation by density differences are shallow, with the sucrose density close to the isopycnic banding density of the lighter particle. As the sucrose density decreases, further resolution is rapidly lost, especially if the ratio S_1/S_2 is small. Separations designed to emphasize $S_{20,w}$ differences are optimal in 10% sucrose. As gradients increase in slope, resolution is lost gradually, especially when S_1/S_2 is large. In homogeneous media resolution can be determined by the ratio of sedimentation coefficients multiplied by the ratio of density differences.

Case 4: $S_1 > S_2$, $\varrho_1 < \varrho_2$. In this case the particle with the larger sedimentation coefficient is the lighter and that with the smaller $S_{20,w}$, the heavier. In

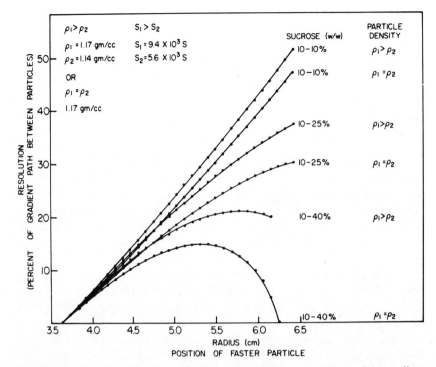

Fig. 5. The separation of two particles for case 3 ($S_1 > S_2$, $\varrho_1 > \varrho_2$) on various gradients compared to the separation of two particles for case 2 ($S_1 = S_2$, $\varrho_1 > \varrho_2$). Sedimentation coefficients and densities used are given in the figure (see explanation in Fig. 1).

contrast to case 3 in which sedimentation coefficients and densities worked together to improve the separation, they work against each other in this case so that in certain gradients and at certain concentrations of homogeneous sucrose media, no separation or very little separation results. First we shall describe the factors determining resolution in homogeneous media and then analyze resolution in density gradients.

A particular homogeneous medium can produce no resolution because the $S_{20,w}$ and density for each particle interact so that boths particle have identical sedimentation rates. For example, in 29.4% sucrose, particles with $\varrho_1 = 1.14$ and $\varrho_2 = 1.17$ and the ratio $S_1/S_2 = 4.0$ do not resolve. To achieve separation it is necessary either to raise or to lower the sucrose concentration. Below the zero resolution concentration separations are achieved by $S_{20,w}$ differences and hindered by density differences. Above the zero resolution concentration separations are gained based on density differences. To analyze separations achieved in homogeneous media we need first to calculate the concentration of sucrose which gives zero resolution.

The sucrose medium giving zero resolution can be computed from $S_{20,w}$ and density values of two particles by the following relationship:

$$\left(\frac{S_1}{S_2}\right)\left(\frac{\varrho_2 - \varrho_m}{\varrho_1 - \varrho_m} \times \frac{\varrho_1 - \varrho_{20,w}}{\varrho_2 - \varrho_{20,w}}\right) = 1 \tag{6}$$

This equation describes the relation between the $S_{20,w}$ and density of the two particles and the medium in which these particles have identical sedimentation rates. It will be recognized that the density term is the ratio of density differences term introduced in case 2. The ratio of sedimentation coefficients and the ratio of density differences determines resolution in homogeneous media. In case, however, the ratio of density differences decreases with increases in the difference between particle densities. When S_1/S_2 equals the ratio of density differences, resolution is zero: both factors cancel each other out. If density is held constant, the ratio of sedimentation coefficients determines the sucrose concentration which does not resolve the particles. For example, when $\varrho_1 = 1.14$ and $\varrho_2 = 1.17$ and S_1/S_2 is 1.2 the zero resolution concentration is 17.7% sucrose; for particles with the same densities but $S_1/S_2 = 3.0$ the sucrose concentration yielding identical sedimentation rates is 29.4%. Thus by using Eq. (6) the concentration of sucrose in which there is no resolution can be calculated.

Separations carried out in homogeneous sucrose media below the zero resolution concentration are based on $S_{20,w}$ differences. Separations are optimal in media such as 10% sucrose in which the density contribution to sedimentation is minimized. Resolution increases or decreases in 10% sucrose as determined by the ratio of sedimentation coefficients times the ratio of density differences. When the ratio of density differences is held constant, resolution improves rapidly with increases in S_1/S_2. For a ratio of density differences of 1/1.2, the separation increases from zero to 57% of the gradient path as S_1/S_2 goes from 1.2 to 2.0. As S_1/S_2 continues to increase from 2.0 to 6.0, resolution increases from 57% to 84%. When the ratio of density differences is changed, the effect on resolution is determined by the value of the ratio of sedimentation coefficients relative to the ratio of density differences. When S_1/S_2 is large relative to the ratio of density differences, resolution is not significantly affected. For a ratio of $S_1/S_2 = 8.0$, resolution decreases from 89 to 86% as the ratio of density differences decreases from 1/1.2 to 1/1.4. Alternately, when the ratio of sedimentation coefficients approaches the ratio of density differences, a dramatic loss of resolution results. For S_1/S_2 of 1.5, resolution decreases from 25% to 8% as the ratio, of density differences decreases from 1/1.2 to 1/1.4. Thus for separations in homogeneous media below the zero resolution concentration, separation is determined by an interaction between the ratio of sedimentation coefficients and the ratio of density differences.

Separations above the zero resolution concentration are based on differences in density and hindered by differences in sedimentation coefficient. The principles are identical to those described above for separations below the zero resolution concentration and will not be described here.

In sucrose gradients such as 10–45% sucrose, the particle with high $S_{20,w}$ and low density sediments faster in the first part of the gradient; the particle with lower $S_{20,w}$ and higher density catches up and sediments past the larger particle as they approach their isopycnic banding densities. This sedimentation pattern is illustrated in Fig. 6. At 29% sucrose both particles have sedimented to the same position in the gradient and resolution is zero. Near this intersection point resolution is very poor.

Because in this case the particles separate initially by rate, come together, and then separate upon isopycnic banding, it is necessary to analyze separation in gradients for this case as a separation problem before and after the intersection point of the particles. Before the intersection point the separation is achieved by sedimentation coefficients and hindered by density. After the intersection point the separation is based on density and hindered by $S_{20,w}$ differences.

In sucrose gradients we analyze particles of selected densities ($\varrho_1 = 1.14$ and $\varrho_2 = 1.17$.) Particular examples of pairs of subcellular particles from brain which have these approximate density values and are classified in case 4 might include the following: large membrane fragments and rough endoplasmic reticulum, synaptosomes and lysosomes, synaptosomes and small mitochondria.

An awareness of the factors determining resolution for case 4 should help in devising a strategy for separating brain particles which fall into this case. In gradients when $\rho_1 = 1.14$ g/ml and $\rho_2 = 1.17$ g/ml, resolution prior to the intersection point is markedly dependent on the ratio of S_1/S_2, increasing with increases in S_1/S_2 and decreasing with decreases in S_1/S_2. Before the intersection point, the particle with the larger sedimentation coefficient and lighter density (S_1, ρ_1) sediments more rapidly. In 10–15% sucrose, resolution increases from 28 to 67% as S_1/S_2 increases from 1.5 to 3.0, and then gradually from 84 to 87% as S_1/S_2 increases from 6.0 to 8.0. Conversely, when S_1/S_2 is 1.2 instead of 1.5, resolution decreases from 28% to only 9%. Besides the ratio of sedimentation coefficients, the slope of the gradient also markedly affects resolution. At a S_1/S_2 value of 1.5, resolution is 28% in a 10–15% gradient compared to 10% in a 10–25% gradient. At a higher value of S_1/S_2 such as 3.0, a similar, but not as marked, effect of gradient slope on resolution exists. In 10–15% sucrose, resolution is 67% compared to 47% in a 10–25% gradient or 24% in a 10–30% gradient. The conclusion is that at density values of $\rho_1 = 1.14$ g/ml and $\rho_2 = 1.17$ g/ml, the separation between the particles is markedly reduced when the ratio of sedimentation coefficients

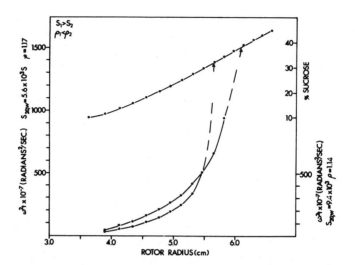

Fig. 6. Sedimentation profile of two particles for case 4 ($S_1 > S_2$, $\varrho_1 < \varrho_2$) on a continuous sucrose gradient (10–40% w/w). At 32% sucrose both particles have sedimented to an identical position in the gradient. $S_1 = 5.6 \times 10^3$ S, $\varrho_1 = 1.17$ g/ml, $S_2 = 9.4 \times 10^3$ normal S, $\varrho_2 = 1.14$ g/ml (see explanation in Fig. 1).

is small and the gradient slope steep.

In summary, separations by $S_{20,w}$ differences decrease with increasing density differences and separations by density differences decrease with increasing $S_{20,w}$ differences. The ratio of sedimentation coefficients times the ratio of density differences determines resolution in homogeneous media as these parameters did in case 3. However, because the ratio of density differences decreases with increases in the differences between particle densities, resolution is lost as the differences between particle densities increases. Resolution is zero in homogeneous media when the ratio of sedimentation coefficients equals the ratio of density differences. In gradients the decrease in resolution is most dramatic when S_1/S_2 is small and the gradient slope is steep. In steep gradients, resolution is very slight when S_1/S_2 is small for particles with density values in the ranged subcellular particles.

The conclusions derived from an analysis of all four cases can be briefly summarized as follows. Separations where $S_1 > S_2$ and $\varrho_1 = \varrho_2$ (case 1) are optimized in very shallow gradients where the density of the gradient is much less than that of the particle. Particles differing in density but not in sedimentation coefficient (case 2) are separated by isopycnic banding. Particles differing in both sedimentation coefficients and density (case 3) can be separated on the basis of either $S_{20,w}$ or ϱ, or both. To effectively utilize both factors and improve the separation, the initial density of the gradient should approach that of the lighter particle. Alternately, to emphasize the $S_{20,w}$ differences between the particles, shallow gradients in which the density of the gradient is much less than that of the lighter particle give good separations. When the sedimentation coefficients differ in an opposite way from the densities (case 4), certain conditions exist in which no separation is achieved because the $S_{20,w}$ and ϱ exactly compensate for each other. Separations need to be performed on either side of this intersection point either by rate or by density, taking advantage of the density in either rate or isopycnic separations. The critical difference between cases 3 and 4 is that if one is ignorant of the parameters in case 4 no separation will result. In case 3 the separation can only be improved by careful consideration of the parameters.*

Although the principles described stand on their own accord, the accurate application of such an approach requires the use of reliable sedimentation coefficients. Because of the complex dependence of the sedimentation coefficient on particle size, shape, and density, sedimentation coefficients might be expected to vary depending on the particular sedimentation conditions. This would negate their usefulness unless some correction factor could be found. In a subsequent section we show that relatively precise sedimentation coefficients can be obtained for certain classes of subcellular particles from brain homogenates in a variety of centrifugation conditions. This suggests the feasibility of this approach. Its use should markedly reduce the number of experiments required to obtain optimum centrifugation conditions.

B. Properties of the Centrifuge Rotor

The degree of separation obtainable from two classes of particles depends not only on the properties of the particles but also on the resolution and precision of the centrifugation technique. The zonal rotor system invented by Norman G. Anderson at Oak Ridge is the latest and most sophisticated in the continued evolution of centrifugation equipment. Zonal rotors are hollow cylinders of various proportions which are filled completely

---

*Basically the same principles used for the separation of particles can be applied to the separation of particle populations. One approach is to select from the range of particles within a population a few $s_{20,w}$ and ρ values from sectors representative of particular portions of the population, e.g., leading, median, and trailing edge. For example, the separation can be analyzed for the resolution of the trailing edge of the faster particle, and the leading edge of the slower particle. Analysis of populations is described more extensively elsewhere (Donyle, Banker, and Cotman, 1972).

with gradient and sample. The gradient and sample are introduced into the rotor through a removable seal while the rotor is running. The seal has an outlet to the center of the rotor and to the edge through septa. This system provides increased resolution, capacity, and flexibility compared with conventional equipment. Thus improvements in subcellular separations are a matter of improving separation design and utilizing the properties available.

Resolution is improved principally because of three factors. First, since the rotor is continually running during loading and unloading, diffusional forces which lead to band broadening are always opposed by a centrifugal field. Disturbances due to gradient reorienting are also minimized. Second, the large gradient volume enables one to collect a very minute portion of the total gradient path in a relatively large solution volume. For example, a 40-ml fraction from a B XV rotor (Anderson *et al.*, 1967a) corresponds to about 1 mm of the 3.5-cm path. Because each zone resides in a relatively large volume, the collection and monitoring through flow cells does not lead to mixing of fractions. Third, the particular geometry of the zonal gradient is more optimal for resolution than the geometry of gradients in centrifuge tubes. As particles sediment in a zonal rotor they undergo radial dilution. They are diluted with increasing volumes of gradient so that particle-particle interactions are minimized and the capacity of the isopycnic zones is increased.

The capacity of the zonal system is large. The quantity of material that can be processed on a given gradient is increased because of the volume of the gradient and the relatively large sample surface of the gradient. The B XV rotor has a gradient volume of about 1300 ml and the B XIV, 450 ml. Thus the volume of the density gradient and quantity of material which can be processed is many times that of conventional instrumentation. In addition, large volumes of sample can be used since the gradient surface area at the sample zone is at least eight times that of the largest high-speed swinging-bucket rotors. For this reason a narrow sample zone can be maintained with relatively large sample volumes.

The zonal system allows increased flexibility. Zonal rotors are now available with the capability for center and edge unloading. In this way particular portions of the population can be removed during a run. These properties can be used to eliminate, for example, preliminary differential centrifugations. "Differential" centrifugation can be carried out from the total homogenate directly in the rotor itself where pelleting is eliminated and sedimentation conditions are excellent because of the thin starting zone and large capacity and stability of the gradient. Center unloading of the microsomal fraction thus minimizes structural damage to the various sensitive particles in the crude mitochondrial fraction. Center and edge unloading properties of zonal rotors would appear to be a particularly useful application of the zonal system to brain subcellular separations.

Zonal centrifugation has certain advantages, but it also has certain limitations. Zonal separations require about the same expenditure of time as separations on continuous gradients carried out in swinging-bucket rotors. However, a central disadvantage of the zonal technique is that only one condition can be run at a time. In addition, separations using expensive gradient material are prohibitively costly because of the large gradient volume required. The resolution is very impressive and the separations are reliable; and when optimal resolution is required zonal centrifugation is the system of choice. Often, for example, we have observed remarkable differences in the morphology of fractions adjacent to one another.

Zonal centrifugation, however, can only improve existing separations by improving the resolution and increasing the quantity of material that can be processed. Like other centrifugation procedures, it is limited by the physical properties of the particles. To cite one example, we investigated the isopycnic banding profile of a crude mitochondrial fraction from brain. There is a slight improvement in the quality of the fractions, but the results are essentially in agreement with those obtained on very narrow density cuts by a variety of investigators (D'Monte *et al.*, 1970; Whittaker, 1968; Metzger *et al.*, 1967) on continuous gradients in conventional rotors. The yields of each fraction in high-resolution separations in conventional rotors are, of course, severely limited. For separations in which the particles are widely separated and the extra capacity is not needed, there is no particular advantage in using the zonal technique.

In summary, we have found zonal centrifugation most useful for subcellular separations as (1) a precise analytical tool for defining and obtaining maximum resolution, and (2) a means of increasing the amount of sample that can be handled in a single run. We have generally found it most satisfactory and economical to "rough out" the general centrifugation conditions for new preparations on conventional instrumentation. Once these are fairly well understood, they can be more precisely defined and confirmed by zonal centrifugation.

III. TECHNIQUES FOR PREPARING AND EVALUATING SUBCELLULAR SEPARATIONS

A. Operation of the Zonal Centrifuge System

A number of different zonal rotors have been designed (Anderson, 1966; Anderson *et al.*, 1964; Anderson *et al.*, 1967; Anderson *et al.*, 1969a;

Anderson *et al.,* 1969b) and are available. The most common are the B XIV and B XV rotors (Anderson *et al.,* 1967a) which are alike except for their total volume capacity. The B XIV holds about 450 ml of gradient and the B XV 1300 ml of usable gradient. Others such as the K II, which holds about 3 liters, are used for batch purifications (Anderson *et al.,* 1969a). The most recent is the B XXIX, which allows for edge as well as center unloading of the sample (Anderson *et al.,* 1969b). This ingenious rotor makes use of a super-ellipse at the edge so that particles that reach the edge collect at the radii extremes and are removed through the septa from these positions.

The procedure for executing zonal centrifugation is as follows:

1.   The rotor is set into a centrifuge chamber adapted for zonal centrifugation. The rotor is started, run to loading speed (about 3000 rev/min), and fitted with its seal. The gradient is pumped into the rotor, introducing the lightest density medium first at the edge so that higher density medium follows and displaces the lighter medium toward the center. A variety of gradient pump devices are available. The simplest and least expensive is an exponential gradient-forming device described by Anderson and Rutenberg (1967). Alternately, programmed gradient pumps are available.

2.   Once the rotor is fully loaded, as evidenced by the emergence of light gradient medium from the center line of the seal, the sample may be introduced into the rotor. We routinely use a 50-ml syringe to load the sample. The syringe is packed in ice to keep the sample cold. Sample size is usually maintained at 100 ml or less, especially for rate sedimentation runs. An overlay of 100 ml is introduced after the sample so that the sample is moved out of the rotor core. The seal is removed, the rotor capped and run to speed.

3.   After the appropriate total force is reached, the rotor is decelerated and brought to 3000 rev/min and the seal replaced on the rotor for unloading. If the rotor stops at this point, the run is lost since with present zonal rotors the gradients mix and will not reorient. To collect the gradient, heavy gradient medium is pumped in at the edge to displace the entire gradient out of the rotor through the rotor core. It is important that the line to the edge of the seal does not contain air, since air will disturb the separation if it enters the rotor and passes through the gradient. Fractions of the desired size are collected, and the separation monitored by following the light scattering absorbance profile at 260 or 280 mμ. The sucrose concentration in each fraction can be measured by refractive index. Refractometers are available which are calibrated to read sucrose concentration directly.

B. Evaluation of Subcellular Separations

1. Use of Analytical Electron Microscopy for Subcellular Fractionation Studies

Electron microscopy has been the most widely used diagnostic test for evaluating the composition of brain subcellular fractions. When executed in an analytical manner it can provide accurate analysis of the fraction obtained. The major advantage of electron microscopy is that it allows determination of the relative composition of the fraction when particular markers for all particles are not well known. For this reason it has served as the unproclaimed absolute standard for fraction purity, especially for brain.

The major difficulty in using this technique is in obtaining data representative of an entire fraction, since it is possible to examine only a very small portion of the sample. Generally an area of no more than about $200\mu^2$ by 0.4μ thick is examined, a total volume of only 0.0008 mm^3! When pelleting procedures are used for sample preparation, layering in the sample is expected on the basis of differences in sedimentation coefficients so that it is difficult to obtain representative data from pellets. Recently we described a method to obtain very thin pellets in which the entir ecross section can be viewed on a single section (Cotman and Flansburg, 1970). This relatively simple approach allows one to obtain representative data on the composition of the entire fraction. The basic outline of this technique is shown in Fig. 7. In this manner the nature of the particles that have sedimentation coefficients at the extremes of a fraction are easily determined.

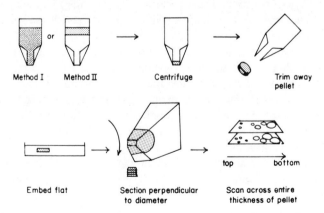

Fig. 7. Outline of the method for sample preparation for electron microscopy. The sample is centrifuged into a thin pellet, cut out of the capsule, embedded flat and sectioned crosswise so that the sections contain the entire thickness of the pellet. (From Cotman and Flansburg, 1970.)

A unique attribute of this technique is that distribution of sedimentation coefficients can be observed.

Once reliable sampling data are obtained, quantitative determination of the amount of contamination contributed by a particle is still difficult to ascertain. For example, one mitochondrion visualized per nine plasma membrane fragments contributes substantially more than 10% mitochondrial protein to the preparation since one mitochondrion contains more protein than one plasma membrane of equivalent size. It is essential to consider the net quantity of a particular material contributed by each structure visualized in the field.

Other limitations of electron microscopy as an assay technique for subcellular fractions are: (1) the uncertainty in identifying all structures; (2) the dependence on embedding and fixation procedures; and (3) the time and technology required for each sample. Because in thin-sectioned preparations one is observing a two-dimensional profile and because all particles of the same type do not appear as "classic" profiles, it is sometimes difficult to interpret micrographs. In addition to electron microscopy, supporting chemical or enzymic data are required to evaluate fraction composition.

2. Use and Limitations of Chemical and Enzyme Markers

Because metabolic pathways are organized to particular subcellular structures, enzymes unique to metabolic sequences have been used as markers to determine the sedimentation behavior of the subcellular structure. In brain one of the central problems in purifying particular classes of subcellular particles has been that there are few specific marker enzymes known for the variety of subcellular components. For example, markers commonly used for synaptosomes, such as acetylcholine or choline acetyltransferase, are not unique to only this portion of the cell. It is reasonable, in fact expected, that dendrite, soma, and axonal membrane fragments contain transmitters in addition to synaptosomes since transmitter molecules are present in portions of the cell other than nerve endings (Kasa *et al.,* 1970; Kravitz *et al.,* 1965). Dendrites, axons, and soma membranes can easily entrap their cytoplasmic interior during homogenization and vesicularization so that vesicles originating from dendrite, axons, and cell bodies carry with them transmitter molecules and other components of the cytoplasm. Nor are certain enzymes, e.g., AChE, found only in one type of particle (Novikoff, 1967). As another example of the lack of specific marker enzymes, an adequate marker for rough or smooth endoplasmic reticulum has yet to be demonstrated.

To a large extent there are only a few marker enzymes because only a few fractions have been sufficiently purified so that they can be surveyed for enzyme content. The effect is cyclic and has made it difficult to determine the optimal conditions to separate particle populations and to find additional marker enzymes. The absence of definitive ways to evaluate the sedimentation properties of many subcellular particles, including subclasses of the same particle, has seriously hindered the progress which is potentially realizable by zonal centrifugation. Recent surveys of the enzyme activities of subcellular fractions from liver (Schneider, 1968) and brain (Hoyer, 1969) are available.

As particular subcellular populations are purified, markers unique to these structures should be enriched. The enrichment from the total homogenate depends on the proportion of the homogenate occupied by the particles. If 20% of the homogenate is mitochondria, for example, as is the case for liver (Leighton et al., 1968), an enrichment of 5-fold indicates homogeneity. Further enrichment can be obtained only if particular classes of mitochondria can be resolved or if the marker is activated as a consequence of an aspect of the procedure. Precise data are not available on the relative composition of brain homogenates, but one of the essential differences between brain and other tissues is its larger content of plasma membranes. In liver plasma membranes make up approximately 5% of the total particulate protein. Neurons, however, have a much larger surface-to-volume ratio than other cells and contain comparatively more plasma membrane. As discussed elsewhere (Cotman and Matthews, 1971; morgan et al., 1971), neuronal plasma membrane constitutes at least 10–20% of the total particulate protein in a brain homogenate. On the basis of this 10–20% estimate, enrichments of 5-to 10-fold are expected for plasma membrane markers. Further enrichments would occur only if the particular marker is confined to a portion of the neuronal surface or to particular populations of neurons or alternatively if the marker enzyme is "activated" by the procedure.

IV. APPLICATION OF ZONAL CENTRIFUGATION TO BRAIN SEPARATIONS

The impact of zonal centrifugation on brain separations has not yet been felt. Zonal centrifugation has been applied to brain in a variety of problems (Cotman et al., 1968; Mahley et al., 1968; Rodnight et al., 1969; Kornguth et al., 1972) but it has not been used extensively. The results have been promising and stand on their own merit, but zonal centrifugation does not in itself solve the problem of preparing pure subcellular fractions from brain.

Clearly, zonal centrifugation will play a major role in preparing highly purified fractions in large quantities. Further developments in the quality of fractions will come with a better understanding of the principles of subcellular separations and the application of these principles as aids in determining experimental conditions. Additional and better markers for subcellular particles and more experience will also have a catalytic effect. With zonal centrifugation, trial and error is uneconomical at best since only one condition can be run at a time, and since many fractions are obtained for assay.

A. Measurements of $S_{20,w}$ Values for Mitochondria and Synaptosomes

Application of theoretical descriptions of particle separation requires knowledge of particle sedimentation coefficients. We computed sedimentation coefficients for mitochondria and synaptosomes during varied running conditions on three different types of sucrose gradients. Mitochondria included both those free and those contained within synaptosomes. For these measurements, synaptosomes were defined by the sedimentation of choline acetyltransferase activity and mitochondria by cytochrome oxidase activity.

To calculate the value of $S_{20,w}$ two measurements are required: (1) isopycnic banding densities and (2) the migration distance of the particle population at different values of total applied force. Accurate measurement of total force requires use of a digital integrator which measures the acceleration, running, and deceleration forces radians squared per second ($\omega^2 t$). Then from the Svedberg equation the sedimentation coefficient can be computed (see Appendix). An isopycnic banding profile for the distribution of cytochrome oxidase and choline acetyltransferase (ChA) is shown in Fig. 8. The enzymic activities spread over a fairly wide range: 90% of the cytochrome oxidase activity sediments past a density of 1.15 g/ml, while 50% is found beyond a density of 1.17 g/ml. Ninety percent of ChA is heavier than 1.09 g/ml, while 50% is found beyond a density of 1.14 g/ml.

Sedimentation coefficients were computed from the location of enzmatic activities achieved at different values of total applied force. Rate zonal separations were performed in a BXV zonal rotor in either 23–45% linear sucrose gradients, 10–45% linear sucrose gradients, or 10–45% linear sucrose gradients with a plateau of 10% sucrose at the beginning of the gradient. $S_{20,w}$ values were computed for the sedimentation of 50% and 90% of the particle populations. In Table IV the values of $S_{20,w}$ obtained are summarized. The sedimentation coefficient for 50% of the cytochrome oxidase population is $9.4 \pm 0.8 \times 10^3$ S and for 50% of the ChA population is $5.6 \pm 0.7 \times 10^3$ S. Thus the $S_{20,w}$ values remain quite constant and are reproducible.

The finding that the apparent $S_{20,w}$ values are relatively constant deserves comment. It would be expected that subcellular particles undergo changes in volume, shape, and density in sucrose gradients. Due to their osmotic properties this may be the case without a change in the sedimentation coefficient. Certain changes in particle configuration and density compensate for one another in the Svedberg equation in such a way that the $S_{20,w}$ can remain constant even though the parameters are changing. Increases in the density of the particle due to osmotic dehydration can be compensated for by an increase in the frictional ratio, θ, due to elongation of the particle in the gradient [Eq. (4)] (de Duve *et al.*, 1959).

Although the $S_{20,w}$ values determined for cytochrome oxidase and choline acetyltransferase are reproducible and relatively independent of the sucrose gradient, the extent to which they depend on homogenization conditions, the animal, or the brain region is not known. To this degree, these values are not meant as absolute values of the $S_{20,w}$, but more as functional parameters to deal with a defined system.

Additional data on other particles and other markers are needed to fully evaluate the generality of obtaining $S_{20,w}$ values which are reproducible and relatively independent of the gradient. Even if $S_{20,w}$ values should change during sedimentation in a particular gradient, it may be possible to

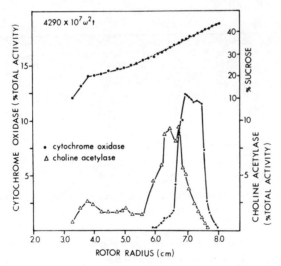

Fig. 8. Isopycnic banding profile of the distribution of cytochrome oxidase and choline acetyl transferase. Homogenates were prepared as previously described (Cotman *et al.*, 1970) and diluted to 10% w/v. Unbroken cells and nuclei were removed by centrifugation in a number 30 rotor to a total applied force of $2 \times 10^7 \omega^2 t$. Centrifugation was performed in a B XV zonal rotor to a total applied force of $4290 \times 10^7 \omega^2 t$.

Table IV. Sedimentation Coefficients ($S_{20,w}$) Computed for Cytochrome Oxidase and Choline Acetyltransferase in Different Sucrose Gradients at Different Total Applied Forces[a]

| Gradient | $\omega^2 t$ $\times 10^7$ | $S_{20,w}$ cytochrome oxidase $\times 10^3$ | | $S_{20,w}$ choline acetyltransferase $\times 10^3$ | |
| | | sedimentation | | sedimentation | |
		90%	50%	90%	50%
10% (300 ml)	167	2.5	9.1	0.72	5.6
Linear 10–45% (900 ml)	345	3.0	10.1	0.76	5.5
Linear 10–45% (1200 ml)	360	4.4	10.1	1.0	4.0
	743	5.3	9.2	1.4	5.6
	756	4.4	8.4		
	1072	5.0	10.0		
Linear 23–45% (1200 ml)	258	1.8	(6.9)		
	279				(7.3)
	410	2.0	8.1		
	506	2.0	10.2		
	510				5.6
	663	2.1	9.6		
	690				6.2
	1138				6.5
Mean		3.3	9.4	1.0	5.6
Standard deviation		±1.4	±0.8	±0.3	±0.7

[a] $S_{20,w}$ values were determined in a B XV zonal rotor for 50% and 90% sedimentation of the recovered enzyme activity. The 50% and 90% values represent the $S_{20,w}$ of a hypothetical spherical particle with a specified density which would sediment to a point in the gradient such that 50% or 90% of the enzyme activity has already migrated past it. The densities for choline acetyltransferase are $\varrho = 1.14$ g/ml, for 50% and $\varrho = 1.09$ g/ml for 90% and for cytochrome oxidase $\varrho = 1.17$ g/ml for 50% and $\varrho = 1.09$ g/ml for 90%. (From Cotman and Doyle, 1972.)

find a function to describe the increase or decrease and incorporate this into computations.

B. Use of Sedimentation Coefficients for Determining Separation Conditions

Since sedimentation coefficients are relatively independent of gradient conditions, they can be used to predict effectiveness of separation on different selected gradients under a variety of conditions. When isolating mitochondria and synaptosomes, it would be advantageous to eliminate preparing a crude mitochondrial fraction and instead work directly with the total homogenate or the supernatant from which the nuclear fraction has been removed. This would eliminate possible particle damage from pelleting and resuspension which is known to occur (Schuberth *et al.*, 1970). With the zonal rotor, differential centrifugations can be executed directly in the rotor. We wished to determine if we could utilize the sedimentation coefficient to establish conditions to separate mitochondria from microsomes. On the basis of the $S_{20,w}$ data obtained for mitochondria we should be able to determine the conditions to sediment 90% of the mitochondria into the gradient. We selected a gradient with a 100-ml plateau of 10% sucrose to provide extra volume for separation under isotonic conditions and for maneuvering the sample back out of the rotor. We wished to determine the force required to sediment 90% of the mitochondrial population from the sample zone to a position 1.5 cm from the rotor center. Since the $S_{20,w}$ for 90% sedimentation of the mitochondrial population is known (Table IV), we could compute the position of this particle at any value of $\omega^2 t$. This calculation is shown in Fig. 9. It can be seen that to move a particle with an $S_{20,w}$ of 3.3×10^3 S from the sample zone to a position 4.9 cm from the rotor center requires 350×10^7 $\omega^2 t$. Figure 10 shows the results of the prediction for sedimentation behavior of brain mitochondria. The mitochondrial population by 345×10^7 $\omega^2 t$ migrated to a position of 4.8 cm, which is very close to the value predicted for 350×10^7 $\omega^2 t$. Thus the microsome

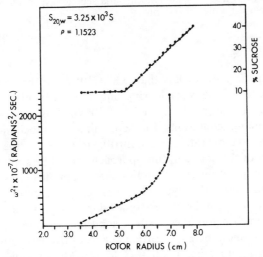

Fig. 9. Graph of the position of a particle in centimeters from the center of the rotor with an $S_{20,w}$ of 3.3×10^3 S ($\varrho = 1.15$) in a 10–45% sucrose gradient with an Inertial 10% sucrose platean as a function of $\omega^2 t$. The computation was carried out as described in the appendix based on the method of Halsall and Schumaker (1969).

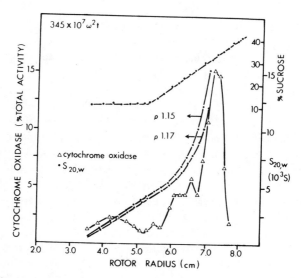

Fig. 10. Rate zonal centrifugation separation on a sucrose gradient to illustrate the value of using experimentally measured $S_{20,w}$ to compute centrifugation conditions. In this experiment we wished to separate a microsome from a mitochondrial fraction by sedimenting 90% of the mitochondria into the gradient. The $S_{20,w}$ measured for the sedimentation of 90% of the mitochondria predicted that at $350 \times 10^7 \omega^2 t$, 90% of the mitochondria should have migrated 4.9 cm from the center of the rotor.

fraction with an $S_{5°,10\%}$ of less than 3.8×10^2 S can be readily removed through the center of the rotor leaving only the crude mitochondrial fraction with an $S_{5°,10\%}$ of greater than 3.5×10^2 S. This approach effectively aids in determining conditions for separating a mitochondrial from a microsomal fraction by rate zonal centrifugation. Since the $S_{20,w}$ values are independent of the gradient, this approach should be applicable to other portions of the population as well and to different gradient designs.

We have also used this type of experimental-theoretical approach to determine separation conditions for purifying synaptosoma mitochondria from synaptosoma membranes. After isopycnic banding of osmotically shocked synaptosomes, there is a certain degree of overlap between synaptosoma membranes and mitochondria (Fig. 11). Mitochondria, assayed by cytochrome oxidase, overlap with membranes, as determined by alkaline phosphatase or acetylcholine esterase. (Alkaline phosphatase is a suitable memberane marker enzyme in this context since it quite accurately gives the same distribution as NaK ATPase, but it is simpler to assay and is not as labile.) Approximately 70% of the total alkaline phosphatase activity over-laps with 90–100% the cytochrome oxidase population.

We wished to determine if this separation could be improved by rate sedimentation. We computed the minimal conditions to approach isopycnic banding of mitochondria in order to determine whether membranes also approach their isopycnic point at these conditions, or if membranes sediment more slowly, allowing for better separation from mitochondria. We measured the isopycnic banding density for 90% of the mitochondrial population and then measured the $S_{20,w}$ experimentally by doing a rate sedimentation run at a low value of $\omega^2 t$. From these data we prepared a plot of $\omega^2 t$ vs the position of sedimentation as carried out above for microsomal separations. These calculations predicted that a total applied force of 1500×10^7 $\omega^2 t$ would move 90% of the mitochondria to a density of 1.13 (29.5% sucrose). The results of this experiment are illustrated in Fig. 12. Ninety per cent of the mitochondrial fraction sediments to a density of 1.133 g/ml (30.4% sucrose). Rate sedimentation improves the resolution of cytochrome oxidase

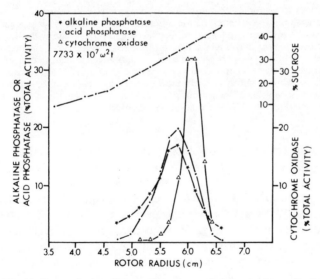

Fig. 11. Isopycnic banding profile of cytochrome oxidase, alkaline phosphatase, and acid phosphatase obtained from osmotically shocked synaptosomes. Synaptosomes were isolated from a crude mitochondrial fraction on a Ficoll-sucrose gradient consisting of 7.5% Ficoll (w/v) in 0.32 M sucrose and 13% Ficoll (w/v) in 0.32 M sucrose (Cotman and Matthews, 1971). Synaptosomes were collected from the 7.5–13% Ficoll-sucrose interface. They were osmotically shocked with 6 mM tris, pH 8.0, and centrifuged on a 12.5–45% sucrose gradient for 7733×10^7 $\omega^2 t$ at 35,000 rev/min in a B XIV zonal rotor.

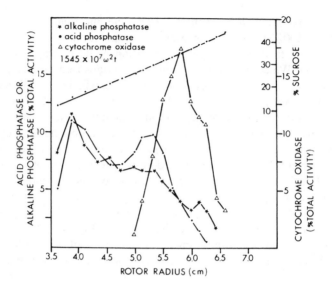

Fig. 12. Rate zonal separation of cytochrome oxidase, alkaline phosphatase, and acid phosphatase obtained from osmotically shocked synaptosomes prepared as described in Fig. 11 on a linear 10–45% sucrose gradient in a B XIV zonal rotor for $1545 \times 10^7 \, \omega^2 t$. Centrifugation conditions were based on those determined by calculations to sediment 90% of the mitochondria to a density of 1.117 (27% sucrose). The sedimentation behavior of mitochondria was close to that predicted and the separation of the various membrane enzymes from the mitochondrial marker cytochrome oxidase was improved.

and alkaline phophastase. Now 27% of the alkaline phosphatase instead of 70% overlaps with the cytochrome oxidase activity. AChE is also more resolved from cytochrome oxidase. Rate sedimentation produces an interesting separation and grouping of acid phosphatase from alkaline phosphatase activity. Acid and alkaline phosphatase are distributed in an identical manner in isopycnic banding, but are partially segregated during rate sedimentation. These separations provide a clear example of the value of rate sedimentation for (1) improving particle separations and (2) evaluating whether or not two enzymes really belong to the same particle. This experiment further demonstrates the utility of combining a theoretical and experimental approach to determine centrifugation conditions.

V. ANALYTICAL DIFFERENTIAL CENTRIFUGATION

Since differential centrifugation is widely used in brain fractionation schemes, both with conventional instrumentation and as a prelude to isopycnic or rate zonal centrifugation, we have determined the separations achieved under various differential centrifugation forces. We survey the extent of sedimentation at various forces, thus defining the minimum force required to initiate and complete the sedimentation of a particular subcellular fraction. In this way a complete profile is obtained, thereby providing data to select conditions to divide particles into classes appropriate to particular applications.

The technique of analytical differential centrifugation involves sedimentation in an angle rotor in defined solution volumes while monitoring the total sedimentation forces with a digital integrator. A suspension of sample is centrifuged to a total applied force accurately measured in $\omega^2 t$ and a defined volume of the supernatant removed for analysis. This supernatant contains the particles which are not sedimented at a particular applied force. This procedure is carried out at a number of forces until all

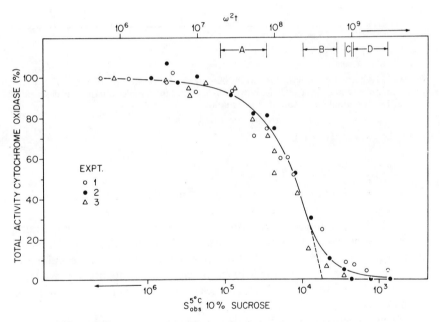

Fig. 13. Sedimentation curve for brain mitochondria. The points (from three separate experiments) represent the percent cytochrome oxidase activity remaining in the supernatant after centrifugation of a 2% brain homogenate (in 10% sucrose) in a No. 30 Spinco rotor for measured integrals ($\omega^2 t$). The curve that fits the data best was obtained by computer computations, utilizing equations described in the section on methods. (Points were deleted where C_f/C_i was less than 10.2% of the enzyme activity.) The dotted projection intercepts the X axis at 5.4×10^3 S, which represents an average sedimentation coefficient for approximately 85% of the mitochondrial population. (From Cotman et al., 1970.)

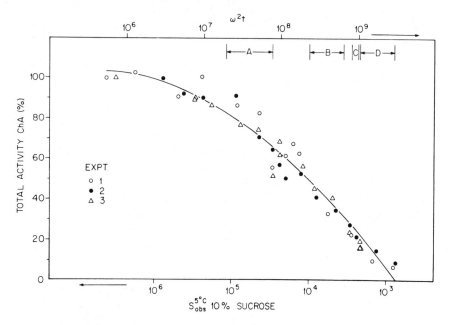

Fig. 14. Sedimentation curve for brain choline acetyltransferase (ChA). The data represent pelletable ChA (C_f/C_i) activity from supernatant samples obtained as described in Fig. 13. The fitted curve follows the equation

$$Y = -102.9 + 74.4 \ln X - 6.7 (\ln X)^2$$

(From Cotman *et al.*, 1970.)

the population is sedimented. Separated samples of the total starting material are used for each data point. The result is a continuous profile of force *vs* per cent of sedimentation, which shows at one end of the spectrum the minimum force necessary to initiate sedimentation, at the other, the minimum force necessary to sediment the entire population. While this technique is quite simple, it has been shown to be precise enough to provide accurate measurements of the sedimentation coefficients of bovine serum albumin, red blood cells, and latex beads.

The sedimentation profile obtained for mitochondria and synaptosomes from rat brain cerebral cortex homogenates is shown in Figs. 13 and 14 (Cotman *et al.*, 1970). The sedimentation of cytochrome oxidase commences at about 2×10^7 $\omega^2 t$ and is about 90% complete at 100×10^7 $\omega^2 t$. No indication of heterogeneity is apparent from the shape of the curvd even though the mitochondrial population is known to be vastly heterogeneous, containing free mitochondria and mitochondria within synaptosomes.

Apparently the sedimentation coefficients of these particles show considerable overlap. Choline acetyltransferase (ChA), a marker for synaptosomes and other neuronal vesicular elements, sediments over a broader spectrum of values than cytochrome oxidase. The sedimentation curve of ChA begins to fall at $1-2 \times 10^7$ $\omega^2 t$ and is 90% complete at 200×10^7 $\omega^2 t$. Thus these data define the precise conditions to sediment a given portion of these populations.

Electron microscopic analysis showed that invariably the fractions sedimented at low forces contained very large mitochondria and synaptosomes (Fig. 15) while the fractions at higher forces contained only very small mitochondria and synaptosomes (Fig. 16). Characteristically, the synaptosomes at these higher $\omega^2 t$ values did not contain mitochondria. The larger

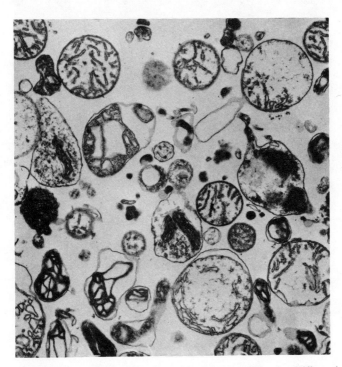

Fig. 15. Fraction collected between 24 and 65×10^7 $\omega^2 t$. Differential centrifugation effectively separates particles of the same density by size. The mitochondria in particular are larger than those seen in the fraction collected between 85 and 102×10^7 $\omega^2 t$ (Fig. 16). The segregation of synaptosomes is not as pronounced; however, synaptosomes in this fraction commonly contain more than one mitochondria while those in the $85-102 \times 10^7$ $\omega^2 t$ rarely contain more than one mitochondrion. ($\times 30,000$ reduced for reproduction 25%).

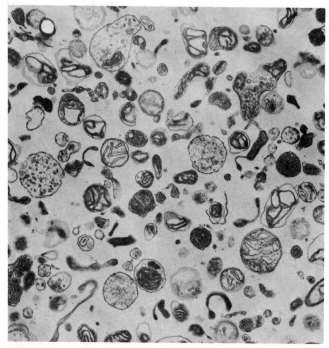

Fig. 16. Fraction collected between 85 and 102 $\times$ 10^7 $\omega^2 t$. This fraction has a prevalence of smaller particles than those in the 24–65 $\times$ 10^7 $\omega^2 t$ fraction (Fig. 15). ($\times$ 30,000 reduced for reproduction 25%).

synaptosomes at 2–67 $\times$ 10^7 $\omega^2 t$ contained one to many mitochondria. In Fig. 17 a summary of the morphological and enzymic analyses on the sedimentation rate of particles from brain homogenates is presented.

Differential centrifugation of brain tissue very effectively separates particles according to sizes, but it does not resolve particle populations. These data illustrate that most brain subcellular particles do not differ widely in their rate sedimentation properties, just as they do not differ widely in their isopycnic banding densities.

VI. CONCLUSIONS AND FUTURE APPLICATIONS OF CENTRIFUGATION TO THE STUDY OF BRAIN

Subcellular separation methods have been invaluable in defining function at a subcellular level in the nervous system. The method itself, however, has had little of the sophistication of the techniques applied to the study

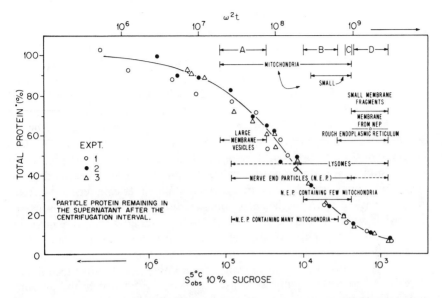

Fig. 17. Summary of morphological and enzymic analysis on the sedimentation of particles from brain homogenates. The size data on the sedimentation range of particular particles (small mitochondria, membrane fragments, rough endoplasmic reticulum, lysosomes, and mitochondria content of NEP) were obtained from morphological analysis. (From Cotman *et al.*, 1970.)

of the fractions. Separation methods in brain have been highly empirical and the conclusions on the composition of the fractions oversimplified. In this paper we have outlined a theoretical basis for separations in gradients and shown that at least in part the necessary quantitative measurements can be made and used as a guide to achieving better separations.

The fractionation of subcellular particles from brain is complex because of the many components and the similarity in the sedimentation properties of these components. There exist many similar particles, particularly membrane fragments of assorted sizes and densities, with overlapping sedimentation properties. To further complicate the task, it is difficult to evaluate the separations achieved because of the absence of markers unique to each particle. In brain the diversity of cell types, both neuronal and glial, which contain specialized subcellular components increases the assortment of particle types even within a particular particle class. The complexity is sufficient so that studies on model systems will provide important information. Such studies for cultured glial cells (Cotman *et al.,* 1971a) and glial and neuron-enriched fractions (Hamberger *et al.,* 1970) have been reported. The use of nervous tissue or closely allied tissues enriched in the particular structures of interest would be extremely beneficial because one is able to start with a more enriched source. Among important recent examples are studies on eel electroplax (Changeux *et al.,* 1969; deRobertis and de Plazas, 1970; Marchbanks and Israel, 1971), retinal rod segments (McConnell, 1965), and secretory vesicles from adrenal tissue (Hillays, 1958; Smith and Winkler, 1967; Trifaro and Dworkind, 1970). One would like to believe that a more favorable tissue exists for isolation of synaptosomes than those commonly used, perhaps a portion of a brain region from a large mammal or from a primitive vertebrate. On the other hand, separation techniques in existing systems can still be improved. However, when the properties of the particles are too similar, it is important to realize this and find a means to modify an appropriate parameter determining sedimentation either by altering the state of the particle directly or the suspending medium or gradient. As discussed in more detail in previous sections (II, A, 1–3), major advances were made in isolation of highly purified organelles from liver homogenates only after modification of particle, gradient, or homogenization was introduced. The isolation of lysosomes in pure form became possible only after techniques were found to make them less dense (deDuve, 1965); rough and smooth endoplasmic reticulum were resolved from each other and other particles after sedimentation coefficients were increased (Dallner and Ernster, 1968); plasma membranes and Golgi apparatus were successfully and unambiguously isolated after appropriate precautions against excess damage by shear were undertaken (Neville, 1960; Morre *et al.,* 1965). Similar concepts and techniques applied to brain would stimulate rapid advances in subcellular fractionation.

The major use of centrifugation techniques for brain to date has been as a preparative tool for subsequent biochemical or structural studies. Centrifugation techniques have not been used as an analytical tool for describing and quantitating changes in the subcellular particles. For example, the alteration in the size and mass of mitochondria or synaptosomes during development could perhaps be accurately determined. Sedimentation analysis has been effectively used to describe changes in the size of mitochondria after cortisone treatment (Loeb and Kimberg, 1970). In agreement with electron microscopic analysis an increase in mitochondrial size was detected. On the basis of sedimentation analysis it could be shown that the differences were due to a net increase in mitochondrial mass and not to swelling. Similar techniques might be applied to brain not only during development but following other functional modifications in brain, such as in selective retrograde degeneration or following treatments where changes in synapse size result (Raisman, 1969). Considerations of the change predicted in the physical properties of the structures would guide the selection of the gradient type and running conditions.

VII. SUMMARY

Subcellular particles separate by centrifugation procedures because of differences in either their sedimentation coefficients or densities or both. Apparent sedimentation coefficients quantitating the rate of particle migration can be measured for classes of brain mitochondria and synaptosomes. These are relatively constant within a gradient and also are independent of the gradient. The success of a separation depends on effectively utilizing and maximizing those differences which exist. A critical variable in optimizing separations is the choice of the most appropriate density gradient. We describe the principles for selecting an appropriate density gradient based on the relationship between particle density (ϱ) and sedimentation coefficient (S). Two-particle separation problems can be reduced to four cases: (1) $S_1 > S_2$, $\varrho_1 = \varrho_2$ (2) $S_1 = S_2$, $\varrho_1 > \varrho_2$ (3) $S_1 > S_2$, $\varrho_1 > \varrho_2$ (4) $S_1 > S_2$, $\varrho_1 < \varrho_2$. Maximum resolution occurs for particles in cases 1 and 3 on flat or very shallow gradients. Changes in gradient design decrease resolution. The loss in resolution is less marked in case 3 than 1 since both S and ϱ work for the separation in case 3. Gradient selection for case 4 is critical since at a certain point S and ϱ exactly compensate for each other and no separation results. Separations meed to be performed on either side of the intersection point. Maximum resolution is obtained experimentally with zonal centrifugation. This technique provides increased capacity, resolution, and flexibility. Its principal limitation is that only one sample can be run at a time and in some cases the extra resolution is not required.

Most subcellular particles from brain appear to fall within a narrow range of densities and sedimentation coefficients, making it difficult to effect a complete separation. Consequently it is essential to understand the basis of these parameters. In this paper, we discuss the factors determining particle density and sedimentation coefficient in relation to subcellular particles. When a separation is essentially optimal for the particular S and ϱ of the particles but the separation is unsatisfactory, it is important to recognize this and seek a means to alter the sedimentation properties of the particle to achieve better separation. This can be accomplished by altering the properties of the particle itself or the interaction of the particle with the gradient. Not only are similar sedimentation properties a major limitation, an equally serious problem is the lack of unique definitive assays to quantitate and characterize the resulting separation. Both these are the central problems that need to be dealt with. The goal of this paper is to provide an understanding of the physical properties of particles underlying a separation by centrifugation and to provide a guide for selecting the optimal centrifugation parameters for particles with known properties.

VIII. APPENDIX

Sedimentation coefficients were computed based on the method described by Bishop (1966) and by Halsall and Schumaker (1969). This method allows one to rapidly compute the sedimentation coefficient and density. It can be easily shown (Halsall and Schumaker, 1969) that

$$S_{20,w}*\omega^2 t = [(\varrho_p - \varrho_{20,w})/\eta_{20,w}] \int_{\ln R_{i-1}}^{\ln R_i} [\eta_m/(\varrho_p - \varrho_m)] \, d\ln R \qquad (7)$$

where $S_{20,w}$ = sedimentation coefficient in water at 20 °C, η = absolute viscosity, ϱ = density in g/ml, ω = angular velocity in radians/sec, t = time in seconds, and R = radial distance from the center of rotation; the subscript, m, refers to medium, p, particle, and w, water. For a particle density gradient profile, the right-hand side of Eq. (7) represents the correction factors for the sedimentation coefficient due to the viscosity and density variation within the gradient. A plot, therefore, of $\eta_m/(\varrho_p - \varrho_m)$ vs. ln R gives a curve beneath which the area is proportional to $\omega^2 t*S_{20,w}$. This area can be computed by trapezoidal integration. The calculation can be readily carried out by a simple program on a desk calculator such as an Olivetti Underwood programmer 101. This program computes the $S_{20,w}$ value or the $\omega^2 t$ value for a particle of known density sedimenting in a density gradient.

Formulas used:

$$S_{20,w} = [(\varrho_p - \varrho_{20,w})/\eta_{20,w}*\omega^2 t]*$$
$$\sum_{\ln R_s}^{\ln R_i} \left[\{[\eta_m/(\varrho_p - \varrho_m)]_i + [\eta_m/(\varrho_p - \varrho_m)]_{i-1}\}/2 \right] (\ln R_i - \ln R_{i-1})$$

or

$$\omega^2 t = [(\varrho_p - \varrho_{20,w})/\eta_{20,w}*S_{20,w}]*$$
$$\sum_{\ln R_s}^{\ln R_i} \left[\{[\eta_m/(\varrho_p - \varrho_m)]_i + [\eta_m/(\varrho_p - \varrho_m)]_{i-1}\}/2 \right] (\ln R_i - \ln R_{i-1})$$

where R_S is the mass center of the sample zone and R_i is the radius at the end of the fraction, when $(R_i - R_{i-1})$ is the width of the fraction in the rotor. The sample mass center for a homogeneous sample is the overlay volume minus the line volume plus one half of the sample volume. (The line volume refers to the volume contained in the lines between rotor core and fraction collection.) The viscosity and density of the medium is calculated from the sucrose

The Olivetti program calculates the area under the curve by trapezoidal integration, multiplies by the conversion factor $(\varrho - \varrho_{20,w})/\eta_{20,w}$, and by $\omega^2 t$ or $S_{20,w}$. Integration of the curve involves a conditional loop that

1. calculates $[\eta_m/(\varrho - \varrho_m)]_i$ and stores this value for the next loop
2. calculates the area under the curve between two points $[\eta_m/(\varrho - \varrho_m)]_{i-1}$ (ln $R)_i$ and $[\eta_m/(\varrho - \varrho_m)]_i$ (ln $R)_{i-1}$.
3. multiplies the area by $(\varrho - \varrho_{20,w})/\eta_{20,w}$ ($\omega^2 t$ or $S_{20,w}$)
4. adds this area to that area previously calculated.

The entries required for this program are in order:
1. ϱ_p, density of particle
2. $\eta_{20,w}$, viscosity of water at 20°C
3. $\varrho_{20,w}$, density of water at 20 °C
4. $\omega^2 t$ or $S_{20,w}$
5. ϱ_m, density of medium at a particular rotor radius, R_i
6. η_m, viscosity of medium at a particular rotor radius, R_i
7. (ln $R)_i$ and (ln $R)_{i-1}$

Initially (ln $R)_{i-1}$ is calculated for the sample mass center and (ln $R)_i$ for the end of the fraction beyond this center. The viscosity and density of the medium is calculated from the sucrose concentration of the fraction by Bishop's program (1966) modified for PDP 12.

The program developed for the Olivetti desk calculator is as follows:

AV	BW	D ↓
MS	MS	C+
b ↑	b ↓	dX
MS	M−	f÷
b ↓	B ↕	eX
MX	MS	E+
F ↕	b ↓	E ↕
MS	MX	E◇
b ↓	B÷	C ↓
M−	C ↕	D ↕
F÷	MS	CW
MS	c ↑	MV
M÷	MS	2.0f ↑
e	C ↓	
	M−	
	d ↕	

ACKNOWLEDGMENT

This work was supported in part by a grant from the National Institutes of Health. The author is grateful to Lynn Doyle and Gary Banker for invaluable discussion and criticism.

REFERENCES

Autilio, L. A., Norton, W. T., and Terry, R. D. (1964) *J. Neurochem.* **11,** 17.

Autilio, L. A., Appel, S. H., Pettis, P., and Gambetti, P. L. (1968) *Biochem.* **7,** 2615.

Anderson, N. G., Price, C. A., Fisher, W. D., Canning, R. E., and Burger, C. L. (1964) *Analyt. Biochem.* **7,** 1.

Anderson, N. G. (ed.) (1966) in *The Development of Zonal Centrifuges and Ancillary Systems for Tissue Fractionation and Analysis*, Natl. Cancer Inst. Monograph **21,** 7.

Anderson, N. G., Waters, D. A., Fisher, W. D., Cline, G. B., Nunley, C. E., Elrod, L. H., and Rankin, C. T. (1967a) *Analyt. Biochem.* **21,** 235.

Anderson, N. G., and Rutenberg, E. (1967) *Analyt. Biochem.* **21,** 259.

Anderson, N. G., Waters, D. A., Nunley, C. E., Gilson, R. F., Schilling, R. M., Denny, E. C., Cline, G. B., Babelay, E. F., and Perarde, T. E. (1969a) *Analyt. Biochem.* **32,** 460.

Anderson, N. G., Nunley, C. E., and Rankin, C. T. (1969b) *Analyt. Biochem.* **31,** 255.

Bentzel, C. J., and Solomon, A. K. (1967) *J. Gen. Physiol.* **50,** 1547.

Berman, A. S. (1966) in *The Development of Zonal Centrifuges and Ancillary Systems for Tissue Fractionation and Analysis* (N.G. Anderson, ed.), Natl. Cancer Inst. Monograph **21,** p. 41.

Bishop, B. S. (1966) in *The Development of Zonal Centrifuges and Ancillary Systems for Tissue Fractionation and Analysis* (N.G. Anderson, ed.), Natl. Cancer Inst. Monograph **21,** p. 175.

Boone, C. W., Ford, L. E., Bond, H. E., Stuart, D. C., and Lorenz, D. (1969) *J. Cell Biol.* **41,** 378.

Brakke, M. K. (1964) *Arch. Biochem. Biophys.* **107,** 388.

Changeux, J. P., Gautron, J., Israel, M., Podleski, T. R. (1969) *Compt. Rend.* **269,** 1788.

Cotman, C. W. (1968) Doctoral dissertation, Department of Chemistry, Indiana University, Bloomington, Indiana.

Cotman, C. W., Mahler, H. R., and Anderson, N. G. (1968) *Biochim. Biophys. Acta* **163,** 272.

Cotman, C. W., Brown, D. H., Harrell, B. W., and Anderson, N. G. (1970) *Arch. Biochem. Biophys.* **136,** 436.

Cotman, C. W., and Flansburg, D. (1970) *Brain Res.* **22,** 152.

Cotman, C. W., and Doyle, L. (1972) In preparation.

Cotman, C. W., and Matthews, D. A. (1971) *Biochim. Biopyhs. Acta* **249,** 380.

Cotman, C. W., Herschman, H., and Taylor, D. (1971a) *J. Neurobiol.* **2,** 169.

Cotman, C. W., Doyle, L. and Banker, G. (1972a) In preparation.

Dallner, G., and Ernster, L. (1968) *J. Histochem. Cytochem.* **16,** 611.

Davis, G. A., and Bloom, F E. (1970) *J. Cell Biol.* **47,** 115.

de Duve, C., Berthet, J., and Beaufay, H. (1959) *Prog. Biophys. Biophys. Chem.* **9,** 325.

de Duve, C. (1965) *Harvey Lect. (1963-1964)* Ser. **59,** 49.

de Robertis, E., and de Plazas, S. F. (1970) *Biochim. Biophys. Acta* **219,** 388.

D'Monte, B., Marks, N., Datta, R. K., and Lajtha, A. (1970) in *Protein Metabolism in the Nervous System* (A. Lajtha, ed.), Plenum Press, New York, p. 185.

Doyle, L. C., Bauker, G., and Cotman, C. W., (1972) in Preparatrod.

Emmelot, P., and Vaz Dias, H. (1970) *Biochim. Biophys. Acta* **203,** 172.

Gamble, J. L., and Garlid, K. D. (1970) *Biochim. Biophys. Acta* **211,** 223.

Graham, J. M., Higgins, J. A., and Green, C. (1968) *Biochem. Biophys. Acta* **150,** 303.

Greenawalt, J. W., Rossi, C. S., and Lehninger, A. L. (1964) *J. Cell Biol.* **23,** 21.

Halsall, H. B., and Schumaker, V. N. (1969) *Analyt. Biochem.* **30,** 368.

Hamberger, A., Blomstrand, C., and Lehninger, A. L. (1970) *J. Cell Biol.* **45,** 221.

Heine, J. W., and Schnaitman, C. A. (1971) *J. Cell Biol.* **48,** 703.

Hillarp, N.-A. (1958) *Acta Physiol. Scand.* **43,** 82.

Hoyer, D. J. (1969) *A Bibliographic Guide to Neuroenzyme Literature,* Plenum Press, New York.

Kasa, P., Mann, S. P., and Hebb, C. O. (1970) *Nature* **266**, 812.
Koening, H., Gaines, D., McDonald, T., Gray, R., and Scott, J. (1964) *J. Neurochem.* **11**, 729.
Kornguth, S. E., Flangas A. L., Geison, R. L., and Scott, G. (1972) *Brain Res.* **37**, 53.
Kravitz, E., Molinoff, P., and Hall, Z. (1965) *Proc. Natl. Acad. Sci. U.S.* **54**, 778.
Kuhar, M. J., Green, A. I., Snyder, S. H., and Gfeller, E. (1970) *Brain Res.* **21**, 405.
Kuhar, M. J., Shaskan, E. G., and Snyder, S. H. (1971) *J. Neurochem.* **18**, 333.
Leighton, F., Poole, B., Beaufay, H., Bandhuin, P., Coffey J. W., Fowler, S., and de Duve, C. (1968) *J. Cell Biol.* **37**, 482.
Leskes, A., and Siekevitz, P. (1969) *J. Cell Biol.* **43**, 80a.
Loeb, J. N., and Kimberg, D. V. (1970) *J. Cell Biol.* **46**, 17.
Mahley, M. S., Day, E., Anderson, N. G., Wilford, R. F., and Brater, C. (1968) *Cancer Res.* **28**, 1783.
Marchbanks, R. M., and Israel, M. (1971) *J. Neurochem.* **18**, 439.
McConnell, D. G. (1965) *J. Cell Biol.* **27**, 459.
Metzger, H. P., Cuenod, M., Grynbaum, A., and Waelsch, H. (1967) *J. Neurochem.* **14**, 99.
Morgan, I. G.,Wolfe, L. S., Mandel, P., and Gombos G. (1971) *Biochim, Biophys, Aefa* **241**, 737,
Morre, D. J., Mollenhauer, H. H., and Chamber, J. E. (1965) *Exp. Cell Res.* **8**, 672.
Neville, D. M., Jr. (1960) *J. Biophys. Biochem, Cytol.* **8**, 413.
Novikoff, A. (1967) in *The Neuron* (H. Hydén, ed.), Elsevier, Amsterdam, p. 255.
Pollak, J. K., and Munn, E. A. (1970) *Biochem. J.* **117**, 913.
Raisman, G. (1969) *Brain Res.* **14**, 25.
Rodnight, R., Weller, M., and Goldfarb, R. S. G. (1969) *J. Neurochem.* **16**, 1591.
Rodriguez de Lores, Arnaiz G., Alberici, M., and de Robertis, E. (1967) *J. Neurochem.* **14**, 215.
Roizman, B., and Spear, P. G. (1971) *Science* **171**, 298.
Schachman, A. K. (1959) *Ultracentrifugation in Biochemistry,* Academic Press, New York, p. 214.
Schneider, W. C. (1968) in *Handbook of Biochemistry* (H.A. Sober, ed.), Chemical Rubber Co., Cleveland, Ohio, p. K3.
Schuberth, J., Sparf, B., and Sundwall, A. (1970) *J. Neurochem.* **17**, 461.
Smith, A. D., and Winkler, H. (1967) *Biochem. J.* **103**, 480.
Spragg, S. P., and Rankin, C. T. (1967) *Biochim. Biophys. Acta* **141**, 164.
Steck, T., and Wallach, D. F. H. (1970) *Methods in Cancer Research* **5**, 93.
Steck, T. L., Straus, J. H., and Wallach, D. F. (1970a) *Biochem. Biophys. Acta* **203**, 385.
Steck, T. L., Weinstein, R. S., Straus, J. H., and Wallach, D. F. H. (1970b) *Science* **168**, 255.
Thines-Sempoux, D., Amar-Costesec, A., Beaufay, A., and Berthet, J. (1969) *J. Cell Biol.* **43**, 189.
Trifaro, J. M., and Dworkind, J. (1970) *Analyt. Biochem.* **34**, 403.
Wallach, D. F. H., and Kamat, V. B. (1964) *Proc. Natl. Acad. Sci.* **52**, 721.
Wallach, D. F. H. (1967) in *The Specificity of Cell Surfaces* (B. D. Davis and L. Warren, eds.), Prentice-Hall, Englewood Cliffs, N. J., p. 129.
Wattiaux-De Coninck, S., and Wattiaux, R. (1969) *Biochem. Biophys. Acta* **183**, 118.
Whittaker, V. P., Michaelson, I. A., and Kirkland, J. A. (1964) *Biochem. J.* **90**, 293.
Whittaker, V. P. (1968) *Biochem. J.* **106**, 412.

Chapter 5

Brain Ribosomes

Claire E. Zomzely-Neurath and Sidney Roberts

Roche Institute of Molecular Biology
Nutley, New Jersey
and
Department of Biological Chemistry
School of Medicine, and the Brain Research Institute
University of California Center for the Health Sciences
Los Angeles, California

I. INTRODUCTION

It is generally believed that specialized function in the central nervous system is closely tied to regulatory mechanisms in protein synthesis in this organ (Roberts 1971). The major site of protein synthesis in the brain, as elsewhere, is the cytoplasmic ribosome. However, methods specifically designed for the isolation of brain ribosomes and detailed investigations of the properties of these preparations are relatively recent developments. Microsomal and ribosomal fractions were first prepared from brain homogenates by centrifugation in a liquid two-phase system (Albertsson *et al.,* 1959) or in sucrose density gradients (Hanzon and Toschi, 1960). Subsequently, several reports appeared which described the application of differential centrifugation procedures to the isolation of microsomal and ribosomal fractions from whole brain or brain regions (Acs *et al.,* 1961; Bondy and Perry, 1963; Datta and Ghosh; 1963*a*; Rendi and Hultin, 1960; Satake *et al.,* 1960; Zomzely *et al.,* 1964). The capacity of these preparations to incorporate amino acids into protein *in vitro* was also demonstrated. These earlier preparations of ribosome fractions from brain consisted mainly of single ribosomes (monoribosomes) and small aggregates. Methods specifically designed for the isolation of polyribosomes from brain tissues and detailed investigations of the properties of these preparations have appeared only within the past few years. (Campagnoni and Mahler, 1967; Mahler and Brown, 1968; Takahashi *et al.*, 1966; Zomzely *et al.*, 1966, 1968).

The various microsomal and ribosomal fractions from brain are grossly similar to analogous preparations from other tissues. However, the brain preparations reveal certain unique characteristics which appear to be related to specialized function *in vivo* (Zomzely *et al.*, 1964, 1966, 1968, 1971). These properties may not be evident in fractions which are not prepared under carefully controlled conditions. Therefore, it is especially important for investigators in this field to be aware of the specific requirements and limitations of the procedures employed for the isolation of ribosomes and other components of protein-synthesizing systems from brain tissues. The following presentation is designed to meet this need.

II. GENERAL CONSIDERATIONS

Electron microscopic studies reveal that a large proportion of the cytoplasmic ribosomes in most mature animal cells are organized into polyribosomal clusters which are closely associated with the endoplasmic reticulum (Palade, 1955). These ribosome aggregates take the form of chains, loops, spirals, circles, and rosettes. Frequently, thin strands thought to be messenger RNA can be observed linking the individual ribosomes. Ribosomes *in situ* are thought to exist in part "free" and in part "bound" to the endoplasmic reticulum or other cellular membranes. Morphologically, free and membrane-bound ribosomes are distinguished on the basis of their apparent proximity to these membranes. Operationally, these classes of ribosomes are defined primarily by the relative ease with which they are prepared free of membrane contamination. Ribosomes which can be isolated only in the presence of a chelating agent (e.g., EDTA), hydrolytic enzymes (RNases or proteases), or a detergent (e.g., sodium deoxycholate) are presumed to exist bound to intracellular membranes with varying degrees of tenacity *in situ* (Palade and Siekevitz, 1956; Petermann, 1964; Rosbash and Penman, 1971). Reconstitution studies *in vitro* support the concept that polyribosomes interact with specific sites on the surface of the endoplasmic reticulum (Ragland *et al.*, 1971).

The degree of aggregation and extent of membrane attachment of cytoplasmic ribosomes in animal cells differ markedly, depending upon the source of these cells and their stage of development (Palade, 1955). Mammalian reticulocytes, specialized for the synthesis of hemoglobin, lack a rough-surfaced endoplasmic reticulum; only free ribosomes are observed and these are mainly in the form of medium-sized aggregates. In contrast, ribosomes of pancreatic zymogen cells occur principally as large polyribosomes which are closely associated with cellular membranes. The state of aggregation of ribosomes and their association with membranes in mature hepatic cells occupy a position which is between these two extremes. Neurons of the mature mammalian brain appear to contain a high proportion of free or loosely bound ribosomes in varying states of aggregation (Ekholm and Hyden, 1965; Merits *et al.,* 1969; Sotelo and Palay, 1968; Zomzely *et al.,* 1971), whereas neuroglia resemble other mature mammalian cells in possessing a greater proportion of membrane-associated polyribosomes (Mugnaini and Walberg, 1964). Ribosomes which are closely associated with the endoplasmic reticulum of mammalian cells are thought to function, in part, as foci for the synthesis of exportable proteins (Siekevitz and Palade, 1960).

Conditions employed for the preparation of ribosome-containing fractions vary with the nature of the fraction desired as well as tissue source (Allfrey, 1959). However, the first step usually consists of gentle homogenization of the tissue in appropriate medium, followed by removal of cell debris, nuclei, and mitochondria at moderate centrifugal speed. This procedure produces the postmitochondrial supernatant fraction, which serves as the starting point for the isolation of ribosome fractions. High-speed centrifugation of this postmitochondrial supernatant fluid, without further treatment, yields the microsomal fraction. Microsomal preparations typically consist of ribosomes attached to the outer surfaces of broken membranes which are largely formed into rounded structures (Palade and Siekevitz, 1956). Ribosomal fractions, freed of these membranes, can be isolated from the postmitochondrial supernatant fraction or from the microsomal fraction by methods detailed below.

Procedures for the preparation of ribosome-containing fractions generally utilize isotonic or slightly hypertonic sucrose (0.25–0.32 M) in the homogenization medium (Hogeboom *et al.,* 1948). These concentrations of sucrose (a) minimize swelling and disruption of subcellular organelles (including the lysosomes which contain RNases and other hydrolytic enzymes), (b) reduce the aggregation of cell components, thereby facilitating their fractionation and (c) result in subcellular fractions with relatively high metabolic activity (Allfrey, 1959; De Duve *et al.,* 1955; Hogeboom *et al.,* 1948). Isolation of ribosome fractions is further favored by the use of buffered media (pH 7.4–7.8) of relatively high ionic strength to decrease contamination by absorbed cytoplasmic proteins (Petermann, 1964). The structural integrity of ribosomes *per se* and of natural aggregates of ribosomes is best maintained by the presence of sufficient Mg^{2+} in the preparation medium to inhibit RNase action and to counteract the tendency of monovalent cations (such as K^+) to displace Mg^{2+} from ribosomal sites of attachment

(Chao, 1957; Petermann and Hamilton, 1957; Petermann, 1964). Appropriate concentrations of Mg^{2+} are especially important for the preparation of ribosome fractions from brain tissue (Zomzely, 1966). The methods which follow were developed originally for the isolation of stable and active ribosome fractions of various types from cerebral cortical tissue of young adult male rats (6–7 weeks old) of a highly inbred Sprague-Dawley strain (Zomzely *et al.,* 1964; 1966). The methods for the isolation of ribosomes and polyribosomes are also applicable to other areas of the brain and to brain tissue from animals at all stages of development (Roberts *et al.,* 1971; Zomzely *et al.,* 1968, 1971).

III. PREPARATION OF MICROSOMAL FRACTIONS

A. Large and Small Microsomes

Animals are sacrificed by decapitation or by exsanguination from the abdominal aorta under light anesthesia induced by the subcutaneous administration of pentobartital sodium in 0.9% NaCl (6 mg per 100 g body weight). The brains are rapidly removed and transferred to Petri dishes containing filter paper moistened with the preparation medium and kept on ice. The dishes are then taken to the cold room (4 °C) for dissection of the brains and for all subsequent manipulations except centrifugation. The tissue is placed in a 50-ml beaker in an ice bath and minced briefly with scissors in a small quantity of medium composed of 0.25 M sucrose, 25 mM KCl, 4 mM Mg^{2+} (as chloride or acetate), and 50 mM tris-HCl buffer, pH 7.4. Mincing facilitates subsequent homogenization of the tissue, which is carried out in 9 parts of medium (v/w) with 5 up-and-down strokes of a Teflon pestle in a glass tube with a smooth inner surface and a clearance of 0.3–0.4 mm. The relatively high ratio of medium to tissue is required to reduce the binding of extraneous proteins to cell structures and to permit efficient recovery of microsomal components during the first centrifugation step. All centrifugation procedures are carried out at 0 °C. The homogenate is centrifuged at 15,000 g for 15 min to remove cell debris, nuclei, and mitochondria. The postmitochondrial supernatant fluid is decanted from the firm pellet and centrifuged at 34,500 g for 30 min to yield the "large" microsome fraction. The resulting supernatant fluid is then centrifuged at 105,000 g for 2 hr to sediment the "small" microsome fraction. This preparation comprises the preponderance of microsomal particles in the initial postmitochondrial supernatant fraction. The microsomal pellets are rinsed 3 times with medium, resuspended, and centrifuged at 105,000 g for 2 hr. The resulting pellets are also washed 3 times with medium and allowed to drain. The

microsomal fractions from rat cerebral cortex can be stored as pellets at
$-60\,^{\circ}\text{C}$ or in liquid nitrogen for at least 4 weeks, without detectable change
in appearance or amino acid-incorporating activity. These pellets consist of
a mixture of free ribosomes, membrane vesicles, and membrane-bound
ribosomes. The yield from rat cerebral cortex is equivalent to about 1 mg
of microsomal protein per gram wet weight of tissue. The ratio of RNA to
protein is approximately 0.3 (see also, Yamagami et al., 1963).

The supernatant fluid obtained after removal of the microsomal fractions contains amino acid synthetases, transferases, and other factors required for amino acid incorporation by ribosomal preparations in vitro.
This postmicrosomal supernatant fraction can be used in amino acid-incorporating systems directly. If stored in small portions at $-60\,^{\circ}\text{C}$, it will
remain active for at least 3 weeks (considerably longer, in the presence of
dithiothreitol or mercaptoethanol). Alternatively, the postmicrosomal fluid
can be used for preparation of the "pH 5 enzyme" fraction (Section V,A).

B. Total Microsomes

A simplified procedure can be used for preparation of a microsomal
fraction which contains both large and small microsomes. The postmitochondrial supernatant fluid is centrifuged directly at 105,000 g for 2 hr.
The resulting pellet constitutes the "total" microsome fraction. This preparation is less stable than the small microsome fraction, presumably due
to the presence of bound degradative enzymes, including RNases and
proteases. Further purification may be achieved by sedimentation of the
total microsomal fraction through 1 M sucrose containing the same buffer
and salts as the preparation medium. Centrifugation at 105,000 g for 3 hr
is required to pellet this fraction.

IV. PREPARATION OF RIBOSOMAL FRACTIONS

Ribosomes of animal cells can be isolated in several forms essentially
free of the membranes which constitute a large part of microsomal fractions.
These membrane-free preparations include (a) heterogeneous populations of
ribosomes and ribosomal subunits in various stages of association and
aggregation ("mixed" ribosomes); (b) ribosomal populations consisting
mainly of heavy aggregates with messenger RNA attached (polyribosomes);
and (c) monoribosomes from which messenger RNA and other factors
essential for protein synthesis have been removed ("stripped" ribosomes).

A. Mixed Ribosomes

Mixed populations of cytoplasmic ribosomes have been used extensively for studies of the basic requirements for amino acid incorporation *in vitro* and the stimulatory action of natural and synthetic messenger RNAs on this process. These "mixed" ribosome preparations are relatively free of extraneous proteins, including the amino acid synthetases and transferases, and therefore require the addition of cell sap or pH 5 enzymes for significant activity. Messenger RNA and transfer RNA are active in these preparations to varying degrees, depending upon the proportion of ribosomes isolated which are deficient in these natural activators.

Preparation of mixed ribosome fractions is relatively simple compared to the procedures required for the isolation of polyribosomes and "stripped" ribosomes. The procedures presented below were developed for the preparation of mixed ribosomes from rat cerebral cortex (Zomzely *et al.,* 1964, 1966) but are equally applicable to other regions of the brain and to brain tissue from other animals.

In the preferred procedure, the total microsomal fraction is obtained and resuspended without further purification in the preparation medium (0.25 M sucrose, 25 mM KCl, 4 mM MgCl$_2$, 50 mM tris-HCl buffer, pH 7.4). This suspension is first centrifuged at 3000 g for 10 min to remove nonspecific aggregates of ribosomes which form during resuspension of the microsomal pellets. Aggregation tends to be more pronounced with brain preparations than with comparable fractions from other sources; e.g., liver. Freshly prepared sodium deoxycholate (5–10% in 50 mM tris-HCl buffer, pH 8.2) is then added to the microsomal suspension to a final concentration of 0.25%. This concentration of detergent is considerably less than that required to liberate the ribosomes from their membrane attachment in other mammalian cells; e.g., liver (von der Decken, 1967). The explanation for this difference appears to reside in the fact that brain ribosomes, especially those of neuronal origin, are less firmly and less extensively attached to cellular membranes (Merits *et al.,* 1969; Zomzely *et al.,* 1971), rather than in a greater sensitivity of these membranes to solubilization by the detergent. The deoxycholate-treated microsomal fraction is centrifuged at 105,000 g for 2 hr. The resulting ribosome pellets are washed 3 times with the preparation medium, resuspended in this medium, and recentrifuged at 105,000 g for 2 hr. These pellets are also washed 3 times and finally the tubes are drained prior to use or storage. The extensive washing procedure is required to remove traces of deoxycholate which may subsequently result in ribosomal breakdown and poor amino acid-incorporating activity. This preparation of mixed ribosomes is stable at −60 °C or in liquid nitrogen for at least 3 months, even though slight

RNase contamination is present (Zomzely *et al.,* 1968). The yield is equivalent to about 0.6 mg RNA per gram wet weight of cerebral cortex.

A simplified procedure may also be used for the preparation of cerebral mixed ribosomes. The postmitochondrial supernatant is treated directly with sodium deoxycholate. In this instance, the final concentration of detergent must be increased to 1 % to ensure complete liberation of ribosomes from the endoplasmic reticulum and other cellular membranes. The mixed ribosome fraction is then isolated as described above. However, the post-microsomal supernatant fraction from this preparation cannot be used as a source of enzymes for amino acid-incorporating studies because of irreversible inactivation of these enzymes in the presence of sodium deoxycholate.

The preparation of mixed ribosomes from brain by either method described above can be carried out with a ratio of homogenization medium to tissue of only 3:1 (v/w), compared to the 9:1 ratio employed in the isolation of microsomal fractions. The subsequent treatment with detergent removes a large portion of the protein contamination which would otherwise be present in ribosomal preparations made from the more concentrated homogenates. However, significant loss of ribosomes into the low-speed pellet occurs under these conditions.

The mixed ribosome preparation is composed principally of ribosomal monomers, dimers, and trimers [Figs. 1 and 2 (a)] with sedimentation values approximating 80 S, 115 S, and 150 S, respectively, in medium composed of 4 mM MgCl$_2$, 25 mM KCl, and 50 mM tris-HCl buffer (pH 7.4). In media of different composition, the sedimentation values and distribution of ribosomal species will vary. The preparations also contain relatively small amounts of larger ribosomal aggregates (Fig. 1). Freedom from gross contamination with extraneous proteins is indicated by ultraviolet extinction spectra and chemical measurements of RNA and protein. These data are given in Table I along with comparable data obtained in other laboratories. Ultraviolet extinction of purified RNA is maximal near 260 nm, whereas protein absorbs maximally at 280 nm; other contaminants generally absorb maximally at shorter wavelengths (235–242 nm) than RNA. Thus, high ratios of RNA to protein as evidenced both by chemical and optical measurements are gross indices of relatively high purity (Petermann, 1964). Nevertheless, the preparations may contain varying amounts of minor contaminants which markedly affect stability and metabolic activity; e.g., degradative enzymes, especially RNases. These can be largely removed by sedimentation of the ribosomes through heavy sucrose following treatment of the microsomal preparation with sodium deoxycholate. Centrifugation is carried out at 105,000 g for 3 hr in medium composed of 1 M sucrose, 4 mM MgCl$_2$, 25 mM KCl and 50 mM tris-HCl, pH 7.4. Attempts to remove or inactivate RNases and other hydrolytic enzymes in tissue pre-

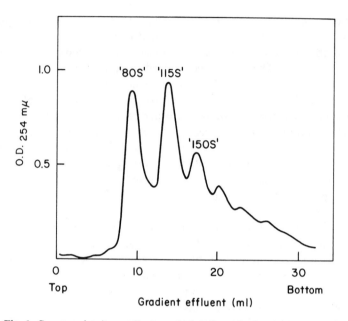

Fig. 1. Sucrose density-gradient analysis of cerebral mixed ribosomes. Ribosomes equivalent to 1.5 mg of ribosomal protein were suspended in 2 ml of medium composed of 4 mM MgCl$_2$, 25 mM KCl, and 50 mM tris-HCl buffer (pH 7.4). The suspension was layered on a linear sucrose gradient (20 to 5%) containing the same buffer and salts and was centrifuged for 3 hr in a Spinco SW 25 swinging-bucket rotor at 25,000 rev/min and 0°C. Absorbance of the effluent collected from the top of the gradient was monitored continuously at 254 nm using the ISCO Model D density gradient fractionator (Instrument Specialties Co.) with the ISCO Model UA ultraviolet analyzer and an external recorder. Positions of ribosomal monomers (80 S), dimers (115 S), and trimers (150 S) are indicated. (Reprinted from Zomzely *et al.*, 1966.)

parations prior to isolation of ribosomes have not met with great success (see Section IV, B).

Resuspension of fresh or frozen pellets of ribosomes from brain or other mammalian tissues usually results in the formation of small quantities of nonspecific aggregates. In some instances, this phenomenon may be due to the presence of protein contaminants or the action of hydrolytic enzymes. However, in the case of brain, even preparations of monoribosomes and subunits which have been highly purified exhibit this property, possibly as a result of their unique sensitivity to variations in ion concentrations, especially Mg^{2+} and K$^+$ (Roberts and Zomzely, 1966; Zomzely *et al.*, 1964). The nonspecific ribosome aggregates can readily be removed by centrifugation at 5000 g for 10 min.

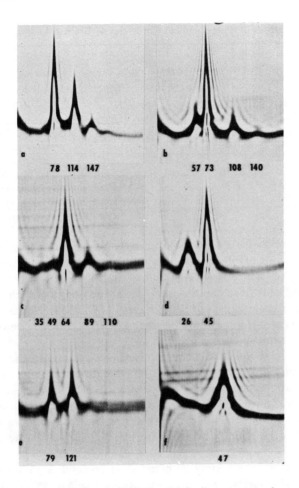

Fig. 2. Sedimentation patterns of cerebral mixed ribosomes. Analyses were carried out in a 12-mm cell in the Spinco model E analytical ultracentrifuge. Temperature of analysis was 20°C except in (c) (13°C) and (d) (6°C). Photographs were obtained using schlieren optics at appropriate intervals after the rotor reached full speed of 29,500 rev/min. Concentrations of ribosomal protein varied from 2 to 3 mg/ml. Sedimentation was from *left* to *right*. $S_{20,w}$ values are shown. (a) Analyzed in 4 mM MgCl$_2$, 25 mM KCl, and 50 mM tris-HCl buffer (pH 7.4). (b) Analyzed in 100 mM KCl, 50 mM tris-HCl buffer (pH 7.4). (c) Dialyzed 16 hr against 1 mM tris-HCl (pH 7.6); analyzed in the same medium. Changes in ribosome conformation and hydration in this medium of low ionic strength were responsible for the low $S_{20,w}$ values for monoribosomes (64 S) and other species. (d) Analyzed in 50 mM KCl, 1 mM tris-HCl buffer (pH 7.6), containing 3 μmoles EDTA/mg ribosomal protein. The chelating agent has reduced the $S_{20,w}$ values of 40 S and 60 S ribosome subunits. (e) Duplicate of sample (d) dialyzed 5 hr at 4°C against 12 mM MgCl$_2$, 100 mM KCl, 1 mM tris-HCl buffer (pH 7.6) and analyzed in the same medium. (f) Dialyzed 40 hr at 4°C against 100 mM KCl, 50 mM tris-HCl buffer (pH 7.4) and analyzed in the same medium. (Reprinted from Zomzely *et al.*, 1966.)

Table I. Physicochemical Properties of Brain Ribosomes

Source	RNA ——— RNA+protein	Extinction ratios		Reference
		260 nm ——— 280 nm	max 260 nm ——— min 235–242 nm	
Guinea pig (whole brain)	0.29–0.32	—	—	Acs *et al.* (1961)
Guinea pig (whole brain)	0.46	—	1.59–1.69	Yamagami *et al.* (1963)
Rat (whole brain)	0.29	—	—	Hanzon and Toschi (1960)
Rat (cortex)	0.45	1.71	1.68	Zomzely *et al.* (1964); Zomzely *et al.* (1966)
Rat (whole brain)	0.45	1.71	1.70–1.80	Datta *et al.* (1964)
Goat (cortex)	0.30	—	1.70	Datta and Ghosh (1963a,b); Petermann (1964)

Cerebral ribosomes cannot be extensively dissociated simply by lowering the concentrations of Mg^{2+} and other ions in the suspension medium [Fig. 2 (b,c)]. This resistance to dissociation is characteristic of ribosomes from eukaryotic cells (Tashiro and Siekevitz, 1965) and contrasts with the ease of dissociation of bacterial ribosomes (Tissierès *et al.,* 1959). However, mammalian ribosomes, including those of cerebral cortex, can be completely dissociated to subunits by treatment with EDTA or some other chelating agent [Fig. 2 (d)]. The 26 S and 45 S components shown correspond to the "40 S" and "60 S" ribosome subunits, with sedimentation values reduced by alterations in hydration and shape in the presence of EDTA and medium of low ionic strength (Zomzely, 1966). Although these subunits can be recombined by dialysis against buffer containing Mg^{2+} [Fig. 2 (e)], the resulting ribosomes exhibit little or no amino acid-incorporating activity (see, however Section VI, C).

Purified RNA can readily be prepared from cerebral mixed ribosomes (Schneider and Roberts, 1968). Ribosomes equivalent to 15 mg protein are suspended in 10 ml of medium containing 8 mM EDTA, 1 % sodium dodecyl sulfate, and 10 mM tris-HCl buffer, pH 7.5. The mixture is first shaken for 15 min with 10 ml of phenol saturated with buffer. The aqueous layer is shaken twice more for 10 min with 5 ml of the phenol-buffer mixture. RNA is then precipitated from the aqueous phase with a final concentration of 0.1 M NaCl and 67 % ethanol. The precipitate is washed, resuspended with water, and finally reprecipitated 3 times with salt and ethanol. This preparation consists principally of 18 S and 28 S RNA (Fig. 3). Small amounts of 4 S transfer RNA and 5 S ribosomal RNA also appear to be present. The mass ratio of the two major species (1:2) indicates that very little breakdown of RNA occurs during the isolation process.

B. Polyribosomes

Cytoplasmic protein synthesis in all cells is presumed to be carried out principally by preformed polyribosomes (Gierer, 1963; Warner *et al.*, 1962). Monoribosomes and ribosome subunits which are liberated after termination of the polypeptide chain or formed in the cell *de novo* appear to require activation before they can be incorporated into polysomes and participate in protein synthesis (Bishop, 1966; Girard *et al.*, 1965; Hogan and Korner, 1968; Joklik and Becker, 1965a, b; Staehelin *et al.*, 1967). Polyribosome fractions which actively incorporate amino acids *in vitro* can readily be isolated from mammalian tissues by the use of discontinuous sucrose gradients (Wettstein *et al.*, 1963), Centrifugation of postmitochondrial supernatant preparations through progressively heavier layers of sucrose effectively concentrates and purifies the larger polyribosomes present. Smaller polyribosomes, monoribosomes, and ribosome subunits are largely left behind in the

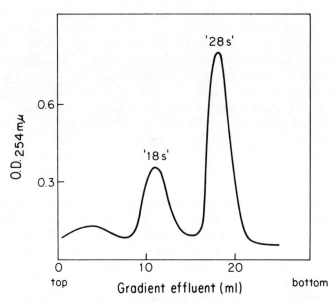

Fig. 3. Sucrose density-gradient pattern of ribosomal RNA from adult rat cerebral cortex. The purified RNA (1 mg) was suspended in 2 ml of buffer composed of 8 mM EDTA, 100 mM NaCl, and 10 mM sodium acetate (pH 5.1) and layered on a linear sucrose density gradient (20 to 5%) containing the same additives. Centrifugation was carried out for 18 hr in a Spinco SW 25 rotor at 22,500 rev/min and 0°C. Absorbance of the effluent was monitored continuously at 254 nm. (Reprinted from Schneider and Roberts, 1968.)

supernatant fluid, along with membranes and membrane-bound polyribosomes if no detergent has been added.

Polyribosomes have been prepared from brain tissues by homogenization in media containing concentrations of Mg^{2+} varying from 2.5 to 12 mM and concentrations of K^+ varying from 25 to 500 mM. However, unlike hepatic preparations, large polyribosomes predominate in brain preparations only when the isolation medium contains about 10–12 mM Mg^{2+} (Zomzely et al., 1966). Free polyribosomes are isolated as a pellet by direct high-speed centrifugation of untreated postmitochondrial supernatant fractions (Bont et al., 1965), whereas polyribosomes which are presumably bound to cellular membranes in situ are also pelleted when a detergent is added to the postmitochondrial supernatant (Wettstein et al., 1963). Endogenous RNase inhibitors in the postmitochondrial supernatant may exert a protective action on the polyribosomes under these conditions (Blobel and Potter, 1966). Thus, polyribosomes cannot readily be prepared from microsomal fractions, because addition of detergent, in addition to solubilizing the membranes and releasing the ribosomes, also results in disruption of the polyribosomal structure.

The method of Munro, Jackson, and Korner (1964), developed for the preparation of hepatic polyribosomes, can also be used for the isolation of fractions from brain which are presumably composed of both free and bound polyribosomes (Zomzely et al., 1966). Homogenization of brain tissue is carried out in 3 volumes (v/w) of medium composed of 0.25 M sucrose, 10 mM magnesium acetate, 40 mM NaCl, 100 mM KCl, and 20 mM tris-HCl buffer, pH 7.6. Only 3 up-and-down strokes of the Teflon pestle are used. The postmitochondrial supernatant fraction is obtained by centrifugation of the homogenate at 12,000 g for 10 min. Freshly dissolved sodium deoxycholate (5 % in 50 mM tris-HCl, pH 8.2) is added slowly with gentle stirring to a final concentration of 1 %. This suspension is layered over a solution of 0.5 M sucrose which was previously layered over a solution of 2.0 M sucrose in the relative proportions of 2:1:1. Both sucrose solutions contain the same buffer and salts as the preparation medium. The discontinuous gradient is then centrifuged at 105,000 g for 4 hr. The clear, colorless pellet obtained is rinsed 3 times with medium. The tube is drained and its inner walls wiped with tissue paper. These polyribosome preparations will retain their initial properties for several months if stored at $-60\,^{\circ}\mathrm{C}$ or in liquid nitrogen (see below).

The unique requirement for high concentrations of Mg^{2+} in the medium employed for the isolation of brain polyribosomes is documented in Fig. 4. In the presence of 10–12 mM Mg^{2+}, stable, active polyribosome fractions can be prepared from cerebral cortex of the adult rat with over 80 % of the particles possessing sedimentation coefficients greater than ribosomal trimers. This value drops to about 50 % when the preparation medium contains only 5 mM Mg^{2+}. The true polyribosomal nature of these cerebral aggregates has

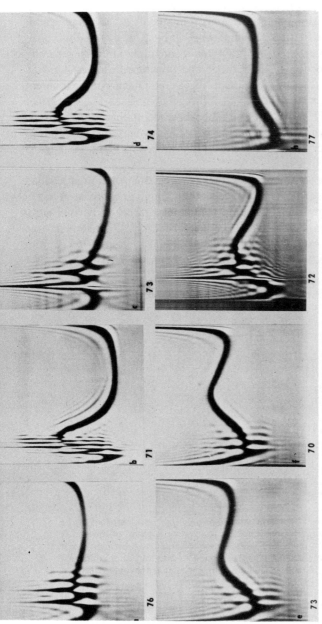

Fig. 4. Sedimentation patterns of cerebral and hepatic polyribosome preparations. Analyses were carried out in a 12-mm cell in the Spinco model E analytical ultracentrifuge at 20°C. Photographs were obtained using schlieren optics at appropriate intervals after the rotor reached full speed of 29,500 rev/min. Concentrations of ribosomal protein varied from 2 to 4 mg/ml. $S_{20,w}$ values are shown for the monoribosomal components. (a) Cerebral ribosomes prepared by method of Wettstein et al.(1963) and analyzed in 5 mM MgCl₂, 25 mM KCl, and 50 mM tris-HCl buffer (pH 7.4). (b) Cerebral ribosomes prepared by method of Munro et al. (1964) and analyzed in 10 mM magnesium acetate, 40 mM NaCl, 100 mM KCl, and 20 mM tris-HCl buffer (pH 7.6). (c) Cerebral ribosomes prepared by method of Wilson and Hoagland (1965) and analyzed in 8 mM MgC₃, 25 mM KCl, and 100 mM tris-HCl buffer (pH 7.5). (d) Cerebral ribosomes prepared by method of Zomzely et al. (1966) and analyzed in 12 mM MgCl₂, 100 mM KCl, and 50 mM tris-HCl buffer (pH 7.4). (e) Hepatic ribosomes prepared by method of Wettstein et al. (1963) and analyzed in 5 mM MgCl₂, 25 mM KCl, and 50 mM tris-HCl buffer (pH 7.4). (f) Hepatic ribosomes prepared by method of Munro et al. (1964) and analyzed in 10 mM magnesium acetate, 40 mM NaCl, 100 mM KCl, and 20 mM tris-HCl. buffer (pH 7.6). (g) Hepatic ribosomes prepared by method of Wilson and Hoagland (1965) and analyzed in 8 mM MgCl₂, 25 mM KCl, and 100 mM tris-HCl buffer (pH 7.5). (h) Hepatic ribosomes prepared by method of Zomzely et al.(1966) and analyzed in 12 mM MgCl₂, 100 mM KCl, and 50 mM tris-HCl buffer (pH 7.4). (Reprinted from Zomzely et al. (1966).)

been demonstrated, including their sensitivity to low concentrations of RNase and their high activity in amino acid incorporation *in vitro* (Zomzely *et al.,* 1968). Hepatic polyribosome fractions, consisting mainly of large aggregates, can be obtained with either 5 or 10 mM Mg^{2+} present in the medium. Preparations of polyribosomes from brain tissue of adult animals generally contain a larger proportion of monomeric and dimeric ribosomes than the corresponding hepatic fractions, presumably as a consequence of the inherent instability of certain messenger RNA-ribosome complexes in the former preparations (Zomzely *et al.,* 1966). Polyribosome preparations can be obtained from either whole brain, cerebral cortical gray matter, or hindbrain-medullary white matter of the adult rat by the procedure outlined (Figs. 5 and 6).

Several factors appear to be critical for the successful isolation of purified polyribosome fractions from brain which contain a high proportion of heavy aggregates, exhibit high levels of amino acid-incorporating activity *in vitro,* and are stable on storage at $-60\,°C$ for several months. First, RNase-free sucrose must be used exclusively. Each batch should be tested for freedom from these enzymes, as well as for interfering substances which absorb at 254

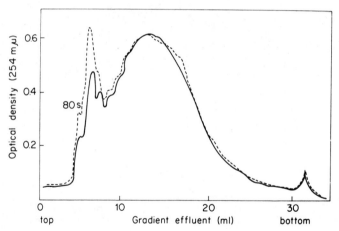

Fig. 5. Sucrose density-gradient profiles of polyribosomes prepared in the presence of 1% sodium deoxycholate from either cerebral cortical gray matter or hindbrain-medullary white matter of adult rats. Polyribosomes equivalent to 0.5 mg protein were suspended in 2 ml of buffer composed of 12 mM MgCl$_2$, 100 mM KCl, and 50 mM tris-HCl, pH 7.6, and layered on a linear sucrose gradient (35 to 15%) containing the same medium. Gradients were centrifuged for $1\frac{1}{2}$ hr in the Spinco SW 25.1 rotor at 25,000 rev/min and 0°C. Absorbance of the effluent was monitored continuously at 254 nm. The position of ribosomal monomers is shown by the designation, 80 S. ————, cerebral cortical gray matter; ⋯⋯⋯⋯, hindbrain-medullary white matter.

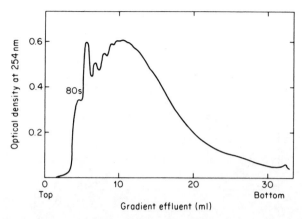

Fig. 6. Sucrose density-gradient profiles of polyribosomes prepared from whole brain of adult rats in the presence of 1 % sodium deoxycholate. See legend to Fig. 5 for explanations.

nm. Double-distilled water should be used throughout. The tris buffer should be filtered to remove sediment. If the final concentration of sodium deoxycholate added to the postmitochondrial fraction is allowed to rise over 1 %, polyribosomal disruption will occur in brain preparations, whereas hepatic preparations appear to be stable at appreciably higher concentrations of this detergent. These differences are presumably related to the greater stability of hepatic polyribosomes, as well as to the greater proportion of membrane-bound polyribosomes in the liver preparations.

Crude preparations of RNase inhibitor fractions from animal tissues, added to cerebral cell-free preparations during isolation of polyribosomes in the presence of 5–10 mM Mg^{2+} using the precautions outlined above, do not seem to improve the final product (Fig. 7). Under different conditions of isolation, polyribosomes may be obtained from brain in the presence of the natural RNase inhibitor fraction (Takahashi *et al.,* 1966), but these preparations are not superior to those depicted in Fig. 7. Comparable studies have not yet been carried out with purified natural RNase inhibitors, which have been obtained from brain and other mammalian tissues (Gribnau *et al.,* 1970; Takahashi *et al.,* 1970). Investigations of synthetic inactivators of RNase, including the polyanions bentonite (Barr and Guth, 1951) and polyvinylsulfate (Fellig and Wiley, 1959), as well as diethylpyrocarbonate (Solymosy *et al.,* 1968), have been disappointing. Carefully purified bentonite (Fraenkel-Conrat *et al.,* 1961; Keller *et al.,* 1963; Petermann, 1964) added to homogenates of rat cerebral cortex at levels which completely inhibit endogenous RNase activity (e.g., 0.5 mg/ml) has little effect on the resulting polyribosomal pattern (Fig. 8) and reduces recovery, presumably as a result of inter-

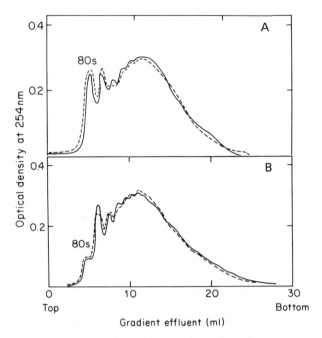

Fig. 7. Sucrose density-gradient analyses of polyribosomes isolated from rat cerebral cortex in the presence or absence of a crude natural RNase inhibitor fraction. Where indicated, one-half of the homogenization medium was replaced by the high-speed supernatant from rat brain. The polyribosomes were prepared using 1 % sodium deoxycholate and suspended in medium composed of 10 mM MgCl$_2$, 25 mM KCl, and 50 mM tris-HCl buffer, pH 7.6. Two milliliters of this suspension (equivalent to 0.3 mg ribosomal protein) were layered on a linear sucrose gradient (35 to 15 %) containing the same medium. The gradient was centrifuged for 1½ hr in a Spinco SW 25.1 rotor at 25,000 rev/min and 0°C. Absorbance of the effluent collected from the top of the gradient was monitored continuously at 254 nm. (A) Cerebral polyribosomes isolated in 5 mM Mg^{2+} by the method of Wettstein *et al.* (1963) in the presence (———) or absence (- - - - -) of the high-speedsupe rnatant from rat brain. (B) Cerebral polyribosomes isolated in 10 mM Mg^{2+} by the method of Munro *et al.* (1964) in the presence (———) or absence (- - - - -) of the high-speed supernatant from rat brain. Similar results were obtained with addition of high-speed supernatants from rat liver. The high-speed supernatants were obtained and employed as described by Blobel and Potter (1967).

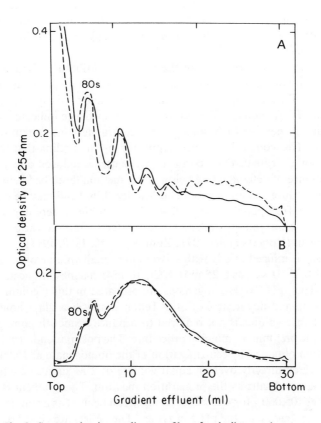

Fig. 8. Sucrose density-gradient profiles of polyribosomal preparations isolated from rat cerebral cortex in the presence or absence of bentonite. (A) Two milliliters of cerebral postmitochondrial supernatant fraction were layered on a linear sucrose gradient (35 to 15%) containing 10 mM magnesium acetate, 40 mM NaCl, 100 mM KCl, and 20 mM tris-HCl buffer, pH 7.6. Centrifugation was carried out for $3\frac{1}{2}$ hr in the Spinco SW 25.1 rotor at 25,000 rev/min and 0°C. (B) Polyribosomes equivalent to 0.2 mg of ribosomal protein were suspended in 2 ml of 12 mM MgCl$_2$, 100 mM KCl, and 50 mM tris-HCl buffer, pH 7.6, and layered on a linear sucrose gradient (35 to 15%) containing the same medium. Centrifugation was carried out for $1\frac{1}{2}$ hr at 25,000 rev/min and 0°C. The postmitochondrial supernatant fractions and purified polyribosomes were prepared by the method of Munro *et al.* (1964) using 1% sodium deoxycholate ———, bentonite present during preparation (0.5 mg/ml homogenizing medium); ------, bentonite absent.

action with basic proteins of the ribosomes (Petermann, 1964). Under comparable conditions, polyvinylsulfate (0.3 mg/ml) causes partial ribosomal breakdown and cannot be readily removed from the polyribosomes. Diethylpyrocarbonate also produces significant breakdown and loss of cerebral polyribosomes.

Omission of detergent from the procedure utilized to isolate polyribosomes from tissue homogenates presumably results in a preparation containing mainly ribosomal aggregates which exist free or loosely bound to membranes *in situ*. As noted above, morphological evidence indicates that a high proportion of neuronal ribosomes in the central nervous system occurs in a free form. This conclusion is also supported by the finding that the yield of polyribosomes from cerebral cortical gray matter is reduced only about 15% in the absence of detergent (see below). The method described below is based on the procedure of Campagnoni and Mahler (1967) and may be used for the isolation of free polyribosomes from whole brain, cerebral cortical gray matter and hindbrain-medullary white matter of rats at various stages of development (Roberts *et al.,* 1971; Zomzely *et al.,* 1968, 1971).

Tissue is minced briefly with scissors in a small volume of medium composed of 0.25 M sucrose, 25 mM KCl, 10 mM magnesium acetate, and 50 mM tris-HCl, pH 7.6. Homogenates are prepared in this medium (3:1, v:w) with 3–4 up-and-down strokes of a Teflon pestle in a glass homogenizing tube. A larger volume is not required to produce a smooth homogenate because of the preliminary mincing procedure. The postmitochondrial supernatant fraction obtained by centrifugation of the homogenate at 15,000 g for 10 min is layered directly over an equal volume of 2 M sucrose containing the same buffer and salts as the preparation medium. This gradient is then centrifuged at 105,000 g for 4 hr. The top layer can be used as a source of activating enzymes, etc., e.g., the pH 5 enzymes. The pellets are rinsed 3 times with medium; then the tubes are drained and their inner walls are wiped with tissue paper. These pellets of free polyribosomes, in common with detergent-treated preparations from the same source, can be stored for several months at −60 °C or in liquid nitrogen without significant alteration in state of aggregation (see for example, Fig. 9) or in amino acid-incorporating activity *in vitro* (Section VI, B).

The yield of polyribosomes from cerebral cortical gray matter of the rat declines during maturation (Table II). However, the proportion of polyribosomes obtained in the absence of sodium deoxycholate remains constant at about 85% of the total polyribosomes isolated throughout development. This value is somewhat smaller for the corresponding preparations from hindbrain-medullary white matter, i.e., about 75%. The total yield of free and membrane-bound polyribosomes from hindbrain-medullary white matter of the rat does not seem to vary after the peak of glial proliferation at 14 days

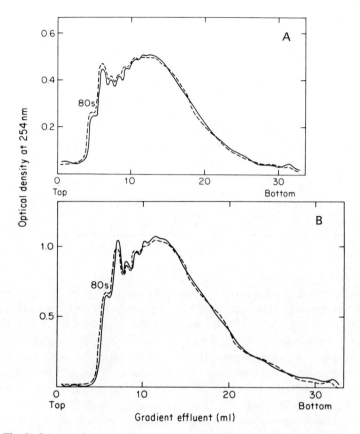

Fig. 9. Sucrose density-gradient analyses of polyribosomes prepared from rat cerebral cortex in the presence or absence of detergent before and after storage at −60°C. Polyribosomes were suspended in medium composed of 10 mM MgCl$_2$, 25 mM KCl, and 50 mM tris-HCl buffer, pH 7.6. Two milliliters of this suspension were layered on a linear sucrose gradient (35 to 15%) containing the same medium. The gradients were centrifuged for 1½ hr in the Spinco SW 25.1 rotor at 25,000 rev/min and 0°C. Absorbance of the effluent collected from the top of the gradient was monitored continuously at 254 nm. (A) Cerebral polyribosomes (0.5 mg ribosomal protein) isolated in absence of detergent. (B) Cerebral polyribosomes (1.0 mg ribosomal protein) isolated in the presence of 1% sodium deoxycholate. ———, freshly prepared; - - - - - -, stored 6 months at −60°C.

of age. All preparations of brain polyribosomes isolated by the procedures described above exhibited high ratios of RNA:protein (1.22–1.50), indicating a considerable degree of purity. These ratios are higher than those obtained by other procedures for the isolation of brain polyribosomes (Dunn, 1970; Takahashi *et al.*, 1966; Yamagami and Mori, 1970).

Table II.   Yields of Polyribosomes Obtained in the Presence and
Absence of Detergent from Different Brain Regions of Rats at
Various Stages of Development[a]

Age of animals	Yield of polyribosomes[b]	
	Detergent-free	Deoxycholate-treated
	(mg protein/g wet weight cortex)	
Days	Cerebral cortical gray matter	
<1	0.328 ± 0.056 (4)	0.392 ± 0.060 (4)
2	0.320 ± 0.045 (3)	0.381 ± 0.055 (3)
14	0.190 ± 0.019 (5)	0.224 ± 0.023 (4)
21	0.200 ± 0.022 (3)	0.238 ± 0.031 (3)
42	0.143 ± 0.014 (8)	0.170 ± 0.021 (6)
	Hindbrain-medullary white matter	
14	0.120 ± 0.010 (6)	0.162 ± 0.011 (6)
42	0.122 ± 0.028 (5)	0.167 ± 0.012 (5)

[a] Reprinted in modified version from Zomzely et al. (1971).
[b] Values shown are means ± standard error, with the number of determinations in parentheses.

Preparations of free polyribosomes from various regions of the brain and at different stages of development exhibit sedimentation patterns and stability properties which are very similar to those obtained with detergent-treated samples from the same source. This phenomenon is illustrated in Fig. 9 (A vs. B) for purified polyribosomes from cerebral cortices of adult rats. Moreover, the distribution of various ribosomal species in the postmitochondrial supernatants from which the polyribosomes are prepared does not appear to be altered by the presence of 1 % sodium deoxycholate (Fig. 10). It seems clear that this concentration of detergent does not result in significant breakdown of brain polyribosomes.

Profound differences in ribosomal aggregation occur in polyribosomal preparations obtained from rat cerebral cortex at various stages of development (Zomzely et al., 1971). Thus, postmitochondrial supernatant fractions from this tissue, either treated with 1 % deoxycholate or untreated, exhibit a decrease in the proportions of heavy aggregates during development (see for example, Fig. 11). Comparable results are obtained with purified polyribosomes from cerebral cortex [Fig. 12 (a, c, e, g,)]. In contrast, ribosomal aggregation in polyribosomal preparations from hindbrain-medullary white matter does not appear to vary significantly between 14–42 days of age in the rat (Fig. 13).

Developmental alterations in aggregation of polyribosomal preparations from rat cerebral cortex are associated with changes in the stability of certain of the larger messenger RNA–ribosome complexes (Zomzely et al., 1971). Thus, polyribosomes obtained from cerebral cortex of the adult rat disaggregate extensively upon exposure to low concentrations of Mg   (Fig. 12).

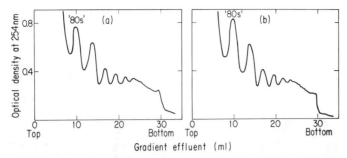

Fig. 10. Influence of detergent on sedimentation profiles of postmitochondrial supernatant fluid obtained from cerebral cortices of adult rats. The postmitochondrial supernatant fluid was prepared in 0.25 M sucrose containing 12 mM MgCl$_2$, 100 mM KCl, and 50 mM tris-HCl buffer, pH 7.6, and was divided into two portions. One portion was untreated. The other portion was treated with sodium deoxycholate (final concentration, 1%) prior to sedimentation analysis. An aliquot of each suspension (2 ml), equivalent to approximately 0.75 g of tissue was layered on a linear sucrose gradient (35 to 15%) containing buffer and salts in the concentrations noted above. The gradients were centrifuged at 25,000 rev/min and 0°C for 4 hr in a Spinco SW 25 rotor. Absorbance of the effluent collected from the top of each gradient was monitored continuously at 254 nm. (a) Detergent free. (b) Deoxycholate-treated. (Reprinted from Zomzely *et al.,* 1971.)

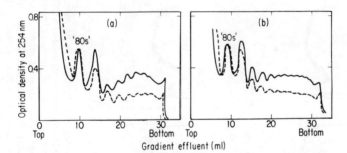

Fig. 11. Sedimentation profiles of postmitochondrial supernatant fluids from cerebral cortices of rats at various stages of development. The postmitochondrial supernatant fluids were prepared without detergent and analyzed as described in the legend to Fig. 10. (a) Cerebral cortical tissue from newborn rats (————) and adult rats (------). (b) From immature (14-day-old) rats (————) and adult rats (------). (Reprinted from Zomzely *et al.,* 1971.)

This instability of certain cerebral polyribosomes *in vitro* is well established by 14 days of age, but is not observed with the corresponding preparations from newborn or 2-day-old animals. Analogous developmental differences in polyribosomal stability are also evidenced during protein synthesis in

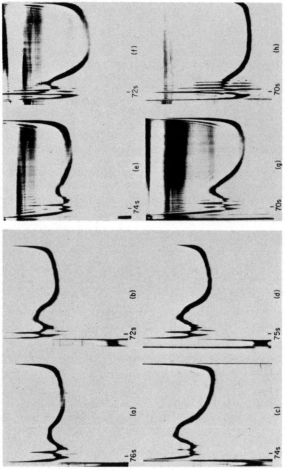

Fig. 12. Sedimentation properties of polyribosomes prepared from cerebral cortices of rats at various stages of development. Polyribosomes were suspended in medium composed of MgCl₂ (1 or 10 mM), 25 mM KCl, and 50 mM tris-HCl buffer, pH 7.6. These suspensions, containing 3–4 mg of ribosomal protein per milliliter, were subjected to sedimentation analysis in a Spinco model E ultracentrifuge. With the use of schlieren optics, photographs of all preparations were obtained at identical intervals after the rotor reached full speed of 29,500 rev/min. $S_{20,w}$ values are shown for the monoribosomal components. (a, c, e, g) Analyses in medium containing 10 mM MgCl₂. (b, d, f, h) Analyses in medium containing 1 mM MgCl₂. (a, b) Cerebral polyribosomes from newborn rats (<1 day old). (c, d) 2-day-old rats. (e, f) Immature rats. (g, h) Adult rats. (Reprinted from Zomzely *et al.*, 1971.)

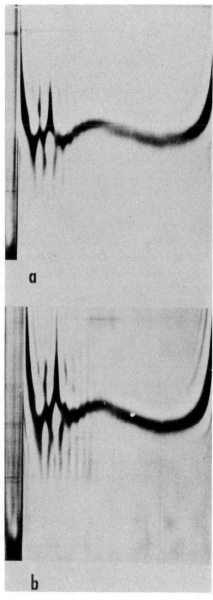

Fig. 13. Influence of development on sedimentation properties of polyribosomes prepared from hindbrain-medullary white matter of the rat. Polyribosomes were suspended in medium composed of 10 mM MgCl₂, 25 mM KCl, and 50 mM tris-HCl buffer, pH 7.6, and analyzed in a Spinco model E ultracentrifuge as described in the legend to Fig. 12. (a) Hindbrain-medullary polyribosomes from immature rats. (b) Hindbrain-medullary polyribosomes from adult rats.

cerebral cortex *in vivo* (see Section VI, B.) Comparable investigations of hepatic polyribosomal systems from the adult rat do not reveal this instability (Zomzely *et al.,* 1966). The decline in stability of certain messenger RNA-ribosome complexes in maturing cerebral tissue is not associated with an increase in RNase activities. Thus, purified cerebral ribosomes do not contain detectable activities of these enzymes (Zomzely *et al.,* 1968, 1971). Moreover,

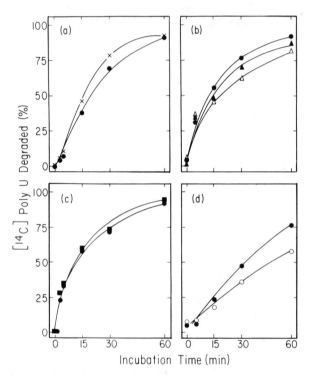

Fig. 14. Ribonuclease activity of postmitochondrial supernatant fractions obtained from cerebral cortical gray matter and hindbrain-medullary white matter of rats at different stages of development. The postmitochondrial supernatants were prepared in 0.25 M sucrose containing 12 mM MgCl$_2$, 100 mM KCl, and 50 mM tris-HCl buffer, pH 7.6. Ribonuclease activity in samples of these suspensions equivalent to 0.65–0.73 mg protein was assayed by a modification (Zomzely *et al.,* 1968) of the method of Barondes and Nirenberg (1962). The assay medium contained 50 nmoles of poly U–^{14}C as polynucleotide phosphorus in a final volume of 1 ml of the medium described above. Incubation was carried out in air at 37°C. Each point represents the average of three closely replicating analyses. Cerebral cortical gray matter: ×, newborn rats; ●, adult rats (42 days old); ▲, 14-day-old rats; ■, 21-day-old rats. Hindbrain-medullary white matter: ○, adult rats; △, 14-day-old rats.

brain homogenates and postmitochondrial supernatant fractions from which polyribosomes are prepared generally contain lower levels of RNase than the corresponding fractions from other tissues. These levels do not appear to vary significantly with brain region or stage of development (Fig. 14). Concentrations of natural RNase inhibitors are unusually high in brain (Roth, 1956), especially in cerebral cortex and may actually increase with age (Suzuki and Takahashi, 1970). Although cerebral polyribosomes may contain occult RNases bound to ribosomal proteins, these enzymes are not active until the ribosomes *per se* have been disrupted, e.g., by urea (Yamagami and Mori, 1970).

C. Stripped Ribosomes

The ribosome preparations described thus far contain varying amounts of messenger and transfer RNA, amino acid synthetases and transferases, and polypeptide chain initiation and termination factors. For this reason, they cannot readily be used for investigations of the basic mechanisms involved in translational events of protein synthesis. Ribosomes essentially devoid of these contaminants ("stripped" ribosomes) can be prepared from cerebral ribosomes by treatment with high salt solutions (Zomzely *et al.*, 1970).

Stripped cerebral ribosomes can be obtained either from preparations of mixed ribosomes or polyribosomes, but not from the microsomal fraction. The ribosomes are suspended in medium composed of 1 mM MgCl$_2$, 0.5 M NH$_4$Cl and 50 mM tris-HCl buffer, pH 7.6, in an amount equivalent to 0.6 gm of tissue per milliliter. This suspension is clarified by centrifugation for 10 min at 5,000 g. The supernatant is removed and recentrifuged if cloudiness appears within 1 hr, then layered on a discontinuous sucrose gradient. This gradient consists of equal parts of a top layer containing the salt-treated ribosomes, a middle layer of 0.5 M sucrose, and a bottom layer of 1.0 M sucrose. All layers contain the same buffer and salts. The gradient is centrifuged at 165,000 g for 6 hr. The resulting pellets are rinsed 3 times in medium composed of 1 mM MgCl$_2$ and 50 mM tris-HCl buffer, pH 7.6. They are stable for 3–4 weeks when stored at $-60\,°C$ or in liquid nitrogen. These preparations of stripped ribosomes consist principally of "80 S" monoribosomes and are free of measurable contamination with RNase. The yield is equivalent to 0.2 mg ribosomal protein per gram of cortex.

V. RIBOSOMAL AMINO ACID-INCORPORATING SYSTEMS

A complete system which is optimal for amino acid incorporation into protein by cerebral ribosomes under standard conditions *in vitro* may be constituted as follows: 0.5–1.0 mg ribosomal protein, 1–4 mg pH 5 enzyme protein, 2 mM NaATP, 0.25 mM NaGTP, 20 mM creatine phosphate (sodium salt), 0.1 mg creatine phosphokinase, radioactive amino acids, 12 mM MgCl$_2$, 100 mM KCl, and 50 mM tris-HCl buffer, pH 7.4–7.6. The final incubation volume is 1 ml (Zomzely *et al.*, 1964, 1968). All additions are made at 0 °C. Variations from these conditions for specific purposes are described below.

A. The pH 5 Enzyme Preparation

The pH 5 enzyme preparation serves as the most practical source of transfer RNAs, activating enzymes, transferases, unlabeled amino acids, etc. required for active incorporation of radioactive amino acids into ribosomal protein *in vitro*. In contrast to the postmicrosomal supernatant fraction (cell sap), from which it is prepared, the pH 5 fraction is stable at −60 °C or in liquid nitrogen for at least a year. Therefore, the same preparation may be used for investigations of induced or natural variations in ribosomal protein synthesis over an extended period. The cell sap *per se* contains inhibitory substances (Munro *et al.*, 1964). When these are removed by passage through Sephadex G-25, amino acids and other essential components of the incubation system are also lost (Mansbridge and Korner, 1963).

The following procedure has been specially adapted for preparation of pH 5 enzymes from brain tissue (Zomzely *et al.*, 1964). The postmicrosomal supernatant fraction prepared in 0.25 M sucrose, 4 mM MgCl$_2$, 25 mM KCl and 50 mM tris-HCl buffer, pH 7.6, is placed in an ice bath in the cold room. If necessary, this fraction is diluted with the same medium to give a 9:1 suspension (v/w). The pH is then adjusted to 4.7 by the slow addition of 1 N acetic acid with constant stirring. The active enzymes from brain are not well precipitated at pH 5.0–5.2. unlike the comparable preparations from liver (Keller and Zamecnik, 1956), or when a more concentrated postmicrosomal fraction is used. The precipitate is allowed to form for 1/2 hr, then is stirred gently, transferred to plastic tubes, and centrifuged at 34,500 g for 15 min. The analogous fraction from liver sediments much more readily. The pellet is rinsed 3 times in cold medium composed of 4 mM MgCl$_2$, 25 mM KCl and 50 mM tris-HCl buffer, pH 7.6, then suspended gently in the same buffer using a glass rod. It is convenient to use a concentration of pH 5 enzymes equivalent to 10 gm of original tissue per 3 ml of buffer. This suspension is centrifuged at 5000 g and 0 °C for 15 min. The supernatant fluid is removed with a capillary pipette and the pH is adjusted to 7.4 with a few drops of 0.2 N KOH. This solution contains 8–12 mg of pH 5 enzyme protein per milliliter. The entire procedure should be carried through without interruption. The pH 5 enzyme preparation should be stored in convenient small volumes to avoid repeated freezing and thawing. However, samples of pH 5 enzymes, frozen at $-60\,°C$ or in liquid nitrogen, can be thawed at least 3 times without any discernible change in activity. The yield of pH 5 enzymes from brain varies with the region and age of the animal, but is generally between 2–4 mg per gram of tissue.

For use in incorporation experiments, the pH 5 enzyme solution should be adjusted to contain the same concentrations of Mg^{2+} and K^+ as the incubation medium. The optimal ratio of pH 5 protein to ribosomal protein is about 2:1 for brain microsomal or ribosomal systems (Zomzely et al., 1964). A higher ratio (4:1) is required for maximal incorporation in brain polyribosomal systems (Zomzely et al., 1968), presumably because essential factors are removed during isolation of the polyribosomes. The ratios of pH 5 enzyme protein to ribosomal protein quoted should not be exceeded because the pH 5 fraction is the major source of RNase activity in these amino acid-incorporating systems (Zomzely et al., 1968, 1971). For this reason, the pH 5 fraction is always added to the incubation medium after the ribosomes, but prior to the addition of exogenous messenger RNA.

B. Ribosomal Factor Protein

Stripped ribosomes require the addition of polypeptide chain initiation and termination factors to exhibit appreciable incorporation of amino acids into protein in vitro (Zomzely et al., 1970). These factors are normally present in other ribosome preparations. A crude preparation of "ribosomal factor protein" may be obtained by the following adaptation (Zomzely et al., 1970) of the method of Ghosh et al. (1967). Cerebral cortical tissue is homogenized in medium containing 0.25 M sucrose, 10 mM magnesium acetate, 60 mM KCl, 1 mM dithiothreitol, and 10 mM tris-HCl buffer, pH 7.6. Ribosomes are obtained by centrifugation at 105,000 g for 2 hr and then resuspended in the same medium to which 1 M NH$_4$Cl has been added. The suspension is allowed to remain for 1 hr prior to removal of the ribosomes by centrifugation at 105,000 g for 2 hr. The supernatant fraction is then adjusted to 70% saturation with (NH$_4$)$_2$SO$_4$. The resulting precipitate is recovered by centrifugation at 5000 g for 15 min, dissolved in medium composed of 1 mM magnesium acetate, 1 mM dithiothreitol, and 10 mM tris-HCl buffer, pH 7.6, and finally dialyzed against this buffer for 12 hr. The dialyzed protein fraction is the source of the ribosomal factors.

C. Amino Acids

Individual amino acids or amino acid mixtures labeled to the highest possible specific activity with [^{14}C] or [^{3}H] are generally employed for studies of amino acid incorporation into protein. These amino acids may be generally labeled or labeled in one or two positions, e.g., L-valine-1-^{14}C, L-leucine-4,5-^{3}H, uniformly labeled L-phenylalanine-^{14}C, etc. Substrate amounts of one or more of the 20 amino acids found in protein may be required for maximum incorporation of radioactive amino acids into protein of certain ribosome systems, including those from brain. However, in the presence of brain pH 5 fractions prepared as described above, addition of substrate amounts of an amino acid mixture results in inhibition of incorporation of labeled amino acids into protein of cerebral microsomal and mixed ribosomal preparations from brain (Samli and Roberts, 1969; Zomzely et al., 1964) and has no effect on this process in the corresponding polyribosome systems. Dialysis of these pH 5 preparations or passage through a column of Sephadex G-25 establishes a requirement for added amino acids. Cerebral ribosome systems may exhibit a requirement for amino acids when pH 5 enzyme fractions are used which have been prepared from brain by different procedures (Campagnoni and Mahler, 1967) or obtained from sources other than brain. Replacement of the pH 5 enzyme fraction with cell sap which has been dialyzed or passed through Sephadex G-25 results in ribosomal amino acid-incorporating systems which are dependent upon added amino acids and possibly other substances.

D. Ribosomes

Utilization of the relatively large amounts of ribosomal protein indicated above (0.5–1.0 mg) permits each incubation tube to be sampled at zero time and at several time intervals during the experiment. This procedure is important since linear kinetics cannot be assumed for the reaction whenever conditions are varied. Triplicate aliquots of each sample should be incubated. When ribosomal material is unavoidedly limited, the amount of ribosomal protein per tube can be reduced to 50–200 μg and the volume of the incubation medium to 0.5 ml or less.

Prior to incubation, the ribosomes are suspended in the medium used for incubation and, if necessary, this suspension is clarified by centrifugation at 5000 g for 10 min. Samples are taken for protein or RNA determination. As noted above, the ribosome suspension is added to the incubation tube before the pH 5 enzyme preparation so that the disruptive action of RNases present in the latter fraction will be minimized.

E. Cerebral Messenger RNA

The isolation of RNA with properties of messenger RNA from cerebral polyribosomes of adult rats (Zomzely et al., 1970) is facilitated by the fact that these preparations are devoid of measurable RNase activity and contain a high proportion of large messenger RNA-ribosome complexes which readily dissociate in media of low Mg^{2+} concentration (Zomzely *et al.*, 1966; 1968).

Polyribosomes equivalent to approximately 12 mg of ribosomal protein are gently suspended with a glass rod in 8 ml of medium composed of 0.3 mM EDTA (sodium salt), 0.001 % polyvinylsulfate, 50 mM KCl and 50 mM tris-HCl buffer, pH 7.6. After 10 min, the suspension is centrifuged for 10 min at 5000 g. The resulting supernatant is layered onto 8 ml of a 0.5 M sucrose solution which was previously layered onto 16 ml of a 2.0 M sucrose solution. Both solutions contain the same buffer and other solutes present in the ribosomal suspension. After centrifugation of the gradient for 16–17 hr at 25,000 rev/min, the top 14 ml are carefully transferred with a capillary pipet to a flask; 3 N NaCl is added with stirring to a final concentration of 0.1 N NaCl. This step is followed by addition of 2.5 volumes of cold absolute ethanol with stirring. The mixture is stored at -20 °C for at least 16–18 hr and then centrifuged for 30 min at 27,000 g using Corex tubes with rubber adaptors. The resulting precipitate is dissolved in 1–2 ml of medium containing 0.001 % polyvinylsulfate and 50 mM tris-HCl buffer, pH 7.6. This solution is treated with NaCl and ethanol, allowed to remain at -20 °C, and centrifuged as described above. The precipitate is subjected to this purification procedure two additional times, then finally redissolved in 50 mM tris-HCl buffer, pH 7.6 and stored at -60 °C or in liquid nitrogen in small volumes at a concentration of 1 mg RNA per milliliter. The yield is 2–3 % of the total polyribosomal RNA.

Special precautions must be taken to avoid RNase contamination during preparation of cerebral "messenger" RNA, including the use of glassware heated to 200 °C for 4 hr. RNase-free sucrose and water, disposable vinyl gloves, etc. The polyvinylsulfate should be colorless and dissolve easily. Properly prepared samples of cerebral messenger RNA have base ratios which are complementary to rat DNA, a high proportion of rapidly labeled molecules which hybridize to homologous DNA, only two peaks on sedimentation analysis with coefficients of approximately 8 S and 16 S, and considerable template activity in amino acid-incorporating systems composed of cerebral stripped ribosomes and crude ribosomal initiating factors (see Section VI, C).

F. Other Additives

Most investigations of ribosome systems derived from animal tissues indicate that addition of an ATP-generating system, as well as ATP *per se*, is necessary for optimal amino acid incorporation. This generally is true for the various types of ribosome-containing systems from brain (Clouet *et al.*, 1966; Lerner and Johnson, 1970; Murthy and Rappoport, 1965; Samli and Roberts, 1969; Takahashi *et al.*, 1966; Zomzely *et al.*, 1964, 1968). However, certain polyribosomal systems may exhibit optimal incorporation in the presence of 5 mM ATP alone (Campagnoni and Mahler, 1967; Dunn, 1970). The ATP-generating systems usually employed include pyruvate kinase plus phosphoenol pyruvate and creatine phosphokinase plus creatine phosphate.

Appropriate concentrations of cations are particularly critical for optimal incorporation of amino acids into protein of brain ribosomal systems. However, magnesium acetate can be substituted for $MgCl_2$ (Campagnoni and Mahler, 1967; Dunn, 1970). Concentrations of Mg^{+2} as low as 8 mM may be as effective as 12 mM (Zomzely *et al.*, 1964). Outside of this range, incorporating activity rapidly decreases. Ammonium chloride may replace KCl as the monovalent cation in cerebral polyribosomal systems (Clouet *et al.*, 1966; Campagnoni and Mahler, 1967; Mahler and Brown, 1968). Sodium chloride is less effective. Relatively high concentrations of the monovalent cation (80–120 mM) are necessary for optimal activity (Roberts and Zomzely, 1966; Zomzely *et al.*, 1964).

The optimum pH for amino acid incorporation by brain ribosomal systems is fairly broad (7.2–7.8). The presence or absence of 0.25 M sucrose seems to be without effect on incorporation.

G. Measurement of Incorporation

Incubation is carried out in small tubes in air at 37°C. The tubes are agitated at intervals. Incorporation is terminated by transferring samples containing 0.1–0.2 mg ribosomal protein to tubes in an ice bath and immediately adding cold trichloroacetic acid containing carrier. The final concentration of the precipitant should be 5% and that of the carrier 0.5 or 1.0%. The lower concentration of carrier is employed for all radioactive amino acids except phenylalanine, which binds with exceptional strength to proteins present in the incubation medium. The samples are allowed to remain in the ice bath for $\frac{1}{2}$ hr, heated at 90°C for 30 min to remove radioactive aminoacyl-tRNAs, and then cooled again in the ice bath. The trichloroacetic acid precipitates are collected on Millipore filters (type AA; pore size 0.8 μ; diameter, 25 mm) and washed on the filters 3 times with 5% trichloroacetic acid containing carrier. This step is followed by successive washes with 5% trichloroacetic acid, ethanol–chloroform (1:1), and chloroform. The Millipore filters are then dried at room temperature, placed in scintillation vials with 5 ml of scintillation solution, and counted in a liquid scintillation counter (Zomzely *et al.*, 1968).

VI. AMINO ACID-INCORPORATING PROPERTIES OF CEREBRAL RIBOSOMAL SYSTEMS

The kinetics of incorporation of amino acids into protein of brain ribosomal preparations vary markedly with the nature of the preparation and the source. However, the overall activity under optimal conditions is comparable to that of the corresponding fraction from other active mammalian tissues, including liver (Zomzely *et al.*, 1964, 1968).

A. Microsomal and Mixed Ribosomal Systems

Amino acid incorporation by microsomal systems obtained from cerebral cortex of the adult rat typically plateaus after about 30 min of

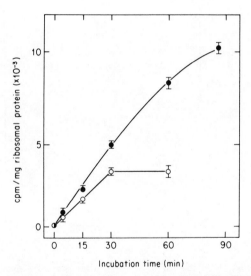

Fig. 15. Kinetics of incorporation of uniformly labeled L-leucine-¹⁴C into protein by microsomal and ribosomal fractions prepared from cerebral cortex of adult male rats. The incubation system contained 1 mg of microsomal or ribosomal protein, 2 mg of pH 5 enzyme protein, 1 μCi (0.16 μmoles) of L-leucine-¹⁴C, 2 mM NaATP, 0.25 mM NaGTP, 20 mM creatine phosphate (sodium salt), 0.1 mg creatine phosphokinase, 12 mM $MgCl_2$, 100 mM KCl, 0.25 mM sucrose, and 50 mM tris-HCl buffer, pH 7.4, in a final volume of 1 ml. Incubation was carried out in air at 37°C. Each value represents the mean $\pm$ S. E. of three analyses. ○ microsomes; ●, ribosomes.

incubation [(Fig. 15) Zomzely *et al.*, 1964]. In contrast, preparations of mixed ribosomes from the same source continue to incorporate amino acids actively for at least twice this period. Since a large fraction of the microsomal protein is membrane protein rather than ribosomal protein, the initial rate of incorporation may actually be greater for the microsomal fraction, if the activity is expressed in terms of RNA rather than protein. The decline in incorporation of amino acids into proteins of microsomal systems after 30 min is probably due to the formation of inhibitory substances (e.g., fatty acids) during incubation (Acs *et al.*, 1962).

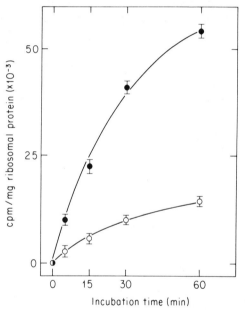

Fig. 16. Kinetics of incorporation of L-phenylalanine-^{14}C into protein by ribosomes and polyribosomes prepared in the presence of 1% sodium deoxycholate from cerebral cortices of adult male rats. The incubation system contained 0.5 mg of ribosomal protein, 2 mg of pH 5 enzyme protein for ribosomes or 4 mg for polyribosomes, 1 μCi of uniformly labeled L-phenylalanine-^{14}C (350 μCi/μmole), 2 mM NaATP, 0.25 mM NaGTP, 20 mM creatine phosphate (sodium salt), 0.1 mg creatine phosphokinase, 12 mM MgCl$_2$, 100 mM KCl, and 50 mM tris-HCl buffer, pH 7.6. The final volume was 1 ml. Incubation was carried out in air at 37°C. Each value represents the mean ± S. E. for three analyses. ○, ribosomes; ●, polyribosomes.

B. Polyribosomal Systems

Amino acid-incorporating activity of cerebral polyribosomal systems is many times greater than that of the corresponding mixed ribosome fractions [(Fig. 16) Zomzely *et al.*, 1968]. The kinetics of incorporation do not appear to be significantly altered by the use of fresh or frozen polyribosomes or by the presence or absence of detergent in the preparation medium (Fig. 17). Of course, functional differences may exist between populations of polyribosomes isolated from the same brain source in the presence or absence of detergent or fractionated on discontinuous sucrose gradients, into "free" and "membrane-bound" components (Andrews and Tata, 1971; Sellinger *et al.*, 1968; Sellinger and Ohlsson, 1969).

Free polyribosomes isolated from different brain regions of the rat or at different stages of development exhibit only minor differences in rates of incorporation of amino acids into protein *in vitro* (Roberts *et al.*, 1971; Zomzely *et al.*, 1971). Thus, the rate of incorporation of L-phenylalanine-^{14}C is similar for cerebral free polyribosomes from newborn, immature, or adult rats, when incubation is carried out in the presence of pH 5 enzymes derived from cerebral cortex of adult animals [Fig. 18(a) and (b)]. Compar-

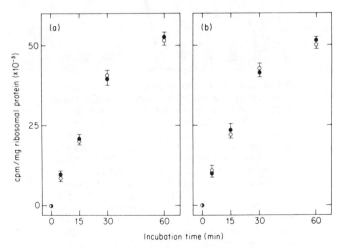

Fig. 17. Influence of freezing and storage on kinetics of incorporation of L-phenylalanine-^{14}C by polyribosomes isolated in the presence or absence of detergent from cerebral cortices of adult male rats. The conditions of incubation were similar to those described in the legend to Fig. 16, except that the amounts of ribosomal and pH 5 enzyme protein were 0.5 mg and 2 mg, respectively. (a) Detergent-treated preparations. (b) Untreated preparations. ○, freshly prepared polyribosomes; ●, polyribosomes stored at −60°C for 6 months.

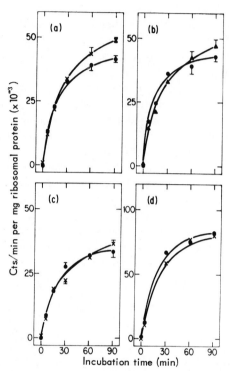

Fig. 18. Kinetics of incorporation of L-^{14}C amino acids into protein by polyribosomes isolated from cerebral cortices of rats at different stages of development. The conditions of incubation were similar to those described in the legend to Fig. 16, with the exceptions noted below. Each sample contained 1.0 mg of ribosomal protein and 4.0 mg of pH 5 enzyme protein. (a) and (b) cerebral polyribosomes from animals of different ages incubated with L-phenylalanine-[14]C (1 μCi, 2.8 nmoles) and cerebral pH 5 enzymes from adult rats. (c) Cerebral polyribosomes from adult and newborn rats incubated with L-phenylalanine-^{14}C and cerebral pH 5 enzymes from newborn rats. (d) Cerebral polyribosomes from adult and newborn rats incubated with an L-amino acid-^{14}C mixture (0.25 μCi, 0.17 μg) and cerebral pH 5 enzymes from adult rats. ●, polyribosomes from adult rats; ×, newborn rats; ▲, immature rats. (Reprinted from Zomzely *et al.*, 1971.)

able results are obtained when the pH 5 enzyme fraction from newborn cerebrum is substituted for the preparation from adult cortex [see, for example, Fig. 18(c)], or when a mixture of uniformly labeled L-[14C] amino acids is substituted for L-phenylalanine-14C [Fig. 18(d)]. Incidentally, comparisons of amino acid-incorporating activity of ribosomal preparations in the presence of different pH 5 preparations or different radioactive amino acids are invalid, because of the impure state of the former and lack of knowledge of variations in endogenous amino acid pools. Amino acid-incorporating activities of polyribosomal fractions prepared from hindbrain-medullary white matter of 14-day-old and adult rats are quite similar to those of the corresponding fractions from cerebral cortical gray matter (Roberts *et al.,* 1971) (Figs. 19 and 20).

Density gradient analysis of cerebral ribosomal preparations from adult animals which have incorporated amino acids either *in vitro* or *in vivo* reveal some interesting differences from other mammalian protein-synthesizing systems. As in these other preparations, incorporation occurs most actively at first into the larger polyribosomes of cerebral systems. However, with time a larger proportion of radioactivity is found associated with smaller

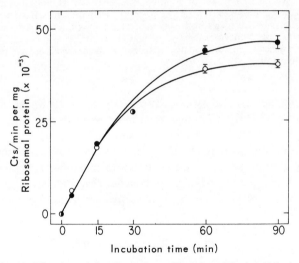

Fig. 19. Kinetics of incorporation of L-phenylalanine-14C into protein by polyribosomes isolated from cerebral cortical gray matter and hindbrain-medullary white matter of immature rats. The pH 5 preparation was derived from cerebral cortices of adult rats. See legend to Fig. 16 for additional explanations. ●, polyribosomes from cerebral gray matter; ○, polyribosomes from hindbrain-medullary white matter. (Reprinted in modified version from Roberts *et al.,* 1971.)

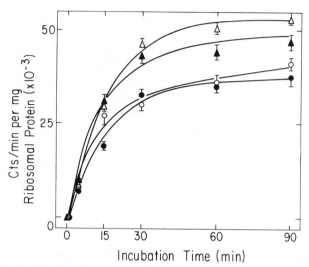

Fig. 20. Kinetics of incorporation of L-phenylalanine-¹⁴C into protein by polyribosomes isolated from cerebral ocrtical gray matter and hindbrain-medullary white matter of adult rats. The pH 5 enzyme preparation was derived from either gray or white matter of adult rats. See legend to Fig. 16 for additional explanations. ●, polyribosomes and pH 5 enzymes from gray matter; ○, polyribosomes from white matter, pH 5 enzymes from gray matter; ▲, polyribosomes from gray matter, pH 5 enzymes from white matter; △, polyribosomes and pH 5 enzymes from white matter. (Reprinted in modified version from Roberts *et al.,* 1971.)

ribosomes in the cerebral systems (Zomzely *et al.,* 1968; see for example Figs. 21 and 22). This finding has been interpreted to mean that (a) certain of the large unstable cerebral polyribosomes in the adult brain undergo dissociation during protein synthesis, and (b) both large and small polyribosomes in this preparation are quite active in amino acid incorporation (Zomzely *et al.,* 1968, 1971). Polyribosome fractions from newborn rat cerebrum do not reveal these unusual properties [(Fig. 23) Zomzely *et al.,* 1971].

C. Purified Ribosomal Systems

Cerebral stripped ribosomes are inactive in amino acid incorporation in an otherwise complete system which includes the pH 5 fraction from cerebral cortical tissue (Zomzely *et al.,* 1970); [Fig. 24(a)]. When saturating amounts of the synthetic messenger poly U are added, polyphenylalanine synthesis proceeds at a rapid and linear rate for at least 90 min. Addition of a cerebral messenger RNA fraction also elicits the incorporation of amino

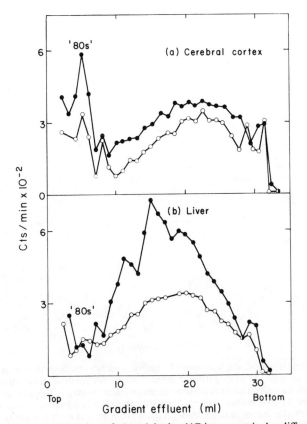

Fig. 21. Incorporation of phenylalanine-^{14}C into protein by different ribosomal species of cerebral and hepatic polyribosomal preparations. The incorporation systems were similar to those outlined in the legend to Fig. 16. After incubation, an aliquot of the medium containing 1.0 mg of ribosomal RNA was diluted to 2 ml and layered on a linear sucrose density gradient (25 to 5%) containing the same buffer and salts as the incubation medium. The gradients were centrifuged in a Spinco SW 25 rotor at 25,000 rev/min and 0°C. The effluent from the top of the gradient was collected as 1-ml fractions for determination of radioactivity. Radioactivity profiles are shown for (a), cerebral polyribosomes, centrifuged for 2½ hr; and (b) hepatic polyribosomes from rats fasted for 18 hr, centrifuged for 2 hr. ○, incubated for 15 min; ●, incubated for 30 min. (Reprinted from Zomzely *et al.*, 1968.)

acids into protein of stripped ribosomes (Zomzely *et al.*, 1970); [Fig. 24(b)]. However, a preparation of chain initiation and termination factors (ribosomal factor protein) must be added to produce appreciable incorporation.

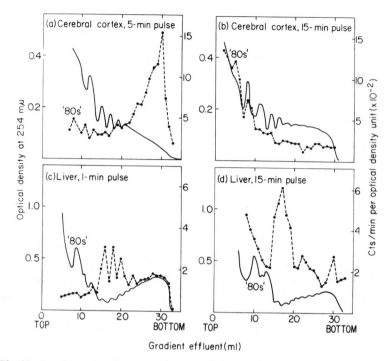

Fig. 22. Protein-synthesizing activities of cerebral and hepatic polyribosomes *in vivo:* relationship to state of aggregation. Cerebral postmitochondrial supernatants were prepared from rats given an intracisternal injection of uniformly labeled L-leucine-^{14}C (10 μCi) 5 or 15 min before autopsy. Hepatic postmitochondrial supernatants were prepared with the use of sodium deoxycholate from rats given an injection via the portal vein of 20 μCi of leucine-^{14}C 1 or 15 min earlier. Postmitochondrial supernatants were layered on linear sucrose density gradients (35 to 15%). The gradients were centrifuged for 4 hr in a Spinco SW 25 rotor at 25,000 rev/min and 0°C. The effluents from the top of the gradient were monitored continuously for absorbance at 254 nm and collected as 1-ml samples for determination of radioactivity. (a) Cerebral cortex, 5 min after injection. (b) Cerebral cortex, 15 min. (c) Liver, 1 min. (d) Liver, 15 min. ——, optical density; ●----●, cpm per optical density unit ($\times 10^{-2}$). (Reprinted from Zomzely *et al.*, 1968.)

Ribosomal factor protein and other RNA fractions from brain (ribosomal RNA, transfer RNA) are completely inactive in this system without added messenger RNA.

Active ribosomal subunits may also be prepared from cerebral tissue which interact with the cerebral messenger RNA fraction, resulting in polyribosomes capable of active incorporation of amino acids (Zomzely-Neurath *et al.*, 1971).

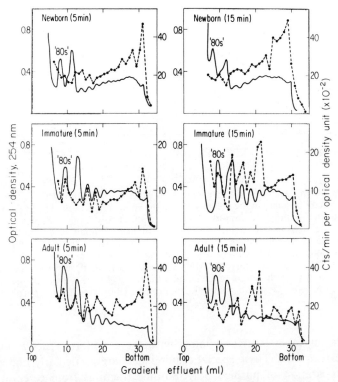

Fig. 23. Protein-synthesizing activities of cerebral cortical polyribosomes *in vivo:* relationship to brain development and ribosomal aggregation. Postmitochondrial supernatant fluids were obtained from cerebral cortices of rats given an intracisternal injection of L-4,5 leucine-³H 5 or 15 min before autopsy. Adult rats received 50 μCi of radioactive amino acid; immature rats and newborn rats received 25 μCi. The postmitochondrial supernatant fluids were prepared without detergent and centrifuged in sucrose density gradients as described in the legend for Fig. 22. ———, optical density; ●----●, cpm per optical density unit ($\times 10^{-2}$). (Reprinted from Zomzely *et al.,* 1971.)

VII. CONCLUSIONS

Isolation of ribosome-enriched fractions from mammalian brain may be accomplished by methods which are basically similar to the procedures developed for liver and other parenchymatous tissues. However, certain technical modifications are necessary to produce preparations which exhibit

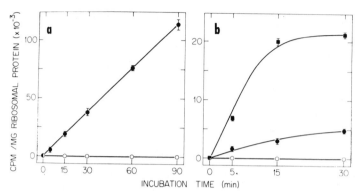

Fig. 24. (a) Kinetics of incorporation of L-phenylalanine-^{14}C by cerebral stripped ribosomes in the presence and in the absence of poly U. The Mg^{2+} content of the incubation medium was 12 mM. $\bigcirc$, without poly U; $\bullet$, with poly U (600 μg per mg ribosomal protein). (b) Kinetics of incorporation of amino acids into protein of cerebral-stripped ribosomes in the presence and in the absence of polyribosomal mRNA preparation. The incubation mixture contained a mixture of 15 [14C] L-amino acids; the Mg^{2+} content was mM. $\bigcirc$, without the mRNA fraction; $\bullet$, with 150 μg of the mRNA fraction; $\blacksquare$, with 150 μg of the mRNA fraction +60 μg of ribosomal factor protein. (Reprinted from Zomzely *et al.*, 1970.)

a high degree of structural integrity and are uniformly active in protein synthesis *in vitro*. These special requirements are particularly important for the preparation of purified polyribosome fractions from cerebral cortical tissue of mature animals. The major precautions include (a) gentle homogenization and fractionation techniques designed to minimize mechanical damage to subcellular organelles and the consequent release of degradative enzymes and protective proteins, (b) utilization of preparation media containing relatively high concentrations of Mg^{2+}, necessary to maintain polyribosome structure in cerebral fractions, and (c) employment of very low concentrations of detergent where membrane removal is desired. The precautions outlined are largely necessitated by the occurrence of a high proportion of unstable, large messenger RNA-ribosome complexes and ribosomes unattached to cellular membranes in maturing neurons of the central nervous system. These characteristics appear during neuronal development and are not seen to the same extent in predominantly glial structures.

The relationship of the unique properties of cytoplasmic ribosomes to protein synthesis in the mature cerebral cortex has been the subject of considerable study. Proteins formed on the unstable cerebral polyribosomes appear to have a very short life. In addition, the synthesis of these proteins is highly responsive to factors which modify the integrity of the unstable polyribosome complexes, including concentrations of ions, cofactors, and substrates in the internal environment as well as perturbations in the external environment (specific stimuli, convulsions, etc.). It is possible that proteins formed on unstable cerebral polyribosomes serve important roles in the specialized functions of neuronal structures. A logical direction for future research involves delineation of the nature of these proteins, the factors involved in regulation of their synthesis, and their specific localization and function in the neuron. One approach to this fundamental problem is the investigation of purified protein-synthesizing systems and natural messenger RNA fractions of neuronal origin which are capable of interacting *in vitro* to produce the specified proteins. Recent developments in methodology, including the successful isolation of stripped ribosomes, active ribosomal subunits, and RNA fractions with the properties of messenger RNA from cerebral tissue, now make this goal seem attainable.

ACKNOWLEDGMENTS

Supported by Grant NS–07869 from the National Institutes of Health. the authors are indebted to Mrs. Carole Feingold for capable bibliographic and secretarial assistance.

REFERENCES

Acs, G., Neidle A., and Schneiderman, N. (1962) *Biochim. Biophys. Acta* **56**, 373.
Acs, G., Neidle, A., and Waelsch, H. (1961) *Biochim. Biophys. Acta* **50**, 403.
Albertsson, P. Å., Hanzon, V., and Toschi, G. (1959) *J. Ultrastruct. Res.* **2**, 366.
Allfrey, V. (1959) in *The Cell*, Vol. 1 (J. Brachet and A. E. Mirsky, eds.) Academic Press, New York, p. 193.
Andrews, T. M., and Tata, J. R. (1971) *Biochem. J.* **121**, 683.
Barondes, S. H., and Nirenberg, M. W. (1962) *Science* **138**, 810.
Barr, M., and Guth, E. P. (1951) *J. Amer. Pharm. Assn.* **40**, 9.
Bishop, J. O. (1966) *Biochim. Biophys. Acta* **119**, 130.
Blobel, G., and Potter, V. R. (1966) *Proc. Nat. Acad. Sci. U.S.* **55**, 1283.
Blobel, G., and Potter, V. R. (1967) *J. Mol. Biol.* **28**, 539.
Bondy, S. C., and Perry, S. V. (1963) *J. Neurochem.* **10**, 603.
Bont, W. S., Rezelman, G., and Bloemendal, H. (1965) *Biochem. J.* **95**, 15c.
Campagnoni, A. T., and Mahler, H. R. (1967) *Biochemistry* **6**, 956.
Chao, F.-C. (1957) *Arch. Biochem. Biophys.* **70**, 426.
Clouet, D. H., Ratner, M., and Williams, N. (1966) *Biochim. Biophys. Acta* **123**, 142.
Datta, R. K., Bhattacharyya, D., and Ghosh, J. J. (1944) *J. Neurochem.* **11**, 87.
Datta, R. K., and Ghosh, J. J. (1963a) *J. Neurochem.* **10**, 363.
Datta, R. K., and Ghosh, J. J. (1963b) *J. Neurochem.* **10**, 285.
Dunn, A. J. (1970) *Biochem. J.* **116**, 135.
De Duve, C., Pressman, B. C., Gianetto, R., Wattiaux, R., and Appelmans, F. (1955) *Biochem. J.* **60**, 604.

Ekholm, R., and Hydén, H. (1965) *J. Ultrastruct. Res.* **13**, 269.
Fellig, J., and Wiley, C. E. (1959) *Arch. Biochem. Biophys.* **85**. 313.
Fraenkel-Conrat, H., Singer, B., and Tsugita, A. (1961) *Virology* **14**, 54.
Ghosh, H. P., Söll, D., and Khorana, H. G. (1967) *J. Mol. Biol.* **25**, 275.
Gierer, A. (1963) *J. Mol. Biol.* **6**, 148.
Girard, M., Latham, H., Penman, S., Darnell, J. E. (1965) *J. Mol. Biol.* **11**, 187.
Gribnau, A. A. M., Schoenmakers, J. G. G., van Kraaikamp, M., and Bloemendal, H. (1970) *Biochem. Biophys. Res. Commun.* **38**, 1064.
Hanzon, V., and Toschi, G. (1960) *Exptl Cell Res.* **21**, 332.
Hogan, B. L. M., and Korner, A. (1968) *Biochim. Biophys. Acta* **169**, 139.
Hogeboom, G. H., Schneider, W. C., and Palade, G. E. (1948) *J. Biol. Chem.* **172**, 619.
Joklik, W. K., and Becker, Y. (1965a) *J. Mol. Biol.* **13**, 496.
Joklik, W. K., and Becker, Y. (1965b) *J. Mol. Biol.* **13**, 511.
Keller, E. B., and Zamecnik, P. C. (1956) *J. Biol. Chem.* **221**, 45.
Keller, P. J., Cohen, E., and Wade, R. D. (1963) *Biochemistry* **2**, 315.
Lerner, M. P., and Johnson, T. C. (1970) *J. Biol. Chem.* **245**, 1388.
Mahler, H. R., and Brown, B. J. (1968) *Arch. Biochem. Biophys.* **125**, 387.
Mansbridge, J. N., and Korner, A. (1963) *Biochem. J.* **89**, 15P.
Merits, I., Cain, J. C., Rdzok, E. J., and Minard, F. N. (1969) *Experientia* **25**, 739.
Mugnaini, E., and Walberg, F. (1964) *Ergeb. Anat. Entwicklung.* **37**, 194.
Munro, A. J., Jackson, R. J., and Korner, A. (1964) *Biochem. J.* **92**, 289.
Murthy, M. R. V., and Rappoport, D. A. (1965) *Biochim. Biophys. Acta* **95**, 132.
Palade, G. E. (1955) *J. Biophys. Biochem. Cytol.* **1**, 59.
Palade, G. E., and Siekevitz, P. (1956) *J. Biophys. Biochem. Cytol.* **2**, 171.
Petermann, M. L. (1964) *The Physical and Chemical Properties of Ribosomes*, American Elsevier Publishing Co., New York.
Petermann, M. L., and Hamilton, M. G. (1957) *J. Biol. Chem.* **224**, 725.
Ragland, W. L., Shires, T. K., and Pitot, H. C. (1971) *Biochem. J.* **121**, 271.
Rendi, R., and Hultin, T. (1960) *Exptl. Cell Res.* **19**, 253.
Roberts, S. (1971) in *Handbook of Neurochemistry,* Vol. V, Part A (A. Lajtha, ed.), Plenum Press, New York, P. 1.
Roberts, S., and Zomzely, C. E. (1966) in *Protides of the Biological Fluids,* Vol. 13 (H. Peeters, ed.), Elsevier Publishing Co., Amsterdam, p, 91.
Roberts, S., Zomzely, C. E., and Bondy, S. C. (1971) in *Cellular Aspects of Neural Growth and Differentiation,* UCLA Forum in Medical Sciences, No. 14, Ch. 20 (D. C. Pease, ed.), University of California Press, Los Angeles, p. 447.
Rosbash, M., and Penman, S. (1971) *J. Mol. Biol.* **59**, 227.
Roth, J. S. (1956) *Biochim. Biophys. Acta* **21**, 34.
Samli, M. H., and Roberts, S. (1969) *J. Neurochem.* **16**, 1565.
Satake, M., Mase, K., Takahashi, Y., and Ogata, K. (1960) *Biochim. Biophys. Acta* **41**, 366.
Schneider, D. and Roberts, S. (1968) *J. Neurochem.* **15**, 1469.
Sellinger, O. Z., and Ohlsson, W. G. (1969) *Life Sci.* **8** (Part II), 1083.
Sellinger, O. Z., Azcurra, J. M., and Ohlsson, W. G. (1968) *J. Pharmacol. Exptl. Therap.* **164**, 212.
Siekevitz, P., and Palade, G. E. (1960) *J. Biophys. Biochem. Cytol.* **7**, 619.
Solymosy, F., Fedorcsák, I., Gulyás, A., Farkas, G. L., and Ehrenberg, L. (1968) *Eur. J. Biochem.* **5**, 520.
Sotelo, C., and Palay, S. L. (1968) *J. Cell Biol.* **36**, 151.
Staehelin, T., Verney, E., and Sidransky, H. (1967) *Biochim. Biophys. Acta* **145**, 105.
Suzuki, Y., and Takahashi, Y. (1970) *J. Neurochem.* **17**, 1521.
Takahashi, Y., Mase, K., and Sugano, H. (1966) *Biochim. Biophys. Acta* **119**, 627.
Takahashi, Y., Mase, K., and Suzuki, Y. (1970) *J. Neurochem.* **17**, 1433.
Tashiro, Y., and Siekevitz, P. (1965) *J. Mol. Biol.* **11**, 149.
Tissières, A., Watson, J. D., Schlessinger, D., and Hollingworth, B. R. (1959) *J. Mol. Biol.* **1**, 221.

von der Decken, A. (1967) in *Techniques in Protein Biosynthesis,* Vol. 1 (P. N. Campbell and J. R. Sargent, eds.), Academic Press, New York, p. 65.

Warner, J. R., Rich, A., and Hall, C. E. (1962) *Science,* **138,** 1399.

Wettstein, F. O., Staehelin, T., and Noll, H. (1963) *Nature (Lond.)* **197,** 430.

Wilson, S. H., and Hoagland, M. B. (1965) *Proc. Nat. Acad. Sci. U.S.* **54,** 600.

Yamagami, S., Masui, M., and Kawakita, Y. (1963) *J. Neurochem.* **10,** 849.

Yamagami, S., and Mori, K. (1970) *J. Neurochem.* **17,** 721.

Zomzely-Neurath, C. E., Moon, H. M., and York, C. (1971) Abstracts. Third International Meeting of the International Society for Neurochemistry, Budapest, p. 38.

Zomzely, C. E., Roberts, S., Brown, D. M., and Provost, C. (1966) *J. Mol. Biol.* **20,** 455.

Zomzely, C. E., Roberts, S., Gruber, C. P., and Brown, D. M. (1968) *J. Biol. Chem.* **243,** 5396.

Zomzely, C. E., Roberts, S., and Peache, S. (1970) *Proc. Nat. Acad. Sci. U.S.* **67,** 644.

Zomzely, C. E., Roberts, S., Peache, S., and Brown, D. M. (1971) *J. Biol. Chem.* **246,** 2097.

Zomzely, C. E., Roberts, S., and Rapaport, D. (1964) *J. Neurochem.* **11,** 567.

Chapter 6

Isolation of Brain Cell Nuclei

Bruce S. McEwen and Richard E. Zigmond

The Rockefeller University
New York, New York

I. INTRODUCTION

In choosing a method for subcellular fractionation, the investigator must first consider the particular question which he wishes to answer. In studies of the subcellular distribution of a substance of almost certain cytoplasmic localization, it is often sufficient to monitor (for purposes of estimating recoveries) the concentration of that substance in a crude "nuclear pellet" obtained by low-speed centrifugation of a sucrose homogenate. From most tissues, however, such a pellet is so heavily contaminated with cytoplasmic debris that it is totally unsatisfactory for situations in which any degree of nuclear localization is a serious possibility. For studies in which determination of nuclear localization of a substance is important, considerable effort must be given to the removal of cytoplasmic particles adhering to nuclei and to purifying the nuclei from such contamination.

This chapter will describe a procedure which has been extensively used in our laboratory for the isolation of cell nuclei from the rat brain. It is basically the same procedure as that described by Løvtrup-Rein and McEwen (1966). The method is particularly useful for the investigation of tightly-bound constituents of cell nuclei, such as macromolecules which bind certain steroid hormones (McEwen *et al.,* 1970; Zigmond and McEwen, 1970). The applicability of this and other nuclear isolation procedures to other types of studies will also be considered in an attempt to show the reader the importance of selecting an isolation procedure to suit his particular experimental requirement.

II. EQUIPMENT

A. Homogenizer

We use a glass homogenizer with a Teflon pestle (A. H. Thomas, Philadelphia, Type A) driven at 1000 rev/min by a variable speed motor. It is essential that the clearance between the pestle and homogenizer tube be adjusted to 0.125 mm on the radius. Since the homogenizer tubes are constant in internal diameter and therefore interchangeable, it is possible, if necessary, to adjust the diameter of the pestle on a lathe.

B. Centrifuges

A high-speed, refrigerated centrifuge, capable of g forces from 850 up to at least 15,000, is necessary for this procedure. The entire isolation can be carried out in such a centrifuge, providing the proper rotors are available (see below). Alternatively, a low-speed (850 g) centrifuge will suffice for the initial isolation steps, providing an ultracentrifuge is also availabel for the final centrifugation step.

C. Centrifuge Rotors

We prefer to use a swing-out rotor for the entire isolation. We have a Lourdes Betafuge (Lourdes Instrument Co., Old Bethpage, N.Y.) equipped with an SBR4 rotor, which holds four 30-ml tubes or eight 3-ml tubes with adaptors. It is possible to use an angle head for the low-speed spins (see below), but a swing-out rotor is essential for the last high-speed spin. When this last spin is performed in a Spinco ultracentrifuge either an SW 25.1 or an SW 50 rotor may be used.

III. SOLUTIONS

Nuclear isolation I (NI): 0.32 M sucrose; 1 mM KH$_2$PO$_4$, pH 6.5; 3 mM MgCl$_2$; 0.25%; Triton X-100 (v/v).

Nuclear isolation solution II (NII): 0.32 M sucrose; 1 mM KH$_2$PO$_4$, pH 6.5; 3 mM MgCl$_2$.

Nuclear isolation solution IIa (NIIa): 0.32 M sucrose; 1 mM KH$_2$PO$_4$ phate, pH 6.5; 1 mM MgCl$_2$.

Nuclear isolation solution III (NIII): 2.39 M sucrose; 1 mM KH$_2$PO$_4$ phate, pH 6.5; 3 mM MgCl$_2$.

Nuclear isolation solution IIIa (NIIIa): 2.39 M sucrose; 1 mM KH$_2$PO$_4$ phate, pH 6.5; 1 mM MgCl$_2$.

Fractionation medium (F): 0.25 M sucrose; 3 mM MgCl$_2$.

Perfusion fluid: Dextran 6% w/v in 0.9% saline (Abbott Laboratories, North Chicago, Ill.).

IV. NUCLEAR ISOLATION PROCEDURES

Sprague-Dawley rats (Charles River Breeding Labs, Wilmington, Mass.), 250–400 g body weight, have been used in our experiments. The animals are killed either by decapitation or by heart perfusion with chilled perfusion fluid. Heart perfusion is accomplished by anesthetizing the animals rapidly with a large dose of sodium pentobarbital (0.4 ml, 60 mg/ml) plus 0.1 ml of heparin (USP, 1000 U/ml) to reduce blood clotting. The chest cavity is opened and the cannula connected to the perfusion bottle is inserted into the left ventricle. The right atrium is cut to allow the blood to flow out, and the perfusion fluid is allowed to flow into the aorta via the heart. We observe very closely the appearance of the ears, eyes, and front paws, and when they become white the perfusion can be terminated. Usually this takes no more than 60 sec, during which time no more than 30 ml of perfusion fluid need have entered the animal. The brain is rapidly removed from the skull, taking care not to damage it, and placed on ice. Without perfusion the brain is pink with noticeable blood vessels and blood clots on the surface; when adequately perfused, it is whitish yellow with no evidence of blood on its surface or in the sella turcica.

A. Whole Brain

The tissue is chilled on ice, minced with scissors, and transferred to the homogenizer tube in portions of 0.5 g. Five milliliters of NI are added and the tissue is homogenized with 20 slow up-and-down strokes and transferred to a chilled tube. (In order to get consistent results, it is important to standardize the motor speed and number of strokes.) The procedure is repeated until all of the tissue is homogenized, and the homogenates are pooled. The pooled homogenate is filtered through two layers of cheesecloth into a 30-ml centrifuge tube and centrifuged for 10 min at 850 g. The supernatant, which includes a fluffy white material, above material rich in lipid and myelin, is decanted and discarded, leaving a tightly packed pellet. The pellet is resuspended in 20 ml of NII, using a stirring rod and a vortex mixer and centrifuged again at 850 g for 10 min. The supernatant is carefully decanted and discarded. The pellet is resuspended as above in 20 ml of NII and centrifuged again at 650 g for 10 min. The supernatant is discarded. The pellet is resuspended in 4 ml of NII, using a stirring rod and a vortex mixer; 25 ml of NIII is added and mixed thoroughly with the nuclear suspension. This mixture is centrifuged for 45 min at 63,600 g (average) in the SW 25.1 rotor of the Spinco ultracentrifuge. Alternatively, we have obtained equally satisfactory sedimentations of nuclei by spinning the mixture at 12,500 g (average) for 90 min in our Lourdes Betafuge. The nuclei sediment to the bottom of the tube as a small, whitish pellet, while cytoplasmic debris and heavily contaminated nuclei float to the surface of the tube as a pellicle. This pellicle is carefully removed and the supernatant is decanted and discarded. It is desirable to swab the interior walls of the tube with cotton or tissue paper to remove bits of the pellicle before attempting to resuspend or transfer the nuclear pellet.

B. Brain Regions

The chilled brain is placed on a chilled glass plate and the desired brain regions are dissected with the aid of a suitable atlas of the rat brain (König and Klippel, 1963); see also (McEwen et al., 1969; McEwen and Pfaff, 1969). The individual brain regions are weighed on a milligram balance and then homogenized in NI, using 20 slow up-and-down strokes. We use between 1 and 2 ml of NI for each 100 mg of wet tissue, but always use a minimum volume of 2 ml for some structures, such as the septum and pituitary, which weigh 10 mg or less. It not necessary to filter the homogenates through cheesecloth; in fact, the loss of volume and tissue precludes our doing so. The homogenates are centrifuged for 10 min at 850 g (average.) The supernatants are carefully decanted and discarded. As was described in IV, A, a white material rich in lipid and myelin should be poured off with this first supernatant, leaving a well-packed pellet. The pellet is resuspended in 2ml of NII and centrifuged again at 850 g (average) for 10 min. The supernatant is carefully decanted and discarded. If the 3-ml capacity tubes are to be used for the high-speed spin, the pellet is resuspended in 0.4 ml of NII, using a vortex mixer; 2.1 ml of NIII are added and mixed thoroughly with the nuclear suspension. This mixture is centrifuged at 12,500 g (average) for 90 min. If the 5-ml tubes of the Spinco SW 50 rotor are to be used, the pellet is resuspended in 0.8 ml of NII and 4.2 ml of NIII are added. The SW 50 rotor is spun at 51,000 g (average) for 45 min. The pellicle is carefully removed, the supernatant is decanted, and the interior walls of the tube are wiped before the nuclear pellet is disturbed.

C. Nuclear Isolation in Combination with Cell Fractionation

In studying the subcellular localization of a substance it is often essential to determine its distribution among cytoplasmic as well as nuclear fractions. To meet this objective we shall briefly describe how we have coupled the standard nuclear isolation with an initial fractionation of the tissue for the isolation of cytoplasmic organelles (McEwen et al., 1970; Zigmond and McEwen, 1970). This tissue is initially homogenized in medium F, because the presence of Triton would disrupt many cytoplasmic organelles and render their isolation impossible. We use between 1 and 2 ml of F for each 100 mg of tissue and homogenize with 20 up-and-down strokes. The homogenate is centrifuged at 850 g (average) for 10 min. This removes cell nuclei and unbroken cells, and the pellet is subjected to procedure IV, A or B described above for direct nuclear isolation from tissue. (The choice of procedure depends, of course, on the mass of the tissue that is being fractionated.) The nuclear yields obtained by this two-step procedure involving two homogenizations are lower by around 20% than those obtained by the application of procedure IV, A or B alone. This is presumably due to the breakage of some additional cell nuclei by the first homogenization step.

The supernatant from the low-speed spin of the homogenate in medium F may be subjected to differential centrifugation to obtain mitochondria, synaptosomes, microsomes, and a soluble fraction. It should be remembered that medium F contains 3 mM MgCl$_2$ to protect nuclei for subsequent isolation, and the effects of these ions should be considered in determining the quality of the fractions so obtained.

D. Nuclear Isolation Without Triton

For certain purposes, discussed in Section X, it is necessary to isolate nuclei without the aid of a detergent. This may be done, using whole rat brain or individual brain regions by procedures described in Section IV, A and B. Instead of medium NI, NIIa is used for the initial homogenization and also for subsequent washes in place of NII. NIIIa is used in place of NIII. The lower magnesium concentration in NIIa and NIIIa improves the appearance and purity of nuclei prepared in the absence of Triton. As can be seen in Fig. 3, the outer nuclear membrane remains intact in nuclei prepared without the aid of detergents and is absent in nuclei prepared with Triton X-100.

V. DETERMINING PURITY OF THE ISOLATED NUCLEAR PELLET

In general there are two methods for measuring the contamination of the nuclear pellet: direct microscopic observation, and determination of enzymes known to be constituents of particular subcellular structures.

A. Light Microscopy

The nuclear pellet is prepared for light microscopy by resuspending it in 0.1 % cresyl violet made up in NII. Good resuspension may be obtained by vortexing the pellet and then rapidly sucking the suspension in and out of a Pasteur pipet. Examination of the stained nuclei under direct transillumination at magnifications of × 160 to 1000 will reveal any gross contamination by cytoplasmic debris, capillaries, or myelin fragments. Phase contrast microscopy is also useful for judging the quality of the preparation Photographs of stained (A) and unstained (B) nuclei prepared by the procedure given Section in IV A are shown in Fig. 1. Aside from a rough evaluation of average purity, light microscopy can be used for counts of nuclear number (using a hemocytometer) and for measurement of nuclear diameters.

B. Electron Microscopy

Accurate morphological determination of contamination requires the electron microscope. We fixed our pellets with 1 % osmium and stained in block with 1 % uranyl acetate. The sections are stained with uranyl acetate and lead citrate (Venable and Coggeshall, 1965). To get a true picture of the amount of contamination in the preparation, it is desirable to examine the top, middle, and bottom of the pellet as demonstrated in Fig. 2, which shows at low magnification the entire thickness of a nuclear pellet obtained after centrifugation in the SW 50 rotor (see Section IV, B). The amount of cytoplasmic contamination is minimal and the contamination is distributed evenly throughout the pellet. Figures 3 (a) and 3 (b) are higher magnification pictures of nuclei prepared in the presence and absence of Triton X-100. It should be noted that Triton has removed the outer nuclear membrane, leaving the inner envelope intact. These pictures also illustrate the heterogeneity of nuclear types found in the brain, as judged by the differences in size of nuclei and density of chromatin as well as by the presence of well-defined nucleoli in certain (presumably neuronal) nuclei.

C. Enzymic Determinations of Purity

Another method of determining the purity of a nuclear preparation is to measure enzymes which have previously been localized in specific subcellular particles. Caution must be exercised in choosing biochemical markers for study in brain tissue,[*] since much of the work on the localization of

---

[*] The *Bibliographic Guide to Neuroenzyme Literature* (Hoijer, 1969) and the *Handbook of Neurochemistry* (Lajtha, 1969, 1970) are good initial sources to consult when one is looking for a particular enzyme marker in brain tissue.

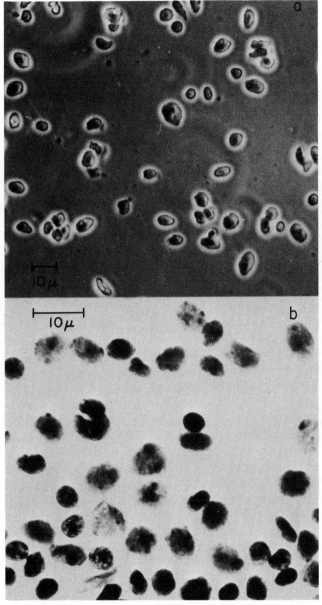

Fig. 1. Nuclear suspensions observed in the light microscope. (a) Phase contrast of unstained suspension in medium NII. (b) Direct transillumination of nuclei suspended in 0.1 % cresyl violet in medium NII. The nuclei were isolated with the use of Triton X-100 as described in Section IV, A.

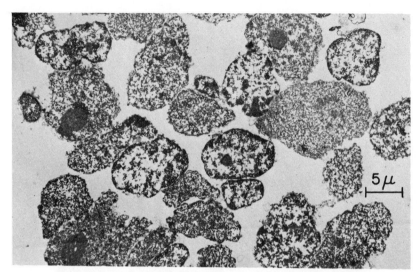

Fig. 2. Low-power electron micrograph of the entire thickness (right to left in photo) of a nuclear pellet from the preoptic-hypothalamic region of the rat brain. The pellet was prepared for microscopy as described in the text.

marker enzymes has been done on the liver and cannot automatically be applied to the central nervous system. For example, glucose-6-phosphatase and cytochrome P450, which are microsomal markers in the liver (de Duve *et al.,* 1955; Klingenberg, 1958) are barely detectable in the brain (Hers and de Duve, 1950; Inouye and Shinagawa, 1965). Aconitate hydratase, an enzyme found in the soluble cytoplasmic fraction of liver, is localized in mitochondria in the cerebral cortex of the rabbit (Dixon and Webb, 1964). Nonspecific esterase, which is highly localized in the microsomal fraction in the liver, appears to be more widely distributed in the brain (Aldridge and Johnson, 1959; Dixon and Webb, 1964).

However, one enzyme has been shown to have the same distribution in the liver and in the brain, namely, cytochrome *c* oxidase, a mitochondrial enzyme (Brody *et al.,* 1952). We have measured this enzyme in a typical nuclear pellet from whole rat brain, using an adaptation of the method of Cooperstein and Lazarow (1951). Table I shows that about 0.06% of the activity of the whole homogenate appeared in the nuclear pellet. The enzyme activity per unit of protein in the nuclear pellet is 0.049 of that of the whole homogenate. These low values are particularly impressive when one considers that the mitochondrial fraction from brain has about 15 times the cytochrome *c* oxidase activity per unit weight of protein as has the whole homogenate (R. E. Zigmond, unpublished observation). This result confirms the

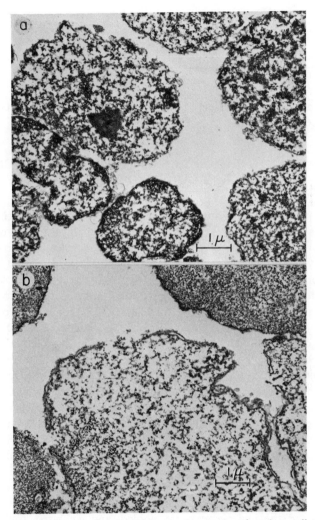

Fig. 3. Higher magnification electron micrographs of nuclear pellets prepared in the presence (a) and absence (b) of Triton X–100. Procedural details may be found in the text. Note absence of outer nuclear membrane in Fig. 3(a).

Table I.   Cytochrome c Oxidase Activity in Nuclear Suspensions from
Rat Brain[a]

	% of enzyme activity	Cytochrome c oxidase Units/mg of protein
Whole homogenate	100	0.164
Nuclei	0.06	0.008
Sum of the remaining fractions	98	0.167

[a] Protein recovery was 98%.

microscopic evidence that there is extremely little mitochondrial contamination of the nuclear pellet.

VI. CHEMICAL ANALYSIS OF THE ISOLATED NUCLEI AND NUCLEAR YIELD PROCEDURE

The nuclear pellet is suspended in 1 ml of cold 0.5 M perchloric acid and transferred quantitatively to a conical centrifuge tube with several additional 1-ml portions of perchloric acid. The nuclear material is sedimented by centrifuging in a clinical centrifuge and the supernatant discarded. The pellet is suspended in 0.3 M KOH (0.5 ml is a convenient volume to use for nuclei from individual brain regions) and the suspension allowed to stand at room temperature overnight or at 37 °C for 2 hr, allowing time for RNA hydrolysis (Munro and Fleck, 1966). Portions (20–50 μl) of the resulting clear solution are analyzed for protein by the method of Lowry et al., (1951) using bovine serum albumin as standard. The remainder is chilled and acidified with 70 μl of 70% (11.65 M) perchloric acid for each milliliter of KOH used. The supernatant is saved. The precipitate, containing protein and DNA and potassium perchlorate is collected by centrifugation and washed once with a volume of 0.5 M perchloric acid equal to that of the supernatant just removed. The supernatants from the acidification and washing steps are pooled and analyzed for RNA by the orcinol method (Munro et al., 1962), using yeast RNA as standard. The DNA pellet material is hydrolyzed in 1–3 ml of 0.5 M perchloric acid at 80 °C for 30 min and the particulate material is collected by centrifugation. This procedure is repeated, and the hydrolyzates are pooled and analyzed for DNA by the diphenylamine method of Burton (1956), using calf thymus DNA as standard. For estimation of recoveries of these substances, tissue samples of the same brain regions are homogenized in cold distilled water and acidified to 0.5 M with concentrated perchloric acid. The acid precipitate is then subjected to hydrolysis in KOH, reacidification, and hot acid hydrolysis as described above for the isolated nuclei.

The results of these determinations are summarized in Table II, which shows results obtained with cell nuclei from seven brain regions and the pituitary, expressed as micrograms of each substance per milligram of the wet tissue from which the nuclei were isolated. The yield of protein, RNA and DNA was very similar for the hippocampus, cerebral cortex, hypothalamus, and amygdaloid region. Higher yields were obtained for nuclei from the cerebellum and this may reflect the high concentration of cell bodies in this region. Nuclei from the midbrain and brainstem sample show lower yields than from any of the above regions. Nuclei from the septum and the pituitary show yields that are different from the other six regions and the variability of the yield is higher, perhaps because of their small size. Table II also shows the mass ratios of protein and RNA to DNA for nuclei from each brain region. The ratio of protein mass to DNA varied from 2.2 (cerebellum) up to 7.5 (septum), while the ratio of RNA mass to DNA varied from 0.08 (cerebellum) up to 0.45 (amygdala). It is interesting that the cerebellum is lowest in both of these parameters, in spite of its unusually high DNA content.

Table II. Composition of Isolated Nuclei from Rat Brain Regions

Structure	Wet mass of tissue (mg $\pm$ SEM)	Nuclear yield (μg/mg wet tissue $\pm$ SEM)[a]			
		Protein	RNA	DNA	% DNA
Hippocampus	136$\pm$8	1.94$\pm$0.02 (3.7)	0.19$\pm$0.04 (0.30)	0.53$\pm$0.04 (1.0)	47
Hypothalamus +preoptic region	123$\pm$5	2.02$\pm$0.20 (3.5)	0.18$\pm$0.06 (0.31)	0.58$\pm$0.07 (1.0)	47
Cerebral cortex[b]	266$\pm$14	2.19$\pm$0.11 (4.8)	0.19$\pm$0.04 (0.41)	0.46$\pm$0.06 (1.0)	45
Amygdala[c]	124$\pm$7	2.20$\pm$0.11 (5.8)	0.17$\pm$0.02 (0.45)	0.38$\pm$0.02 (1.0)	38
Cerebellum	300$\pm$9	6.92$\pm$0.84 (2.2)	0.26$\pm$0.03 (0.08)	3.15$\pm$0.23 (1.0)	61
Midbrain+brainstem	346$\pm$12	1.41$\pm$0.17 (3.3)	0.19$\pm$0.02 (0.21)	0.43$\pm$0.06 (1.0)	45
Septum	14$\pm$1	3.59$\pm$0.41 (7.5)	0.20$\pm$0.03 (0.42)	0.48$\pm$0.07 (1.0)	42
Pituitary	11$\pm$1	9.72$\pm$2.57 (4.7)	0.44$\pm$0.13 (0.21)	2.05$\pm$0.55 (1.0)	31

[a] Means are based on values for four to five determinations on each structure. Figures in parentheses represent the mass ratio of protein or RNA to DNA, based on the average yields which are given. % DNA refers to the percentage of tissue DNA recovered in the nuclear pellet and is an indication of the nuclear yield (see text).
[b] Posterior portion.
[c] With overlying cortex.

The yield of nuclei is of great importance for many kinds of biochemical studies. The best indication of the yield is the percentage of tissue DNA recovered in the isolated nuclei, since only a few percent of total tissue DNA occurs in the mitochondria (Gibor and Granick, 1967); the rest is found exclusively in the cell nuclei. The last column of Table II presents the recovery of DNA in each of the eight kinds of isolated nuclei, expressed as the percentage of total tissue DNA that we recovered in the nuclei. These recoveries are quite similar for all of the brain structures (38–48 %), with the exception of the cerebellum, for which the recovery is somewhat greater (61 %).

The extent to which the nuclear population isolated by these procedures represents accurately the population of nuclei found in the whole tissue is an open question. We are of the opinion that the nuclear population isolated by our procedure is at least representative of the nucleus population in the tissue although it may not reflect the exact proportion of nuclear types originally present. Recent support for this assertion is that the distribution of nuclear size for a structure such as the hippocampus is basically bimodal, with peaks of 5.5 and 7.8 μm; moreover, some small numbers of nuclei are observed with diameters in the range of 9–15 μm, indicating that even extremely large nuclei characteristic of hippocampal pyramidal neurons are able to survive the isolation procedure. (McEwen et al., 1972a)

In the original description of this procedure (Løvtrup-Rein and McEwen 1966), it was noted that prolonged exposure to Triton X-100 and excessive homogenization tended to destroy the larger cell nuclei, and for that reason both the duration of exposure to Triton and the degree of homogenization were minimized. It should also be noted that other investigators (Hadjiolov et al., 1965) have reported a loss of nuclei of smaller size during their isolation experiments, and it is conceivable that this may occur in our method.

VII. OTHER METHODS FOR ISOLATING BRAIN CELL NUCLEI

Other procedures have been reported which employ detergents for nuclear isolation. Hadjiolov et al. (1965) used Triton X-100 and Cemulsol NPT 12, another nonionic detergent, to isolate clean nuclei from the cat brain cortex in yields of 25–32%. Casola and Agranoff (1965) have reported the use of a mixture of deoxycholate and Tween 40, originally described by Penman (1966) for HeLa cells, in isolating nuclei from the goldfish brain. Rappoport et al. (1963) used Triton X-100 to isolate nuclei from the developing rat brain.

A number of other aqueous isolation procedures have been reported which do not use detergents (Sporn et al., 1962; Bondy and Roberts, 1964;

Bondy and Waelsch, 1965; Kato and Kurokawa, 1967; Dutton and Mahler, 1968). In all of them, the tissue is homogenized in isotonic, buffered sucrose solutions containing divalent cations, and the nuclei are subsequently purified by centrifugation through dense sucrose (2 M or greater) solutions. Yields reported for these procedures vary between 11 % (Sporn et al., 1962) and 30 % (Kato and Kurokawa, 1967). The nuclei are largely free of visible cytoplasmic contamination, although the electron microscope reveals the presence of the outer nuclear membrane. In two published procedures (Borkowski et al., 1970; Mandel et al., 1967) the tissue is homogenized directly in the dense sucrose solutions, and nuclei are purified directly by centrifugation.

Two of the most difficult problems with all methods of nuclear isolation in aqueous media are the loss of soluble nuclear substances and the translocation of cytoplasmic substances to nuclei during isolation. Examples of these difficulties are cited by Allfrey (1959). Methods for estimating the magnitude of these two problems include autoradiography of intact cells and the addition to tissue homogenates of substances suspected of adsorbing to nuclei in order to ascertain the degree of binding during nuclear isolation. Both of these techniques have been used in our laboratory in studies of steroid hormone binding in vivo to brain cell nuclei (Section X, A).

A completely different strategy for nuclear isolation, which minimizes these problems of loss and exchange, is the nonaqueous technique. This technique was first described by Behrens (1935), developed by Allfrey and Mirsky and collaborators (1969), and utilized by them and by Siebert (1961), and most recently by Kuehl (1967). In this method, tissue is frozen in liquid nitrogen and lyophilized, and then disrupted in petroleum ether by means of a ball mill or other grinding apparatus. Nuclei are then purified from cytoplasmic debris by isopycnic centrifugation through mixtures of cyclohexane and carbon tetrachloride. Considerable evidence indicates that this procedure minimizes the loss of soluble nuclear constituents which often occurs in aqueous nuclear isolation procedures and prevents the exchange of components between nuclei and the cytoplasm. Nonaqueous nuclei from brain and other tissues contain ATP and other nucleoside triphosphates, and metabolites and enzymes of the glycolytic pathway and citric acid cycle (see Section X, A). These substances are difficult to detect in nuclei isolated from such tissues by aqueous procedures. Such findings indicate the extensive loss of such materials that frequently occurs during aqueous isolation. Although it is essential for demonstrating that certain water-soluble molecules are normally present in cell nuclei, the method is limited by the fact that lipid-soluble substances are extracted during the isolation procedure and some enzymes are inactivated.

VIII. SEPARATION OF NUCLEAR TYPES

Each cell type in the brain has characteristic nuclei which can be recognized in the light microscope in intact tissue sections and in broken cell suspensions of fresh brain tissue (Glees, 1955; Nurnberger, 1958). Neuronal nuclei are generally the largest, with a clear nucleoplasm and one or more distinct and often very large nucleoli; astroglial nuclei are also large, with denser nucleoplasm than neurons and multiple inclusions which resemble small nucleoli but are less distinct; oligodendroglial nuclei are smaller, with denser nucleoplasm than astroglia, and they also appear to have nucleolarlike inclusions; microglial nuclei are small and elongated in shape, with extremely dense nucleoplasm that obscures observation of internal structure in the light microscope. There are, of course, many nuclei which are hard to identify either because of size or because of the density of the nucleoplasm. This is particularly true of the cerebellum (McEwen *et al.,* 1972*a*). According to Nurnberger (1958), the clearly identified neuronal nuclei constitute around 15% of the nuclear population of the rat brain, with a range of 10% (hypothalamus) up to 24% (cerebral cortex).

A number of published reports indicated that in a centrifugal separation of nuclei in hypertonic sucrose, it is the oligodendroglial and microglial nuclei which migrate most rapidly, leaving the neuronal and astroglial nuclei near the top of the gradient. In the procedure originally described by Løvtrup-Rein and McEwen (1964) and again recently by Løvtrup-Rein (1970 a,b) and Løvtrup-Rein and Grann (1970) nuclei suspended in 2.0 *M* sucesos containing the ionic composition of medium NIII (Section III) are layered on a discontinuous gradient of 2.8, 2.6, 2.4, 2.2, and 2.0 *M* sucrose and centrifuged at 75,000 *g* (average) for 30 min. Three fractions are obtained at the interfaces between layers, which are enriched in three nuclear types: astrocytic (top), neuronal (middle), and oligodendroglial and microglial (bottom). Burdman and Journey (1969) reported separations of nuclei using discontinuous gradients of 2.6, 2.4, and 2.2 *M* sucrose, into the same three enriched fractions. These authors report that their fractions each contain about 20% contamination by nuclei of the other types. Burdman and Journey (1969) also report that they find astroglial nuclei moving ahead of the neuronal nuclei. This discrepancy suggests that small differences in handling of the nuclear suspension may be very important to the behavior of these two nuclear types and indicate that it may be impractical to routinely separate neuronal from astrocytic nuclei by these techniques.

Another method for fractionating brain cell nuclei into neuronal and glial types has been reported by Kato and Kurokawa (1967) and used by them (1970). This procedure also relies on the differential sedimentation of nuclei in dense sucrose: glial nuclei migrate more rapidly than neuronal.

The reported purity for the large (neuronal and astroglial) nuclei is 72–83%
while for the small (oligodendroglial and microglial) nuclei the purity is
between 94 and 99%.

IX. PROPERTIES OF CELL NUCLEI

No chapter on the isolation of cell nuclei from brain would be complete
without a summary of the important biochemical events which occur in
cell nuclei. Since a recent chapter by Allfrey (1970) has covered the topic
in great detail, we shall only outline the major considerations as they are
believed to apply to nuclei in all animal cells.

A. Energy Metabolism (Conover, 1967; McEwen, 1967; Allfrey, 1970)

Cell nuclei contain ATP and other nucleoside triphosphates and have
the ability to generate ATP for biosynthetic reactions by means of the
glycolytic pathway, which contains two substrate-linked phosphorylation
steps. In addition to the glycolytic pathway, cell nuclei from all tissues so
far studied by nonaqueous procedures contain enzymes and metabolites of
the citric acid cycle. Although nonaqueous nuclei are not suitable for demonstrating the integrated function of aerobic glycolysis in generating ATP,
studies on nuclei isolated in 0.25 M sucrose from the calf thymus gland have
demonstrated the conversion of labeled glucose, acetate, and pyruvate to
$C^{14}O_2$, and have in addition demonstrated the existence of nuclear ATP
synthesis linked to an electron transport chain which is similar in many
respects to that in mitochondria. Recent spectral evidence suggests that
cytochromes of the a, b, and c types are present in thymus nuclei and may
be located in the inner nuclear envelope. Such a system should be capable of
acting as a terminal oxidase, transferring electrons to oxygen. Studies on
liver nuclei have so far failed to show the presence of cytochromes other
than type c, and so the generality of nuclear oxidative phosphorylation
remains to be established.

B. Protein Synthesis (Allfrey, 1970)

Cell nuclei from many cell types contain amino acid activating enzymes,
transfer RNA, ribosomes, ATP, and amino acids. Nuclei isolated from
thymus, Novikoff hepatoma, and intestinal mucosa and HeLa cells are able
to incorporate radioactive amino acids into protein by reactions dependent
on the intranuclear pools of these essential constituents. Evidence will be
discussed in the next section that isolated brain cell nuclei incorporate

amino acids into protein *in vitro*. Kinetic analysis of the labeling of nuclear proteins in diverse cell types has revealed that incorporation into certain classes of nuclear protein occurs so rapidly (within seconds in some cases) as to be explicable only by intranuclear synthesis. In addition, nuclear amino acid incorporation in the intact cell appears to be less susceptible than cytoplasmic incorporation to puromycin inhibition. However, not all nuclear proteins are synthesized in the nucleus, and certain vital aspects of cell function depend on the entry of cytoplasmic proteins into the nucleus, as will be indicated below.

C. RNA Synthesis (Allfrey, 1970)

As noted above, all but a few percent of the DNA of the cell resides in the nucleus. Since all RNA synthesis occurs along a DNA template, most of the RNA in the cell is produced within the nucleus, utilizing the intranuclear nucleotide pool. The enzyme or enzymes which catalyze RNA synthesis are known as RNA polymerases, and recent evidence suggests that there may be two forms of this enzyme in mammalian tissues differing both in intranuclear localization and sensitivity to the divalent cations Mg^{2+} and Mn^{2+} (Jacob *et al.*, 1969; Jacob *et al.*, 1970; Roeder and Rutter, 1970).

D. DNA Synthesis (Allfrey, 1970)

DNA replication, like that of RNA, occurs along a DNA template. Although the enzyme, DNA polymerase, is not localized exclusively within the cell nucleus, the process of DNA replication is certainly a nuclear process. It should be emphasized that DNA replication occurs almost exclusively within a specific period in the cell cycle and, furthermore, that some somatic cells, such as neurons, cease DNA synthesis and cell replication at a certain point in their differentiation.

E. Modification of Nuclear Macromolecules (Allfrey, 1970)

Certain reactions occurring within the nuclei of interphase cells appear to be important to the process of activating and deactivating the genome. These transformations include the acetylation and methylation of histones and the phosphorylation of histones and other chromosomal proteins. The mechanism by which these reactions or the products of these transformations participate in the regulation of genomic activity is not yet clearly understood.

F. Nucleocytoplasmic Interactions

Many cellular functions result from the interaction of the nucleus and the cytoplasm. As noted above, the nucleus is the source of most cellular RNA (messengers, ribosomes, and transfer RNA) with which all proteins are synthesized. In addition, the nucleus is the source of NAD, since it contains the enzyme, NMN-ATP adenyltransferase, which condenses NMN and ATP to form NAD (Allfrey, 1970). Since NAD and NADP are essential to cellular oxidations, it seems likely that the nucleus participates in the regulation of cellular oxidative processes.

Interactions in the opposite direction—i.e., cytoplasmic effects on the nucleus—are of equal importance to cellular function, as the following examples clearly demonstrate. The classic experiments of Goldstein (1965) with amoebas demonstrated the rapid entry of labeled cytoplasmic protein into unlabeled nuclei transplanted into labeled cytoplasm and also demonstrated the preferential exchange of labeled nuclear protein with unlabeled nuclei when labeled nuclei are transplanted into an unlabeled cell. More recently, cell fusion experiments from the laboratory of Harris (1970) have shown that nuclei from dormant cells such as nucleated avian erythrocytes can be reactivated, increasing in protein content, nucleolar size, and RNA synthesis, when such nuclei are placed in the cytoplasmic environment of an active cell in tissue culture. The histones also present an intriguing example of nucleocytoplasmic interaction: while lysine-rich histones can be synthesized within isolated cell nuclei (Allfrey, 1970), a number of classes of histones are also formed in the cytoplasm at the time of DNA replication within the nucleus (Gallwitz and Mueller, 1967; Robins and Borun, 1967). These proteins then enter the nuclei to complex with the newly formed DNA. A final example of cytoplasmic effects on nuclear function deals with the action of certain steroid hormones on genomic activity. Hormones such as estradiol, testosterone, and aldosterone stimulate RNA and protein synthesis within their respective target tissues (Jensen et al., 1969; Liao et al., 1969; Swaneck et al., 1969). In interacting with these tissues, these hormones bind to stereospecific proteins which most probably are located in the cytoplasm of the target cells. The hormone is then transferred to the cell nucleus by an unidentified temperature-dependent process where it is also found to be associated with a binding protein (Jensen et al., 1969). In at least one case —that of the estradiol-binding protein of the uterus— it seems almost certain that the nuclear-binding protein is derived from the cytoplasmic protein (Jensen et al., 1969).

X. USES OF ISOLATED BRAIN CELL NUCLEI

The purpose of this section is to outline typical neurochemical studies which have utilized isolated brain cell nuclei. We shall attempt to be illustrative rather than exhaustive in our coverage and to point out the underlying rationale for and the problems involved in each kind of study.

A. Steroid Hormone-Binding Macromolecules in Brain Cell Nuclei

The major use in our hands of the nuclear isolation procedure described in this chapter has been to demonstrate that two steroid hormones, corticosterone and estradiol, bind stereospecifically to limited-capacity binding sites in the cell nuclei of certain brain regions (McEwen *et al.*, 1970; Zigmond and McEwen, 1970). These studies were performed on brains of animals given the radioactive steroid hormone *in vivo* and have depended on two principal factors: the ability to isolate purified cell nuclei from brain regions weighing between 10 and 400 mg and the abilitiy of the steroid-hormone complex and of the hormone-binding macromolecule itself to withstand the nuclear isolation procedure and remain attached to the nucleus. We have succeeded in showing that two hormones each concentrate in cell nuclei in different brain regions: estradiol concentrates primarily in cell nuclei in the hypothalamus and amygdala (Zigmond and McEwen, 1970); corticosterone concentrates primarily in cell nuclei from the hippocampus, amygdala, and cerebral cortex (McEwen *et al.*, 1970). Recent autoradiographic evidence has confirmed the localization of both hormones in neuronal cell nuclei of these brain regions (Stumpf, 1968; Anderson and Greenwald, 1969; Gerloch and McEwen, 1972). Since the isolation procedure employs Triton X-100, which removes most membranes and other lipoid material, it is not surprising that little, if any, hormone adsorbs 'to the nuclei during the isolation procedure. This was shown directly by adding labeled estradiol or corticosterone to an unlabeled brain homogenate and then isolating nuclei. Essentially no hormone was recovered in the nuclear pellet.

B. Study of Other Nuclear Components after *in Vivo* Labeling

As in our steroid-binding studies, the two requirements for most other *in vivo* labeling studies on brain cell nuclei are that the isolated nuclei be as pure as possible and that the constituents under investigation be strongly associated with the nuclei so as to withstand the stresses of the isolation procedure. These criteria have been met in several studies of the histones of brain cell nuclei (Dingman and Sporn, 1964; Piha *et al.*, 1966), which provide a clear indication of the relative metabolic inertness of histones in brain and of the rather constant ratio between histone and DNA in many tissues. A number of papers have also dealt with the RNA labeled *in vivo* from brain cell nuclei isolated without the aid of detergent. For example, Zemp and co-workers (1966) have described the pattern of labeled mouse brain nuclear RNA, showing that it differs clearly from cytoplasmic RNA in sucrose gradients. Similar experiments on rat and rabbit brain nuclei have been reported by Løvtrup-Rein (1970b) and Løvtrup-Rein and Grann (1970).

On the other hand, highly purified nuclei isolated with Triton X-100 are not suitable for such analysis of RNA. Casola and Agranoff (1968) found extensive breakdown of nuclear RNA in such nuclei prepared from goldfish brain. They did successfully isolate high molecular weight RNA from nuclei isolated with the aid of Tween 40 and deoxycholate (Casola and Agranoff, 1968), and their findings should be carefully considered in making a choice of a nuclear isolation technique for future studies of nuclear RNA.

A third important nuclear component, the nonhistone proteins, has been receiving increasing attention in laboratories interested in genomic regulation (Paul and Gilmore, 1968; Kleinsmith *et al.,* 1970). Little work has been published on these proteins in brain cell nuclei, but the study of such proteins prepared from nuclei isolated by procedures described in this chapter should present no problems because they are not easily extractable.

C. Study of Nuclear Enzymes

Two enzymes unique to cell nuclei have received considerable attention in the brain. Kurokawa *et al.,* (1967) reported the unequal distribution of the enzyme NMN-ATP adenyltransferase in neuronal and glial cell nuclei of the guinea pig brain. Another enzyme, RNA polymerase, has been studied by a number of laboratories (Barondes, 1964; Bondy and Waelsch, 1965; Dravid and Duffy, 1969; Kato and KuroKawa, 1970). Both enzymes are so highly localized to cell nuclei that there is no particular advantage in using nuclei of extreme purity. Rather, in view of the adverse effects of Triton X-100 referred to above, isolation methods not employing this or any detergent are to be preferred. In fact, the cited studies on these two nuclear enzymes have been made on brain nuclei prepared by utilizing only purification through (2 *M* or greater) sucrose to eliminate most cytoplasmic contamination.

D. Study of Biosynthetic Reactions in Isolated Brain Nuclei

Several reports indicate that isolated brain cell nuclei can incorporate amino acids into nuclear proteins (Burdman and Journey, 1969; Løvtrup-Rein, 1970a). Both reports have stressed the low level of incorporation into nuclei isolated with Triton X-100. The finding suggests that Triton has deleterious effects on the metabolic apparatus responsible for the incorporation; it may also indicate, however, that the small amount of endoplasmic reticulum removed by the Triton is important for the incorporation. However, both of these studies suggest that the incorporation is a nuclear process: one study has shown, by autoradiography, incorporated radioactivity within isolated nuclei (Burdman and Journey, 1969); the other study has shown a dependence of such incorporation in nuclei on sodium ions, which is believed to be a characteristic unique to nuclear protein synthesis (Løvtup-Rein, 1970a).

XI. SUMMARY OF SOME OF THE FACTORS AFFECTING NUCLEAR ISOLATION AND THE CHOICE OF ISOLATION PROCEDURES

Factors that affect the yield and quality of the nuclei isolated from nervous tissue may be summarized as follows. As stated previously (Løvtrup-Rein and McEwen, 1966), the optimum pH for nuclear isolation in sucrose solutions lies between 6 and 7; pH in excess of 7 results in gelation of the nuclei and prevents successful isolation free of cytoplasm. A lower pH is deleterious to the preservation of nuclear metabolism and tends to extract large amounts of soluble nuclear constituents, as is the case with isolations of liver cell nuclei in citric acid (Allfrey, 1959). The divalent cation concentration is also critical. Absence of such divalent cations as Ca^{2+} or Mg^{2+} leads to swelling (Anderson and Wilbur, 1952) and gelation of nuclei during isolation. Excessive divalent cation causes the nucleoplasm to condense and become granular (Maggio *et al.*, 1963). The presence of sucrose or a similar sugar in the isolation medium, although not tested directly for brain, is known to be important for preserving the permeability characteristics of the nuclear envelope and for maintaining endogenous nuclear metabolic reactions in other tissues (Allfrey, 1959). Finally, the choice of homogenizer is of great importance. We prefer a coaxial homogenizer, with a loose-fitting Teflon pestle (clearance: 0.125 mm on the radius is optimal in our hands), although homogenizers of many types have been used for the isolation of nuclei (Allfrey, 1959).

The purity of the final nuclear preparation is a function of two steps in isolation. The most generally used step is centrifugation in dense sucrose solutions (2 M or greater) during which the cytoplasmic debris floats to the top of the centrifuge tube, while the nuclei sediment to the bottom. The other step is the use of detergents in the initial homogenization of the tissue. As stated in Section X, Triton X-100 is of limited use because it tends to promote degradation of RNA and because it is deleterious to endogenous metabolic activity of the isolated nuclei such as the incorporation of labeled amino acids. Other nonionic detergents, such as Tween 40, Nonidet P 40, and Triton N 101 (Hadjiolov *et al.*, 1965; Casola and Agranoff, 1968; Berkowitz *et al.*, 1970) may not share this disadvantage. However, the use of a detergent such as Triton X-100 is desirable in studies where the stability of RNA or of amino acid incorporation is not important, since this detergent assists in the removal of cytoplasmic contamination and the outer nuclear membrane. Another distinct advantage of detergents in nuclear isolation is that they tend to increase the nuclear yield. The method reported in this chapter gives yields of 38–61 % for various brain regions while other methods not employing detergent give yields of 11–30 %. As we have indicated in Section XI, A, purity and high yield have been extremely valuable in studies of hormone binding to brain cell nuclei.

It should finally be stated that the only adequate standard for nuclear composition is the nonaqueous isolation procedure described in Section VII. The absence of a substance or a metabolic reaction from cell nuclei isolated in aqueous media is no proof that the substance or the process is not normally present in cell nuclei. Likewise, the presence of a substance in aqueous cell nuclei must be regarded with caution until the possibility of adsorption of these substances during the isolation procedure has been ruled out.

ACKNOWLEDGMENTS

Research for this paper has been supported by USPHS research grants NS 07080 to Bruce S. McEwen and MH 13189 to N. E. Miller. Richard E. Zigmond has been supported by a training grant in behavioral sciences, GM 01789.

We wish to thank Mrs. Sally Zigmond for preparation of electron micrographs, and Mrs. Carew Magnus, Miss Linda Plapinger, and Mrs. Gislaine Wallach for their excellent technical assistance.

REFERENCES

Aldridge, W. N., and Johnson, M. K. (1959) *Biochem. J.* **73**, 270.
Allfrey, V. G. (1959) in *The Cell*, Vol. 1 (J. Brachet and A. E. Mirsky, eds.), Academic Press, New York, p. 193.

Allfrey, V. G. (1970) in *Protein Biosynthesis* (C. B. Anfinsen, Jr., ed.), Academic Press, New York, p. 247.
Anderson, C. H., and Greenwald, G. S. (1969) *Endocrinology* **85**, 1160.
Anderson, N. G., and Wilbur, K. M. (1952) *J. Gen. Physiol.* **35**, 781.
Barondes, S. H. (1964) *J. Neurochem.* **11**, 663.
Behrens, M. (1938) in *Handbuch der biologischen Arbeitsmethoden* (E. Abderhalden, ed.), Bd. V, Abt. 10, II, Seite 1363. Urban and Schwarzenberg, Berlin and Vienna.
Berkowitz, D. M., Kakefuda, T., and Sporn, M. B. (1970) *J. Cell Biol.* **45**, 851.
Bondy, S. C., and Roberts, S. (1964) *Biochem. J.* **115**, 341.
Bondy, S. C., and Waelsch, H. (1965) *J. Neurochem.* **12**, 751.
Borkowski, T., Berbec, H., Brzuskiewicz, H. (1965) *Acta Biochimica Polonica* **12**, 143.
Brody, T. M., Wang, R. I. H., and Bain, J. M. (1952) *J. Biol. Chem.* **198**, 821.
Burdman, J. A., and Journey, L. J. (1969) *J. Neurochem.* **16**, 493.
Burton, K. (1956) *Biochem. J.* **62**, 315.
Casola, L., and Agranoff, B. W. (1968) *Brain Res.* **10**, 227.
Conover, T. E. (1967) *Current Topics in Bioenergetics* **2**, 235.
Cooperstein, S. J., and Lazarow, A. (1951) *J. Biol. Chem.* **189**, 665.
Dingman, C. W., and Sporn, M. B. (1964) *J. Biol. Chem.* **239**, 3483.
Dixon, M., and Webb, E. (1964) *The Enzymes*, Academic Press, New York, p. 629.
Dravid, A. R., and Duffy, T. E. (1969) *Brain Res.* **16**, 516.
Dutton, G. R., and Mahler, H. R. (1968) *J. Neurochem.* **15**, 765.
de Duve, C., Pressman, B. C., Gianetto, R., Wattiaux, R., and Applemans, F. (1955) *Biochem. J.* **60**, 604.
Gallwitz, D., and Mueller, G. C. (1969) *Science* **163**, 1351.
Gerlash, J., and McEwen, B. S. (1972) *Science* in press.
Gibor, A., and Granick, S. (1967) *Progress in Nucleic Acid Research and Molecular Biology*, Vol. 6, p. 143.
Glees, P. (1955) *Neuroglia: Morphology and Function*, Blackwell Scientific Publications, Oxford.
Goldstein, L. (1965) *Symp. Intern. Soc. Cell Biol.* **4**, 79.
Hadjiolov, A. A., Tencheva, Z. S., and Bojadjieva-Mikhailova, A. G. (1965) *J. Cell Biol.* **26**, 383.
Harris, H. (1970) *Cell Fusion*, Harvard Univ. Press, Cambridge, Mass.
Hers, H. G., and de Duve, C. (1950) *Bull. Soc. Chim. Biol.* **32**, 30.
Hoijer, D. J. (1969) *A Bibliographic Guide to Neuroenzyme Literature*, Plenum Press, New York.
Inouye, A., and Shinagawa, Y. (1965) *J. Neurochem.* **12**, 803.
Jacob, S. T., Sajdel, E. M., and Munro, H. M. (1970) *Biochem. Biophys. Res. Commun.* **38**, 765.
Jensen, E. V., Suzuki, T., Numata, M., Smith, S., and DeSombre, E. R. (1969) *Steroids* **13**, 417.
Kato, T., and Kurokawa, M. (1967) *J. Cell Biol.* **32**, 619.
Kato, T., and Kurokawa, M. (1970) *Biochem. J.* **116**, 599.
Kleinsmith, L. J., Heidema, J., and Carroll, A. (1970) *Nature* **226**, 1025.
Klingenberg, M. (1958) *Arch. Biochem. Biophys.* **75**, 376.
König, J. F. R., and Klippel, R. A. (1963) *The Rat Brain*, Williams and Wilkins, Baltimore.
Kuehl, L. (1967) *J. Biol. Chem.* **242**, 2199.
Kurokawa, M., Kato, T., and Inamura, H. (1967) *Proc. Japan Academy* **42**, 1217.
Lajtha, A., ed. (1969–1970) *Handbook of Neurochemistry*, Vols. 1–3, Plenum Press, New York.
Liao, S., and Fang, S. (1969) *Vit Hormones* **21**, 17.
Liao, S., Sagher, D., Lin, A. H., and Fang, S. (1969) *Nature* **223**, 297.
Løvtrup-Rein, H. (1970a) *Brain Res.* **19**, 433.
Løvtrup-Rein, H. (1970b) *J. Neurochem.* **17**, 853.
Løvtrup-Rein, H., and Grann, B. (1970) *J. Neurochem.* **17**, 845.
Løvtrup-Rein, H., and McEwen, B. S. (1966) *J. Cell Biol.* **30**, 405.

Lowry, O. H., Rosebrough, N. J., Farr, A. L., and Randall, R. J. (1951) *J. Biol. Chem.* **193**, 265.

McEwen, B. S. (1967) Ph. D. Thesis, Rockefeller University, 1964. *Dissertation Abstracts* **27**, 3436B.

McEwen, B. S., and Pfaff, D. W. (1970) *Brain Res.* **21**, 1.

McEwen, B. S., Weiss, J. M., and Schwartz, L. S. (1969) *Brain Res.* **16**, 227.

McEwen, B. S., Weiss, J. M., and Schwartz, L. S. (1970) *Brain Res.* **17**, 471.

McEwen, B.S, Plapinger, L., Magnus, C., and Wallach, G. (1972*a*) *J. Neurochim.* in press.

McEwen, B. S., Zigmond, R. E., and Gerlach, J. (1972*b*) in *Structure and Function* of *Nervous Tissue,* Vol. VI (G. H. Bourne, ed.), Academic Press, New York.

Maggio, R., Siekevitz, P., and Palade, G. E. (1963) *J. Cell Biol.* **18**, 267.

Mandel, P., Dravid, A. R., and Pete, N. (1967) *J. Neurochem.* **14**, 301.

Munro, H. N., and Fleck, A. (1966) *Meth. Biochem. Anal.* **14**, 113.

Munro, H. N., Hutchison, W. C., Ramaiah, T. R., and Nielson, F. J. (1962) *Brit. J. Nutr.* **16**, 387.

Nurnberger, J. I. (1958) in *Biology of Neuroglia* (W. F. Windle, ed.), C. C Thomas, Springfield, Ill., p. 193.

Paul, J., and Gilmour, R. S. (1968) *J. Mol. Biol.* **34**, 305.

Penman, S. (1966) *J. Mol. Biol.* **17**, 117.

Piha, R. S., Cuenod, M., and Waelsch, H. (1966) *J. Biol. Chem.* **241**, 2397.

Rappoport, D. A., Fritz, R. R., and Morcaczewsi, A. (1936) *Biochim. Biophys. Acta* **74**, 42.

Robbins, E., and Borun, T. W. (1967) *Proc. Nat. Acad. Sci., U.S.* **57**, 409.

Roeder, R. G., and Rutter, W. J. (1970) *Proc. Nat. Acad. Sci., U.S.* **65**, 675.

Siebert, G. (1961) *Biochem. Zeit.* **334**, 369.

Sporn, M. B., Wanko, T., and Dingman, W. (1962) *J. Cell Biol.* **15**, 109.

Stumpf, W. E. (1968) *Science* **162**, 1001.

Swaneck, G. E., Highland, E., and Edelman, I. S. (1969) *Nephron* **6**, 297.

Venable, J. H., and Coggeshall, R. E. (1965) *J. Cell Biol.* **25**, 407.

Zemp, J. W., Wilson, J. E., Schlesinger, K., Boggan, W. O., and Glassman, E. (1966) *Proc. Nat. Acad. Sci., U.S.* **55**, 1423.

Zigmond, R. E., and McEwen, B. S. (1970) *J. Neurochem.* **17**, 889.

Section II
PROPERTIES OF INTACT NEURAL TISSUES

Chapter 7

Ventriculocisternal Perfusion as a Technique for Studying Transport and Metabolism Within the Brain

Joseph D. Fenstermacher

Office of the Associate Scientific Director for Experimental Therapeutics
National Institutes of Health
National Cancer Institute
Bethesda, Maryland

I. INTRODUCTION

Ventriculocisternal (VC) perfusions were first performed by Leusen (1948, 1950) in work on the influence of cerebrospinal fluid (CSF) cations on the vasomotor system of anesthetized dogs. Feldberg and his group in London modified Leusen's procedure and used it to examine the effects of drugs on cerebrospinal fluid flow and composition in cats (Bhattacharya and Feldberg, 1958a, b; Feldberg and Sherwood, 1954). In the first quantitative studies with the VC perfusion technique, Pappenheimer and co-workers (Heisey *et al.*, 1962; Pappenheimer *et al.*, 1961, 1962) examined the dynamics of CSF formation and the molecular exchange of material in the cerebrospinal fluid system of unanesthetized goats. Their application of the technique and equations for the kinetics of transport in the perfused ventricular system were subsequently adopted by many other investigators interested in CSF physiology and pharmacology. In an attempt to determine the size of the brain extracellular space (ECS), Rall *et al.* (1962) performed VC perfusions on dogs and, at the conclusion of the perfusion, serially sampled the periventricular tissue. Their results demonstrated that there is a sizable ECS in the brain and suggested that a more accurate assessment of CSF-brain exchange could be made by including tissue sampling as a part of the technique. Since the work of Rall *et al.*, there have been no basic changes or additions to the VC perfusion methodology. At present, ventriculo-cisternal perfusion experiments are used to study drug metabolism by the brain and the transport of various materials between CSF, brain, and blood.

Figure 1 illustrates the VC perfusion system. An inflow needle is placed in the anterior horn of each lateral ventricle. An outflow needle is positioned in the cisterna magna. The lateral ventricles and the third and fourth ven-tricles plus a portion of the subarachnoid space can then be perfused by pumping a suitable fluid through the system. At the end of the perfusion period, the brain is removed and coronal sections are made. The periven-tricular tissue can then be readily located, sampled, and analyzed for the test material. This technique has been employed in studies with rhesus monkeys, dogs, goats, cats, rabbits, and rats. Successful placement of the needles and establishment of a well-flowing perfusion system is achieved

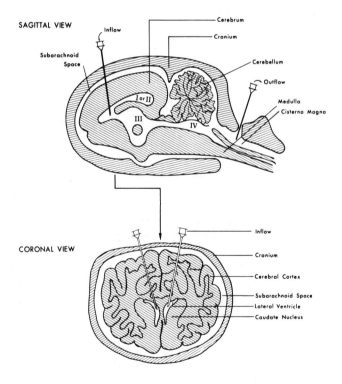

Fig. 1. Two diagrammatic views of the ventriculocisternal perfusion system.

in about 90 % of all attempts; however. the percentage of useful experiments is less than this. For the types of experiments performed in our laboratory, several checks are employed to assess the physiological condition of the animal, the adequacy of tissue perfusion, and the proper geometrical orientation of the sample series. The stringency of these criteria reduces the number of experiments which actually yield useful data to 60–70 % of all attempts.

II. METHOD

A. General Surgical Procedures

The species most commonly used in VC perfusion studies are rhesus monkeys, goats, dogs, cats, rabbits, and rats. The size of the brain in these animals ranges from 90 to 100 g (monkey, goat, and dog) to 1.6 g (rat). Since only the periventricular tissue is perfused, the amount of brain material that can be studied is a small fraction (10–20 %) of the total. Because the ventricles are larger in monkeys, dogs, and goats, a successful perfusion is much easier to achieve in these animals. Ease of perfusion and amount of tissue are two reasons for selecting the larger animals for VC perfusion; however, economic factors may make the smaller animals attractive. Besides the obvious difference in the price of the animals, lesser amounts of perfusion fluid and test material are required. The cat is a good compromise species for use in VC perfusion experiments because of its intermediate size (brain weight = 30 g).

All experiments are acute, thus necessitating the use of anesthetics and the monitoring of the physiological condition of the animal throughout the experimental period. (Anesthetic agents have physiological and metabolic effects on CSF and brain. Several specific reports concerning this (Ashcroft et al., 1968; Lorenzo et al., 1968) have appeared in the literature.) Anesthesia is generally induced with i.p. or i.v. administered pentobarbital (30 mg/kg). Cannulation of the femoral vein and artery are performed using polyethylene tubing filled with heparinized saline. Subsequent doses of anesthetic or other materials are infused through the indwelling femoral vein catheter. Systemic arterial pressure is continuously monitored and arterial blood samples periodically obtained by way of the arterial catheter. Arterial blood pH and plasma composition, e.g., osmolarity, are determined on these samples. In addition, body temperature is maintained at 37 °C by using a rectal temperature probe connected in series to a relay and an electric blanket placed under the animal's chest and abdomen. It is unnecessary to artificially respire these animals when properly attended.

B. Placement of Inflow and Outflow Needles

To perfuse as much of the ventricular system as possible, the inflow needles are usually placed in the lateral ventricles and the outflow needles at the cisterna magna, a widened portion of the subarachnoid space just above the fourth ventricle. Within the lateral ventricles there are two possible sites for the inflow needle, the anterior horn (rostral to the foramen of Monro) and the posterior portion of the body (caudal to the foramen of Monro). Placement of the needle in the anterior horn allows for the perfusion of the caudate nucleus; positioning the needle in the body allows for the perfusion of the tail of the caudate and the superior surface of the thalamus. If the needle is placed near the foramen of Monro, very little of the tissue surrounding the lateral ventricles will be perfused. In the larger animals, inflow needles can be placed in the right and left lateral ventricles and both perfused simultaneously. This increases the chances of successfully perfusing at least one lateral ventricle and enlarges the amount of tissue that can be sampled. For rats only a single inflow needle can be employed.

The anesthetized animal is placed in the head holder of a stereotaxic instrument. The frontal and parietal bones are exposed by a midline scalp incision and lateral displacement of the underlying connective tissue and muscle. Skull holes are prepared using a dental drill and size 11 dental burrs. The drill is held by a special attachment for the electrode holder of the stereotaxic device. With such an attachment the holes can be drilled down to the dura mater with a minimum of trauma to the underlying brain tissue. The stereotaxic parameters of these holes for six species are presented in Table I. After the skull holes are made, the inflow needle is attached to the electrode holder. The appropriate needle sizes for the various species are listed in Table I; they should be either short-beveled or blunt-tipped and have a stylet.

Before attempting to position the tip of the inflow needle in the ventricle, a cisternal puncture is made. A short-beveled hypodermic needle with the hub removed and a 20-inch piece of polyethylene tubing on its stem is used for this. The outflow needle sizes are listed in Table I. The puncture is made by aiming the needle at a point between the occiput and the first cervical vertebra and slowly advancing the needle through the skin and musculature at the base of the skull until the tip of the needle passes through the dura and lies in the cisterna magna. Proper placement is determined by gently sucking on the open end of the tubing while the needle is being forced through the tissues. When the cisterna has been successfully entered, CSF will begin to flow through the outflow line. A small sample of clear CSF should be taken for osmotic analysis. A similar volume of artificial CSF should be run back into the cisterna to avoid partial collapse of the ven-

Table I. Stereotaxic Parameters and Needle Sizes for VC Perfusion

Species	Position in lateral ventricle	Anterior (A) or posterior (P) (mm)	Lateral from midline (mm)	Down from dura (mm)	Inflow needle (gauge)	Outflow needle (gauge)
Goat	Body	P 10[a]	15	14	20 spinal	18
Dog	Anterior horn	A 30[b]	3	17	20 spinal	19
	Body	P 5[b]	12	15	20 spinal	19
Monkey	Anterior horn	A 18[b]	2.5	14	22 spinal	19
	Body	P 3.5[b]	10	18	22 spinal	19
Cat	Anterior horn	A 15[b]	2.5	12	20 spinal	20
	Body	A 1.0[b]	10	10	20 spinal	20
Rabbit	Body	P 6[a]	6.5	6	25 hypo	25
Rat	Body	P 1.0[a]	1.0	3	26 hypo	26

[a] Relative to coronal suture.
[b] Relative to external auditory meatus.

tricular system. The outflow tubing is now firmly secured in position by taping it to part of the stereotaxic device, and its end is temporarily clamped. If this sampling of the cisternal fluid seems to cause ventricular collapse and difficulty in properly placing the inflow needles in the ventricles, the osmotic activity determination can be made on a sample of plasma since the osmolalities of plasma and CSF are approximately equal.

Following the placement of the cisternal needle, the inflow needles with stylets in place are lowered to a depth 1–2 mm above that indicated in Table I. At this point the stylet from one needle is removed, and that needle is connected to a 20–30-inch piece of plastic extension tubing which has been filled with red-colored artificial CSF. Phenol red dye is used to give this color. By holding the end of the tubing 5–10 cm above the top of the skull, a slight hydrostatic pressure is generated at the tip of the needle. The needle is advanced in small (0.5 mm) increments. When the tip of the needle enters the ventricle, the artificial CSF will begin to flow from the tubing into the ventricle. The outflow line is immediately opened, and the line's open end placed about 5 cm below the height of the external auditory meatus. Fluid should drip freely from the outflow. If the inflow needle is in the lateral ventricle, the fluid coming out of the tubing will turn red in 10–20 sec. If it does not do so, the tip of the inflow needle is not in the lateral ventricle, and the outflow line should be immediately clamped. (The supracallosal subarachnoid space is fairly close to the lateral ventricle. It is possible to have a "false" flow if the needle tip is here; in this case the appearance time of the dye at the cisterna magna is on the order of several minutes.) The inflow needle is then advanced further until the fluid in the inflow tubing begins to run into the system again. The outflow line is opened, and the color check on the effluent solution is repeated. The advancing of the inflow needle must be done cautiously since lowering the needle too far will carry the tip past the lateral ventricle and into the underlying tissue. If the fluid does not run properly after moving the needle 1–2 mm below the depth listed in Table I, the needle should be reamed out with the stylet, the plastic tubing containing the color test solution reconnected to the needle, and the needle slowly withdrawn to the starting level. This cycle of lowering-reaming-raising is to be repeated until the proper flow is obtained. If unsuccessful after several tries or if successful, try the other inflow cannula. The procedure is the same as for the first; however, the perfusion fluid in the second line should contain trypan blue. Again the rapid appearance of the dye, this time blue, in the outflow fluid indicates proper placement of the needle in the lateral ventricle. Pappenheimer *et al.* (1962) suggest a different test; however, we have found the appearance time to be more reliable.

C. Perfusion Solution

The concentrations of protein and potassium and the pH of mammalian cerebrospinal fluid are low compared to plasma; the osmotic activity of the CSF is approximately equal to that of the plasma. The composition of the perfusion fluid, therefore, should resemble that of the endogenous CSF. A comparison of plasma, CSF, and perfusate is presented in Table II. The concentrations of the various compounds in g/liter for the synthetic CSF are as follows: NaCl, 7.4; KCl, 0.22; NaH_2PO_4, $2H_2O$, 0.075; $NaHCO_3$, 2.2; $CaCl_2$, 0.2; $MgSO_4$.7 H_2O, 0.1. glucose, 0.65; and urea, 0.2. Large volumes of the perfusate, e.g., 5 liters, can be made in advance, sterilized by Millipore filtration, placed in small bottles, and stored in a refrigerator. It will keep well for several months when treated in this manner.

For most studies it is essential to have the perfusion fluid osmotically balanced to the endogenous CSF. We have found a simple way of achieving this. Divide the stock solution (osmolality = 300 mosm) into three parts and add the appropriate amounts of NaCl to two of the three portions to achieve an osmolality of about 307 and 314, respectively. By combining any two of these solutions, one can precisely match perfusate and CSF osmolality over the range of 300–314 mosm.

Before preparing the perfusion solution for a given experimental animal, the osmolality of the freshly drawn CSF or plasma (Section II, B) is determined, and a perfusion solution of similar osmolality is made. This is warmed in a water bath to 50–60 °C. The materials to be studied are then added plus enough trypan blue to make the solution dark blue. The trypan blue in the artificial CSF will stain the perfused brain tissue and indicate which areas have been well perfused. A gas mixture of 95% O_2-5% CO_2 is bubbled through the fluid for 5–10 to bring the pH to 7.35.

The perfusion solution should always contain some sort of a reference material which will indicate the condition of the tissue, the adequacy of

Table II.   Composition of Plasma, CSF, and Perfusion Fluid

	Plasma	CSF	Perfusate
Na (mEq/kg H_2O)	158	155	155–162
K (mEq/kg H_2O)	4.6	3.0	3.0
Ca (mEq/kg H_2O)	5.5	3.0	3.6
Mg (mEq/kg H_2O)	1.4	1.8	0.8
Cl (mEq/kg H_2O)	122	134	135–142
Urea (mmoles/kg H_2O)	4.5	3.3	3.3
Glucose (mmoles/kg H_2O)	6.3	3.5	3.6
Osmolality	305	308	300–314
pH	7.4	7.3	7.35

the perfusion, and the possible errors of the tissue sampling. An extracellular marker such as sucrose or inulin is excellent for this purpose. The concentration or activity of the test and reference materials in the perfusate depend on the amount of tissue to be sampled, the concentration of the material in the sample, the duration of the perfusion, and the sensitivity of the method of analysis. For our work with radioactive materials, we perfuse for 1–6 hr, obtain 10–20-mg samples of tissue and count them by liquid scintillation spectroscopy. To obtain the necessary tissue counts for an extracellular-type material, a specific activity for the perfusion fluid of 1 μC/ml for ^{14}C labeled compounds and 5 μC/ml for ^{3}H labeled compounds is required.

D. Procedure for Perfusion

Glass syringes of the appropriate size are equipped with 30–40-inch pieces of Tygon tubing and filled with the perfusion fluid. The loaded syringes are placed in a constant speed infusion pump which is used to drive the perfusate from the syringes to the inflow needles at the desired rate. For most studies it is necessary to quickly achieve a certain concentration of the test material within the ventricular sytem and to maintain this level reasonably constant for the duration of the experiment. This can be done by perfusing the system rapidly for the initial 10–12 min (priming rate) and continuing thereafter at a slower perfusion rate (maintaining rate). The absolute values of these pump rates are determined by the volume of the ventricular system, the rate of CSF production, and the exchangeability of the test materials between perfusate and tissue. Table III lists typical pump rates for several species. These rates should be modified to fit individual experimental situations.

The pressure in the system can be easily monitored by connecting a pressure transducer into the inflow line with a T-tube. The open end of the outflow line is usually placed 5 cm below the level of the external auditory meatus. With the outflow pressure set at this level and the pump rates listed in Table III, the pressures measured in the inflow line and within the ventric-

Table III. Typical Perfusion Pump Rates

	Priming (ml/min)	Maintaining (ml/min)
Goat	1.5	0.75
Monkey	0.4	0.2
Dog	0.4	0.2
Cat	0.2	0.1
Rabbit	0.1	0.05
Rat	0.06	0.03

ular system are 25–35 and 0–5 cm H_2O (relative to the external auditory meatus), respectively.

The temperature of the artificial CSF should be 35–40 °C. To achieve this, the perfusate is warmed prior to beginning the perfusion as previously mentioned in Section II,C. During the perfusion the temperature of the inflowing fluid is maintained around 37 °C by the radiant heat from a light placed close to the inflow tubing just above the head of the animal.

Samples of the inflow solution are taken directly from the end of the inflow line before and after the perfusion period. The outflow fluid is collected in small flasks or tubes which are sealed with parafilm to minimize evaporation. The outflow containers are changed at regular intervals, e.g., every 15 min. The inflow and outflow fluids are analyzed for the test and reference materials and for osmotic activity. In addition, samples of systemic venous blood are obtained periodically and determinations of the concentrations of the perfused materials and the osmotic activity in the plasma made. All fluid analyses are performed in duplicate.

E. Duration of Perfusion

The duration of perfusion ranges form 1 to 6 hr. Usually 1 hr of perfusion is necessary to obtain adequate tissue levels of the labeled material; after 5–6 hr of perfusion and anesthesia, the animal's general condition begins to deteriorate. The concentration of the various isotopic materials in the tissue depends on the time to establish a steady state in the ventricular system, the concentration attained within the ventricular fluid at the steady state, the rate of movement of the material into the brain extracellular fluid, the amount taken up by the cells, and the amount lost from the tissue to the circulating blood. For materials which accumulate in cells, e.g., amino acids and K^+, the apparent concentration of material in the tissue may be as much as five to ten times that in the perfusate. Greater amounts and deeper penetration (3–5 mm) of such materials into periventricular brain tissue will be found with the longer perfusion times. For materials which cross the capillary wall readily, e.g., 3-0-methyl-D-glucose and tritiated water, their concentration in the tissue will be low and the depth of penetration slight (2 mm or less). Longer periods of perfusion will not yield higher concentrations or deeper penetration.

F. Tissue Sampling

One to 2 min prior to the termination of the experiment, the inflow and outflow needles are removed, the electrode holders taken off the stereotaxic device, and the tissue around the calvarium cut down and reflected.

The animal is killed with an overdose of anesthetic. By cutting around the outer border of the calvarium with an autopsy saw and prying upward in the saw kerf with a periosteal elevator, the calvarium is separated from the remainder of the skull and removed. The olfactory nerves are cut, and the anterior portion of the cerebrum raised. Proceeding caudally, the cranial nerves are snipped with a curved scissors; the medulla severed at its junction with the spinal cord; and the brain lifted out of the cranium. The brain is placed on several cotton sponges and bisected by separating the cerebral hemispheres and carefully cutting through the corpus callosum, the diencephalon, and the medulla. The lateral ventricles of each brain half are opened by placing a forceps in the foramen of Monro and teasing away the tissue anterior and posterior to the foramen. If the perfusion has been successful, much of the tissue around the lateral, third, and fourth ventricles will be stained blue. Areas of the brain damaged by the placement of the needles or the perfusion should be noted and not used in the subsequent sampling of the tissue. The brain halves, with the sagittal or cut surface up, are placed on cold 3 × 4-inch glass plates. Using a set of tongs, the glass plates with the attached brain halves are submerged in liquid nitrogen for 20–30 sec to partially freeze and harden.

The frozen tissue can now be handled in several ways depending on the goals of the experiment. By using a device like a cork borer, a cylinder of tissue running form the perfused surface into the brain can be punched out and sectioned into individual samples. An alternative approach is to cut each hemisphere into a series of 3–5-mm-thick coronal sections. Pieces of periventricular tissue from well-perfused areas (darkly stained) can then be readily trimmed from these sections. A modification of the coronal slice sampling procedure is often used in transport studies in which a simple uniform geometrical orientation of the tissue sample series is necessary for analysis of the data (Fenstermacher *et al.*, 1970; Levin *et al.*, 1970). In this case, flat ventricular surfaces are located on the coronal sections. Strips of tissue running perpendicularly to these flat surfaces are cut, and these strips are sectioned into a series of 0.5-or 1.0-mm-thick slices by a multibladed knife. Regardless of the method of sampling, a piece of brain from a remote unperfused area should be obtained in order to estimate the tissue "background" for that particular experiment.

To prevent postmortem movements or changes in the test material, two things are essential–speed and freezing the tissue. With a team of two or three people, the time from the death of the animal to the freezing of the brain halves is under 3 min, and all sampling can be finished within 10 min of the termination of the perfusion. Once the coronal sections or tissue plugs have been made, the material being handled must be kept frozen by dipping in liquid nitrogen for 5–10 sec whenever it begins to thaw.

G. Analysis of Data

All samples of perfusate, plasma, and brain are placed in appropriate vials or containers at the time of sampling and analyzed. Subsequent handling of the data depends upon the experimental design. In general, one or all of the following calculations will be made: the CSF secretion rate, the tissue distribution space, and the tissue concentration profile.

The CSF secretion rate is calculated from the concentration of a relatively nondiffusible, inert tracer material in the inflow and outflow perfusate using the following formula:

$$V_{CSF} = V_I (C_I/C_O - 1) \qquad (1)$$

in which V_{CSF} = CSF secretion rate; V_I = perfusion pump rate; C_I = concentration of tracer material in inflow perfusate; and C_O = steady-state concentration of tracer material in outflow perfusate (Heisey et al., 1962). Although a large, essentially nondiffusible marker such as blue Dextran 2000 (Pharmacia; Uppsala, Sweden) is best for this determination, extracellular markers, e.g., inulin and sucrose, can be used with a fair degree of accuracy. The values of V_{CSF} obtained should agree reasonably well with the published values for that species if the experiment has been properly performed (see Davson, 1967, for a summary of CSF secretion rates in various animal species).

The conversion of all tissue data to tissue concentrations and tissue distribution spaces and the construction of the tissue concentration profile are straightforward; the analysis of the distribution spaces and the concentration profiles is complex. The tissue concentration is calculated by dividing the amount of material found in a sample by the weight of that particular tissue sample and must be corrected for tissue and/or blood residual levels if appreciable.

The tissue concentration profile is constructed from a serial set of tissue sample data by plotting the individual tissue concentrations as a function of the distance from the perfused surface to the midpoint of each sample, e.g., in a series of 0.5-mm-thick slices, the appropriate distance for the separate samples in the series would be 0.25 mm, 0.75 mm, 1.25 mm, etc. (Such a plotting procedure assumes that the change in tissue concentration with the change in distance is linear across any tissue slice. Schantz and Lauffer (1962) report that this is a good approximation for thin slices, 1.0 mm or less, and does not lead to significant averaging errors.)

The apparent distribution spaces are calculated by dividing the tissue sample concentrations by either the inflow (for samples obtained near the inflow site), the inflow-outflow average (for samples obtained midway along the perfusion path) or the outflow (for samples obtained near the outflow site), concentrations. As will be discussed briefly in the next paragraph, the distribution spaces measured by VC perfusion must not be considered as distribution spaces in the usual sense.

Following a ventriculocisternal perfusion, the amount of a given material found in a tissue sample depends upon: the duration of the perfusion; the geometrical relationship between tissue and perfusate (e.g., the distance from the perfused surface to the tissue sampling site); the permeability of the ependyma; the mechanism(s) of material transport within the brain parenchyma (e.g., diffusion and solvent drag); the distribution of the material within the brain parenchyma (extracellular, intracellular, or both); the metabolism and/or binding of the material by the brain cells; and the permeability of the brain capillary complex to the material. Because of the number of variables in this system, the analysis of the apparent distribution spaces and the tissue concentration profiles are complex and beyond the scope of an article on methodology. A full theoretical and experimental treatment of the ventriculocisternal perfusion system is currently being prepared for publication.

H. Use of Drugs

There are two possible routes—intravenous and intraventricular—available for administering drugs and inhibitors to the brain. Drugs that are infused into the systemic circulation must be able to cross the blood–brain barrier to be effective within the central nervous system. To study the effects of a drug injected into or perfused through the ventricles, the opposite situation must hold for that agent. It must diffuse into the periventricular brain tissue and *not* be removed appreciably by transport across the blood–brain barrier into the general circulation. The differences in these two routes of administration are not always appreciated.

III. EQUIPMENT NEEDS

The essential equipment for doing ventriculocisternal perfusions are a stereotaxic device with two electrode holders, a dental drill, a constant speed infusion pump, and an autopsy saw. Pressure tranducers with a recorder, an osmometer, pH meter, and electric heating pad are needed to monitor the animal's life signs and maintain a sound preparation. In addition, the usual laboratory and surgical equipment, e.g., needles, hemostats, and syringes, are used.

IV. VARIATIONS OF THE TECHNIQUE

Methods for carrying out repeated ventriculocisternal perfusions have been described. The animal species and the published descriptions are: goats, Pappenheimer, et al. (1962); rabbits, Moir and Dow (1970); and rats, Hayden, et al. (1966) and Goodrich et al. (1969).

Techniques for perfusing the cranial subarachnoid space have also been developed. Ommaya et al. (1969) have reported an elaborate procedure for monkeys in which the cranium is partially removed and replaced with a plastic dome. For details concerning this method, see the original article. Levin et al. (1970) have successfully perfused the subarachnoid space of various mammals by placing the inflow needles in the supracallosal subarachnoid space and the outflow needle at the cisterna magna. This technique is identical to that described in this article with the exception of the stereotaxic parameters for the inflow needles and the rates of perfusion. The stereotaxic parameters for four species are listed in Table IV. The inflow perfusion rates for subarachnoid perfusion should be about two times the ventriculocisternal perfusion rate for a particular species as listed in Table III.

V. CONCLUSIONS

Ventriculocisternal perfusions have been used successfully for studies of drug action and metabolism within the brain and of transport between CSF, brain, and blood. Further valuable work in both of these areas can be performed using this technique. In addition, ventriculocisternal perfusion studies can be applied to many important neurochemical, neurophysiological, and neurohormonal problems.

Table IV.   Inflow Needle (s) Stereotaxic Parameters for Subarachnoid Space Perfusions[a]

Species	Number of inflow needles	Distance anterior from ear bar (mm)		Distance down from dura (mm)
		Rostral needle	Caudal needle	
Monkey	Two	15	5	9–10
Dog	Two	42	32	8–10
Cat	Two	19	10	9–10
Rabbit	One	32	—	2.5

[a] All needles are positioned at the midline. This table was adapted from Table I, Levin et al. (1970).

ACKNOWLEDGEMENTS

The experimental method presented in this article is the product of several years of collaboration with Drs. David P. Rall, Victor A. Levin, and Clifford S. Patlak. The author gratefully acknowledges their numerous contributions.

REFERENCES

Ashcroft, G. W., Dow, R. C., and Moir, A. T. (1968) *J. Physiol.* **199**, 397.
Bhattacharya, B. K., and Feldberg, W. (1958a) *Brit. J. Pharmacol.* **13**, 156.
Bhattacharya, B. K., and Feldberg, W. (1958b) *Brit. J. Pharmacol.* **13**, 163.
Davson, H. (1967) *Physiology of the Cerebrospinal Fluid,* Little, Brown and Co., Boston, p. 120.
Feldberg, W., and Sherwood, S. L. (1954) *J. Physiol.* **123**, 148.
Fenstermacher, J. D., Rall, D. P., Patlak, C. S., and Levin, V. A. (1970) in *Capillary Permeability,* (C. Crone and N. A. Lassen, eds.), Munksgaard, Copenhagen, p. 483.
Goodrich, C. A., Greehey, B., Miller, T. B., and Pappenheimer, J. R. (1969) *J. Appl. Physiol.* **26**, 137.
Hayden, J. F., Johnson, L. R., and Maickel, R. P. (1966) *Life Sci.* **5**, 1509.
Heisey, S. R., Held, D., Pappenheimer, J. R. (1962) *Am. J. Physiol.* **203**, 775.
Leusen, I. (1948) *Arch. Int. Pharmacodyn.* **75**, 422.
Leusen, I. (1950) *J. Physiol.* **110**, 319.
Levin, V. A., Fenstermacher, J. D., and Patlak, C. S. (1970) *Am. J. Physiol.* **219**, 1528.
Lorenzo A. V., Hammerstad, J. P. and Cutler, R. W. P. (1968) *Biochem. Pharmacol.* **17**, 1279.
Moir, A. T. B., and Dow, R. C. (1970) *J. Appl. Physiol.* **28**, 528.
Ommaya, A. R., Boretos, J. W., and Beile, E. E. (1969) *J. Neurosurg.* **30**, 25.
Pappenheimer, J. R., Heisey, S. R., and Jordan, E. F. (1961) *Am. J. Physiol.* **200**, 1.
Pappenheimer, J. R., Heisey, S. R., Jordan, E. F., and Downer, J. deC. (1962) *Am. J. Physiol.* **203**, 763.
Rall, D. P., Oppelt, W. W., and Patlak, C. S. (1962) *Life Sci.* **2**, 43.
Schantz, E. J., and Lauffer, M. A. (1962) *Biochemistry* **1**, 658.

Chapter 8

The Estimation of Extracellular Space of Brain Tissue *in Vitro*

Stephen R. Cohen

*New York State Research Institute for Neurochemistry
and Drug Addiction
Ward's Island, New York, New York 10035*

Dedicated to my children, Meryl and Eric.

I. INTRODUCTION

The measurement of extracellular space in central nervous tissue presents unresolved difficulties in both methodology and interpretation of data. Van Harreveld's book (1966a) contains an excellent discussion of the problem. There is still no consensus on whether there is any appreciable extracellular space in living brain. Measurements by reputable workers range from little or none, that is, 5% at most, through a moderate amount, about 10%, to the same as other soft tissues, say 15–30%, or even higher. Brain slices and other *in vitro* central nervous system preparations have appreciable extracellular space which may be 60% or more of the final wet weight, when measured by marker methods. Because these preparations are invariably swollen —possibly because of the dearth of connective tissue in brain—this finding is compatible with the absence of an appreciable extracellular space *in vivo*. The swelling *in vitro,* and the blood–brain barrier *in vivo*, make it impossible to check *in vitro* and *in vivo* measurements against each other. The measured extracellular space *in vitro* depends on both the extent of swelling, which in turn depends on the preparation and its treatment, and on details of the method of measurement used. There can be large discrepancies between

results by different workers for what appear to be the same or similar preparations. None of the methods in use have been shown unequivocally to
measure the extracellular space, either *in vivo* or *in vitro*, of central nervous
tissue. With the best, we have reason to believe that the measured space is a
reasonable approximation to the true extracellular space; with some others
we are hard put to guess what the measured "space" might represent.

The largest number of methods for measuring extracellular space in
tissues of all types, including central nervous tissue, are so-called "marker"
or "chemical" methods. In these, some identifiable substance, preferably one
that is presumably confined to noncellular water, is allowed to enter tissue.
The extracellular space is then calculated from its concentration in the tissue,
or, less often, from the kinetics of its exit from the tissue.

This chapter is primarily concerned with the estimation of *in vitro*
extracellular space from the penetration of a suitable marker substance into
central nervous system preparations. The procedure for brain slices and the
method of computing results that are used in our Institute are given in detail.
Various common extracellular space marker substances are described,
compared, and evaluated. The phenomenon of the "second marker space,"
which may reflect a qualitative difference between extracellular space measured at blood temperature, and extracellular space measured at 0°C, and
other phenomena that may affect the interpretation of marker spaces are
discussed. Several alternate bases for expressing tissue spaces are listed
(e.g., percent wet weight, ml/g dry weight), and methods given for trans-
forming from one to another. Markers and conventions for defining extracellular space for different purposes are recommended where possible, because
the extracellular space depends upon the marker and convention adopted.
Finally, because several methods for expressing results depend on knowing
the water content of tissue, a procedure for measuring the water content of
brain slices is described, and a method is given for correcting the observed
dry weight of tissue for the weight of dried solids from the medium.

A brief critique of four other methods for measuring extracellular space
in central nervous tissue is appended. These various methods are not equivalent; and the choice of a method should not be governed entirely by ease of
procedure, familiarity with techniques, and available equipment.

II. ESTIMATION OF THE EXTRACELLULAR SPACE
FROM THE PENETRATION OF "EXTRACELLULAR
SPACE MARKERS" *IN VITRO*

A. General Considerations

If a tissue is incubated with a marker until all the extracellular space,
and only the extracellular space, contains maker at the same concentration

as in the incubation medium, and if there is no binding of marker to tissue, then the fraction of extracellular space is equal to the ratio of the concentration of marker in the tissue to the final concentration of marker in the medium. Equilibration of tissue with a marker has been widely used on a variety of nonnervous tissues with satisfactory results. (This method has also been used *in vivo* on nonnervous tissues by introducing a nonmetabolizable marker into the bloodstream. Because of the blood–brain barrier, this cannot be done on central nervous system tissue.) In central nervous tissue,

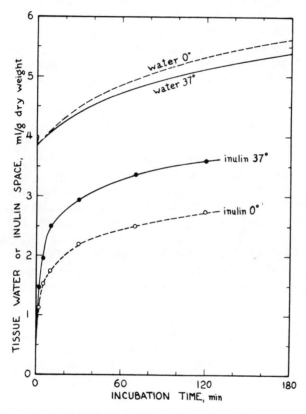

Fig. 1. Water content and inulin space of mouse cerebrum slices. Slices 0.0416 cm thick, prepared from one cerebral hemisphere without olfactory lobe of a 6- to 8-week-old Swiss mouse of either sex were placed in 5 ml of oxygenated tris-buffered Krebs-Ringer medium (Table II) at 0°C containing ^{14}C-inulin and carrier, and incubated at either 37° or 0°C. For incubation with inulin at 37°C for 5 min or less, slices were placed in 4.5 ml of inulin-free medium, preincubated at 37°C for 5 min, then 0.5 ml of medium containing ^{14}C-inulin and carrier was added and slices were incubated for the indicated period. Inulin was omitted from the determinations of tissue water. The difference in tissue water at 37° and 0°C may reflect experimental error (from Cohen *et al.*, 1968).

problems arise in the choice of a marker, and in the interpretation of the *second marker space* (pp. 187–191); it is also difficult to ensure complete penetration of the extracellular space with negligible penetration into cells. Other tissues, which in general deteriorate less during prolonged incubation, can be incubated for 24 hr or more, if necessary, until the marker space and total water no longer change with time. Prolonged incubation is rarely feasible with nervous tissue. Preparations may swell indefinitely during an incubation of several hours without showing any sign of approaching a limit (Fig. 1). In such cases, equilibration of extracellular space with marker may be assumed when the nonmarker space (total tissue water — marker space) no longer decreases with time (Fig. 2). If such a time cannot be found, the time required for equilibration may be estimated from equilibration times for the same marker in similar preparations and conditions in a medium where there is evidence of equilibration. In the author's experience, 20–30 min is the minimum time for equilibration with inulin, and incubation for 1 hr provides a large margin of safety. Note, however, that because of tissue swelling, marker spaces after 1 hr are often significantly larger than after 30 min (Fig. 1).

Although measurements of marker penetration are usually used to calculate the extracellular space in a preparation at the end of the incubation period, a series of such measurements for different incubation periods can be extrapolated back to zero incubation time to estimate the extracellular space in freshly killed tissue. By extrapolation of data for 0.10-cm-thick slices for rat brain, Allen (1955) estimated the marker space before incubation to be 0.17 ml/g tissue for ferrocyanide ion, and 0.145 ml/g tissue for inulin, values which are in concordance with estimates of *in vivo* extracellular space from conductance measurements, and from perfusion with artificial cerebrospinal fluid containing an extracellular space marker.

The measured marker space of brain slices, and similar preparations, contains a contribution from labeled marker in the film of medium adhering to the surface. By measuring the water content as function of slice thinness (reciprocal thickness) and extrapolating to zero thinness (infinitely thick slices), the film of adherent medium on cut surfaces of mouse cerebrum slices was estimated to be 0.00054 cm thick at 0 °C, and 0.00078 cm thick at 37 °C.* For slices nominally 0.0416 cm thick this surface film contributes a

---

* Slices ranging from 0.0156 to 0.0676 cm in nominal thickness were prepared from cerebral hemispheres less olfactory lobes of 6- to 8-week-old Swiss mice of either sex, as described by Blasberg and Lajtha (1965). The slices from one hemisphere (approximately 100–150 mg) were placed in 5 ml of oxygenated, standard HEPES- (N-2-hydroxyethylpiperazine-N'-ethanesulfonic acid)-buffered medium (Table II) at either 37° or 0°C, shaken just long enough to separate them completely (about 1 to 2 sec), then filtered off, frozen in solid carbon dioxide, and their dry weight determined as described in Section III (S. R. Cohen, work in progress).

tissue space of 0.13 ml/g dry weight at 0 °C and 0.19 ml/g dry weight at 37 °C. Since fresh mouse cerebrum contains 4.0 ml of water/g dry weight (20% dry weight), the relative error from this film is 3 and 5% respectively. (This estimated surface film is a maximum value that contains contributions from superficial swelling at the cut surfaces. The lower viscosity and surface tension of water at 37 °C should produce a thinner film than at 0 °C. The greater thickness may be due to greater swelling and deterioration of the cut surfaces.) More error is introduced by rinsing the preparation with unlabeled medium. Rinsing a similar preparation of 0.0416-cm-thick mouse cerebrum slices for 3 sec reduced the inulin space by 0.4 to 0.5 ml/g dry weight, which is equivalent to a film thickness of about 0.002 cm, $2\frac{1}{2}$ to 4 times the estimated maximum thickness of the surface film.*

B. Extracellular Spaces and Markers

1. "Ideal" Markers

An ideal "extracellular space marker" for central nervous system tissue should: (1) dissolve in aqueous media, (2) freely enter all extracellular liquids, (3) be completely excluded from cells, (4) diffuse rapidly into tissue, (5) have a sufficiently small molecular size to enter easily into microchannels and other fine extracellular structures, (6) be unaffected by metabolic processes, (7) be nontoxic, (8) not affect tissue metabolism, (9) not be native to the tissue, (10) be neither adsorbed nor absorbed by tissue or, in *in vitro* preparations, by cut surfaces, (11) be easily determined, and (12) in *in vivo* and *in situ* studies, not be removed from interstitial and cerebrospinal fluids by ependyma, membranes, choroid plexi, and similar structures. It is difficult to show that a given marker substance meets these requirements; none are known to meet all. In particular, there is no satisfactory way to demonstrate a substance fulfills requirements 2 and 3, which are absolutely essential for most marker methods. There is some evidence, mostly by autoradiography, that several widely used markers, including inulin, sucrose, dextran, D-mannitol, and sulfate, may enter some cellular compartment in nervous tissue under certain conditions (Nicholls and Wolfe, 1967; Brown *et al.*,

---

* Slices 0.0416 cm thick were prepared from cerebral hemispheres less olfactory lobes of 6- to 8-week-old Swiss mice, incubated at 37°C for 0.5–120 min in oxygenated, tris-buffered Krebs-Ringer medium (Table II) containing labeled inulin and carrier, then filtered with section on Whatman No. 50 hardened filter paper in a Büchner funnel, as previously described (Cohen *et al.*, 1968). Slices were rinsed by pouring 10 ml of inulin-free medium over them in the funnel, then draining rapidly with suction. They were frozen, weighed, homogenized, and counted, and the inulin space determined as described in Section III. Spaces were compared with spaces in similar but unrinsed preparations (Blasberg, Levi, and Lajtha, unpublished observations).

1969; Lehrer, 1969; Fenstermacher *et al.*, 1970a). Evidence for the exclusion of a marker from cells is indirect. If several marker substances indicate approximately the same space, this is presumed to be evidence that they all measure the same tissue compartment, which, hopefully, is the extracellular space. The commonly used extracellular space markers are probably widely accepted as reliable because they *are* commonly used, and because their molecular dimensions, properties, and structure make it unlikely *a priori* that they can enter cells.

2. Common Marker Substances

The most common marker substances are various nonmetabolized carbohydrates, such as inulin, sucrose, raffinose, mannitol, sorbitol, and dextran. Others are ions, including chloride, bromide, iodide, thiocyanate, sulfate, sodium, and, surprisingly, potassium; enzymes, usually peroxidase; and other proteins, such as ferritin, and radioiodinated- or fluorescence-labeled albumin.

The most widely used marker in both central nervous tissue and other tissue is inulin, a polysaccharide from various plant species. This is a linear fructose polymer with an initial glucose residue. Like other natural polysaccharides, it has a range of chain lengths. The number average molecular weight of commercial inulin is most often 5000 to 5500 (30 to 34 hexose residues), but may range from 500 (3 residues) to 21,000 (130 resideues), depending on the natural source, season of the year, and subsequent treatment (Phelps, 1965.) The polymer is stable in neutral and moderately basic solutions, but is degraded by acid. The ease of solution in water increases markedly with temperature (Phelps, 1965). It is difficult to dissolve at room temperature, but solutions containing 1–2% by weight can be easily prepared by gentle heating, and, once made, can be chilled without precipitating. The solubility of different preparations can differ greatly (Phelps, 1965). Inulin is commonly labeled either by adding a $-^{14}COOH$ group to the initial glucose residue, or by converting 5% or less of the hydroxyl groups to tritiated methoxy groups. (See Section III, B, Note 2, p. 196.)

Inulin has been reported to penetrate neurons in leech nerve cord (Nicholls and Wolfe, 1967), and cat sympathetic ganglia (Brown *et al.*, 1969). Contrary to some statements, the adsorption on cut surfaces, which has been inferred from a comparison of inulin spaces and protein marker spaces (Pappius *et al.*, Pappius, 1965) is not a serious artifact when inulin is used with brain slices. The localization of protein marker at cut surfaces that is observed in histological preparations probably represent precipitation during fixation and tissue preparation.

Sucrose is also extensively used as a marker. It is not metabolized by brain tissue, and equilibrates faster than inulin. Using autoradiography,

Lehrer (1969) has found some indication of penetration of sucrose into neurons in the puffer fish *(Spheroides maculatus)* central nervous system. The trisaccharide, raffinose [O-α-D-galactopyranosyl-(1→6)-O-α-D-glucopyranosyl-(1→2)-β-D-fructofuranoside] offers an interesting compromise between inulin and sucrose. It does not appear to be metabolized by nervous tissue. Because of its larger molecules there is less possibility of cellular penetration than with sucrose, while its smaller molecular size compared with inulin permits more rapid and complete equilibration with extracellular fluid. Because labeled raffinose is not available, its use is limited by the necessity for a chemical determination. (See p. 198, Note 15, for references to methods.) The sugar alcohols, D-mannitol and D-sorbitol, are unsatisfactory. Mannitol enters cells under certain conditions (Brown *et al., 1969*) and sorbitol is a minor constituent of central and peripheral nervous tissue (Sherman and Stewart, 1966; Stewart *et al., 1967*). The high molecular weight ($>20,000$) dextrans that have been used have no advantage over inulin, but may indicate a low space because of incomplete penetration and slow diffusion.

Although ions are extensively used to measure extracellular space, they are *a priori* poorer choices than inert carbohydrates, other things being equal, because there is less reason to believe that they cannot cross cell membranes in the absence of specific transporters. Many anions that are excluded from a good fraction of the tissue water may penetrate some cellular water either *in vivo* or *in vitro*. To the extent that they are excluded by a negative membrane potential and the Gibbs-Donnan equilibrium, they may penetrate cells in various *in vitro* preparations or in pathological conditions where these barriers are lower. For brain slices and similar preparations, and for *in vivo* perfusions, the most commonly used anions are thiocyanate, chloride, and sulfate. Thiocyanate and chloride are unsuitable. The thiocyanate space *in vitro* is usually appreciably higher than the inulin space, and is extremely sensitive to details of preparation, making comparisons of results by different workers less meaningful than with most other common markers. Thiocyanate binds to many proteins including serum albumin (Rosenbaum and Lavietes, 1939; Pollay *et al., 1968*). *In vivo*, thiocyanate is rapidly removed from cerebrospinal fluid by the choroid plexi; this must be corrected for, or overcome by saturating the transport system with an excess of thiocyanate ions or by using an inhibitor. *In vitro* chloride spaces at body temperature have been reported to be similar to thiocyanate spaces. Measurements at 0 °C are not available. Although tissue chloride is largely extracellular, chloride is present within cells in significant concentrations, and therefore the tissue chloride "space" should not be equated with the extracellular space. The partial exclusion of Cl⁻ ions from cellular water is almost certainly the result of a negative membrane potential and the Gibbs-Donnan equilibrium coupled with continuous pumping of entering sodium ions out of the cells, rather than any inherent barrier to crossing cell membranes. Sulfate may be as suitable an anionic marker as any. In isotonic medium (Cohen and Lajtha, 1970), and by perfusion *in vivo,* sulfate spaces are similar to those indicated by carbohydrates. If the tonicity of the medium is altered by varying the NaCl content, the sulfate space, compared with carbohydrate spaces, changes (Cohen and Lajtha, 1970), which suggests that electrostatic forces are at least partly responsible for the exclusion of sulfate from cells. Iodide has frequently been used both *in vivo* and *in vitro,* but has no real advantages. Unless prevented, it is rapidly removed from *in vivo* and *in situ* preparations by the choroid plexi. The low intracellular sodium ion content of living nervous tissue is due to continuous excretion of entering Na^+ by the $Na^+ - K^+$-pump. The intracellular Na^+ content of brain slices is much higher, even when precautions are taken to minimize alterations from living tissue. Radioisotopes of Na^+, K^+, and Cl^- have been used to estimate the extracellular space by kinetic analysis of efflux data under steady-state conditions, a method which is insensitive to cellular penetration (Section IV, A). The anion $^{60}Co\text{-}EDTA^{2-}$ has been used to measure extracellular space in smooth muscle (Brading and Jones, 1969), but has not been tried in neural tissue.

Enzymes and other proteins are poor choices. Their large size compared with inulin means a longer incubation time for equilibration with extracellular fluid, and more complete exclusion from microchannels and other extracellular structures of macromolecular dimensions; and their many highly polar groups may promote tissue binding. Entry of peroxidase (Becker *et al.,* 1968) and ferritin molecules [94 Å diameter (Farrant 1954)] (Rosenbluth and Wissing, 1964; Brightman, 1965; Selwood, 1970) into neuronal and glial cell bodies and processes shows that the principal argument for such large molecules, the supposition that they are more completely excluded from cells, is false.

3. Effect of Marker, Incubation Temperature, Incubation Medium, and Other Factors on the Marker Space

The *in vitro* marker space depends greatly upon the marker, the incubation temperature, and the incubation time, as well as the species, the medium, and details of preparation and technique. Typical spaces for a variety of central nervous tissue preparations and conditions are listed in Tables I and II. To aid in the comparison of various markers, the percentage increase in the space compared to the inulin space under the same conditions is given in Table I.

Many workers have found that the space shown by carbohydrate markers both *in vitro* and *in vivo* varies inversely with the molecular size of the marker, for example, inulin space < raffinose space < sucrose space < sugar alcohol spaces, for a wide variety of preparations and conditions (Table I; Table II; Cohen and Lajtha, 1970; Cohen *et al.*, 1970). This relation is not peculiar to brain tissue, but occurs in many tissues, including muscle (Barr and Malvin, 1965; Page, 1965; Goodford and Leach, 1966; Law and Phelps, 1966; Brading and Jones, 1969) and lens (Thoft and Kino-shita, 1965). Bourke and Tower (1966) report identical sucrose and inulin spaces in cat cerebral cortex slices, and Ames and Nesbett (1966) report the mannitol and inulin spaces to be the same in rabbit retina. In HEPES-(N-2-hydroxyethylpiperazine-N'-2-ethanesulfonic acid) -buffered isotonic medium the sulfate space of mouse cerebrum slices is greater than the sucrose space but less than the spaces shown by the sugar alcohols, D-mannitol and D-sorbitol (Table I; Cohen *et al.*, 1970). In a similar HEPES-buffered medium made hypotonic by reducing the NaCl concentration by 65 mM the sulfate space of the same preparation is less than the insulin space (Table II), while in a similar HEPES-buffered medium made hypertonic by increasing the NaCl concentration by 400 mM, the sulfate space is about the same as the spaces indicated by D-mannitol and D-sorbitol (Cohen and Lajtha, 1970). Chloride and thiocyanate spaces are generally appreciably higher than inulin or sucrose spaces. Other properties of the marker molecule besides size and charge may be important. In some media the spaces indicated by the structural isomers, D-mannitol and D-sorbitol, are appreciably different (Cohen and Lajtha, 1970).

The penetration of an extracellular space marker depends on the incubation temperature. In a variety of media the spaces indicated by inulin, sucrose, D-sorbitol, D-mannitol, and sulfate are greater at 37 °C than 0 °C, even when total tissue water is the same at both temperatures. Figure 1 shows this effect for inulin. Cohen and co-workers have concluded that this increased penetration of markers at 37 °C represents entry of the markers into a distinct tissue compartment, which they call the *second marker space* (Cohen *et al.*, 1968; Cohen and Lajtha, 1970; Cohen *et al.*, 1970). To a first approximation, they consider the second marker space to act like a tissue compartment which is permeable to extracellular space markers at 37 °C but impermeable at 0 °C. [Varon and McIlwain's (1961) data for guinea pig cerebral cortex slices show penetration by inulin of the second space at 37 °C and exclusion at 20 °C (Cohen *et al.*, 1970).] In several media the D-glutamate space of mouse cerebrum slices at 0 °C is equal to the inulin space at 37 °C (Cohen *et al.*, 1968; Cohen and Lajtha, 1970; Cohen *et al.*, 1970). This has been interpreted as showing the continuing existence at 0 °C of a tissue compartment corresponding to the 37 °C inulin space. In spite

Table I. *In Vitro* Marker Spaces in the Central Nervous System

Preparation	Incubation time (min)	Incubation temperature (°C)	Conditions	Marker	Space, % initial wet wt.	% Increase over inulin space	Reference
Mouse cerebrum[a]	60+10	37	0.0416-cm-thick slices in standard HEPES-buffered medium (Table II)	Inulin	66		
				Sucrose	75	14	
				D-Mannitol	84	27	Cohen et al. (1970)
				D-Sorbitol	84	27	
				Sulfate	76	15	Cohen and Lajtha (1970)
				Thiocyanate	94	42	
Mouse cerebrum[a]	60+10	0	0.0416-cm-thick slices in standard HEPES-buffered medium (Table II)	Inulin	56		
				Sucrose	67	20	Cohen et al. (1970)
				D-Mannitol	72	29	
				D-Sorbitol	73	30	
				Sulfate	69	23	Cohen and Lajtha (1970)
				Thiocyanate	107	91	
Mouse cerebrum[a]	20+10	37	0.0416-cm-thick slices in high-salt HEPES-buffered medium (Table II)	Inulin	80		
				Sucrose	89	11	Cohen and Lajtha (1970)
				D-Mannitol	95	19	
				D-Sorbitol	97	21	
				Sulfate	92	15	
				Thiocyanate	114	42	
Cat cerebral cortex	65	37	First slice, 0.045–0.05 cm thick, in bicarbonate-buffered medium containing 27.4 mM K$^+$	^{14}C-Inulin	40		
				Raffinose	46	15	Bourke and Tower (1966)
				^{14}C-Sucrose	45	12	
	60			Chloride	64	60	
	65			Thiocyanate	64	60	

Table I (Continued)

Preparation	Incubation time (min)	Incubation temperature (°C)	Conditions	Marker	Space, % initial wet wt.	% Increase over inulin space	Reference
Rat cerebral cortex	60	38 (oxygenated in ice)	0.05-cm-thick slices in bicarbonate-buffered Ringer medium	Inulin	54		Pappius et al. (1962)
				Sucrose	74	37	
				Thiocyanate	85	57	
				Protein	47	-13	
Cat subcortical white matter	60	38	Over 0.05-cm-thick slices in bicarbonate-buffered Ringer medium	Inulin	50		Pappius et al. (1962)
				Sucrose	80	60	
				Thiocyanate	90	80	
Frog whole brain (Rana pipiens)[b]	30	room temperature (?)		Inulin (A)	15.8	-9	Bradbury et al. (1968)
				Inulin (B)	17.3	(standard)	
				Sulfate	22.0	27	
				Sucrose	22.1	28	
				^{36}Cl	24.4	41	
				^{24}Na	27.9	63	

[a] Incubation was for 60 min or 20 min with marker after a 10-min preincubation without marker, both at the indicated temperature. Spaces were computed from values in references assuming an initial dry weight of 20.7%.
[b] Two samples of inulin were used with B giving consistently larger spaces than A. I have arbitrarily taken B as the standard.

Table II.   37°C Spaces and Second Marker Spaces in Mouse Cerebrum Slices[a]

Medium	Marker	Marker space at 37°C (ml/g dry wt. or dry tissue)	Second space at 37°C	Second space as % of marker space	Reference
Standard	Inulin	2.18	0.51	16	Cohen et al.
HEPES-buffered	Sucrose	3.65	0.44	12	(1970)
(isotonic)	D-Mannitol	4.05	0.58	14	
	Sulfate	3.65	0.36	10	
Low-salt	Inulin	3.32	0.68	21	Cohen and
HEPES-buffered	Sucrose	3.44	0.53	16	Lajtha
(hypotonic)	D-Mannitol	4.31	1.06	25	(1970)
	Sulfate	2.75	0.16	9	
High-salt	Inulin	4.65	0.94	20	Cohen and
HEPES-buffered	Sucrose	5.19	1.01	19	Lajtha
(hypertonic)	D-Mannitol	5.72	1.24	22	(1970)
	Sulfate	5.43	0.92	17	
Choline chloride	Inulin	3.38	0.07	2	Cohen and
HEPES-buffered	Sucrose	5.07	0.94	18	Lajtha
(hypertonic)	Sulfate	4.32	0.38	9	(1970)
Tris-buffered, modified	Inulin	3.37	0.94	28	Cohen et al.
Krebs-Ringer					(1968)

[a] Slices, 0.0416 cm thick, were prepared from cerebral hemispheres, without olfactory lobes of 6- to 8-week-old Swiss mice of either sex. All spaces were measured after 10 min preincubation without marker followed by 60 min incubation with marker, except the spaces in modified Krebs-Ringer medium, which were measured after 70 min incubation with marker and no preincubation. Values in high-salt and choline chloride media were corrected for the excess nonvolatile solids from medium, in dried tissue (pp. 202–203). *Media:* Standard HEPES-buffered: 119 mM NaCl, 5.0 mM KCl, 0.75 mM CaCl$_2$, 1.2 mM MgSO$_4$, 1.0 mM NaH$_2$PO$_4$, 25 mM HEPES, 12 mM NaOH, and 10 mM glucose; low-salt HEPES-buffered, 54 mM NaCl, otherwise like standard medium; high-salt HEPES-buffered; 519 mM NaCl, otherwise like standard medium; choline chloride HEPES-buffered: standard HEPES-buffered medium with 400 mM choline Cl added; Krebs-Ringer: 128 mM NaCl, 5.0 mM KCl, 2.7 mM CaCl$_2$, 1.2 mM MgSO$_4$, 5 mM Na$_2$HPO$_4$, 50 mM tris-tris·HCl buffer adjusted to pH 7.4 at room temperature, and 10 mM glucose.

of large changes in total tissue water and marker space depending on the composition and tonicity of the incubation medium, the second space, after correction for any difference in total water content at the two temperatures, is for the most part between 0.5 and 1.0 ml/g dry tissue (Table II), and, as Fig. 2 shows, only slightly affected by incubation time. Obviously the fraction of the 37 °C marker space contributed by the second space (Table II) varies widely. The second marker space has been demonstrated *in vitro* only in slices of mature mammalian brain, and possibly in chick brain (Levi and Lattes, 1970) by comparing measurements made at 37 °C and 0 °C. Except for the subarachnoid perfusion studies by Fenstermacher et al., (1970a) that show somewhat less penetration of sucrose and mannitol at

15 °C than at 37 °C (Table IV), there are no data for or against a second space effect in living brain.

Unlike other markers, thiocyanate shows a greater space at 0 °C than at 37°C possibly because of greater binding by tissue proteins at the lower temperature (Cohen and Lajtha, 1970).

In media containing 27 mM K$^+$ ion, Bourke and Tower (1966) reported a significantly smaller sucrose or inulin space in cat cortex slices incubated for 65 min if marker was present only during the final 20 min. After 2 hr of incubation, the sucrose space was the same whether sucrose was present

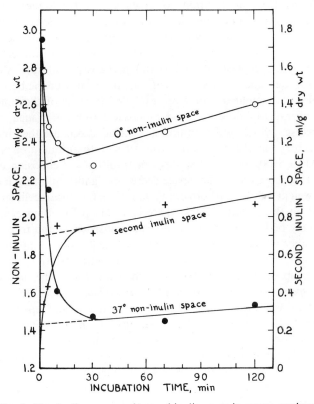

Fig. 2. Non-inulin spaces and second inulin space in mouse cerebrum slices. The non-inulin space at each temperature is the difference between the total tissue water and the inulin space, both measured at that temperature. The second inulin space is the difference between the inulin space at 37°C and the inulin space at 0°C. These spaces are calculated from data in Fig. 1. (From Cohen *et al.*, 1968.)

throughout the period or added only after 40 min of preincubation. These observations may indicate decreasing permeability of some tissue compartment during the course of incubation.

C. Recommended Markers and Conventions

Because of the phenomena described above—the dependence of the observed space on the marker selected, the dependence of the space on the incubation temperature (the second marker space phenomenon), and the decreased permeability of the marker space, in some cases, upon prolonged incubation—the measurement of *in vitro* extracellular space by penetration of markers involves, in addition to problems of technique, important, unresolved questions of interpretation. Among markers, cations are unacceptable because of the strong likelihood of passage through cell membranes. Although there is less evidence for the penetration of anions into cells, most, with the possible exception of sulfate and perhaps perchlorate, should be mistrusted for the same reason. Inert carbohydrates may be the best choices. If high molecular weight dextrans are excluded because of their molecular bulk and low rates of diffusion, and monosaccharides and sugar alcohols such as fructose, xylose, and mannitol are excluded because they may enter cells, satisfactory markers can range from sucrose to an inulin of molecular weight 5000 to 5500, with no basis except tradition for choosing one over another; yet, because the marker space decreases significantly with increasing molecular weight of the carbohydrate, the observed "extracellular" space will depend on this choice. Unless there is a reason for using a particular marker, it may be best, for convenience and consistency, and to permit the greatest number of comparisons with published data, to use inulin. At best the selection of a marker substance is to a great extent arbitrary. For clarity the measured space should be designated the *inulin space,* the *sucrose space,* the *sulfate space,* etc., rather than the *extracellular space.* All computed quantities that require a knowledge of the extracellular space, such as intracellular and extracellular concentrations of amino acids, ions, etc., should be considered, and referred to as operationally defined or conventional values rather than "true" values, and the method used to measure the "extracellular" space should be stated explicitly.

The problem raised by the second marker space is more vexing. The *in vitro* marker space of mature mammalian brain tissue incubated at 37 °C (body temperature) contains the second marker space, and the marker space of such tissue incubated at 0 °C does not. Therefore these two spaces are qualitatively different. Because the physical tissue compartment corresponding to the second marker space is not known, it is impossible to say which space better represents the "true" extracellular space. Because no substance is known to be excluded at 37 °C from the second space, it seems reasonable, as well as consistent with current practice, to use the 37 °C marker space without correction for the second space as the conventional functional extracellular space at 37 °C. The proper convention for the functional extracellular space at 0 °C is less clear. Data for the uptake of D-glutamate by brain slices at 0 °C and some uptake data for L-lysine (Cohen *et al.*, 1968; Cohen and Lajtha, 1970; Cohen *et al.*, 1970) indicate that for these amino acids the functional extracellular space at 0 °C should include the second marker space, even though carbohydrate markers and sulfate ions are excluded from the second space. This same functional extracellular space might well be used for other amino acids since they enter tissue at 0 °C to the same or a greater extent. With this convention, the extracellular space at 0 °C is taken to be the marker space at 37 °C corrected for any difference in total tissue water at these two temperatures (see pp. 203–204 and Fig. 4); not the 0 °C marker space. At present there is no indication of whether or not the functional extracellular space at 0 °C, for any other tissue components, such as K^+, Na^+, or Cl^-, should include the second marker space. A typical example of the effect of the second marker space on θ_{in}, the calculated relative intracellular concentration of a substrate (that is, the ratio of the intracellular concentration to the concentration in the medium) is shown by Fig. 3. The intracellular and tissue concentration are linearly related by $\theta_{in} = (100/S_{in})\theta_{tis} - (S_{ex}/S_{in})$, where S_{in} and S_{ex} are the intracellular and extracellular water compartments respectively in percent of tissue final wet weight, and θ_{tis} is the observed relative tissue concentration. [$S_{in} + S_{ex}$ = total tissue water space $\equiv 100 - (\%$ dry weight).] At high tissue levels of substrate the intracellular concentrations calculated on these two bases approach a constant ratio, $\theta'_{in}/\theta_{in} = S_{in}/S'_{in}$ (1.23 for the example shown), where *primed* quantities are based on including the second marker space in the extracellular space, and *unprimed* quantities are based on the extracellular space observed at 0°; the difference between θ'_{in} and θ_{in} increases steadily. At equilibration of substrate with all tissue water without concentrative uptake, $\theta_{tis} = (100 - \%$ dry weight)/100 (0.85 for the example shown), and $\theta'_{in} = \theta_{in} = 1$; and at lower relative tissue concentrations reflecting partial exclusion of substrate from tissue water, $\theta'_{in} < \theta_{in}$. Estimation of the functional extracellular space from a marker space in systems other than mature mammalian brain, or at intermediate temperatures, must be done with extreme caution, because virtually nothing is known about the second space in such cases.

The decision to include, exclude, or ignore the existence of the second space, like the choice of a marker, defines a *conventional* extracellular space which bears an unknown relation to the so far unmeasurable "true"

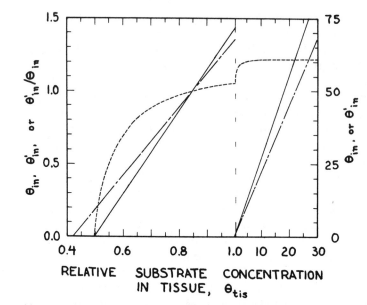

Fig. 3. The effect on computed intracellular concentrations of including the second marker space in the functional low-temperature extracellular space. —— – —— θ_{in}, relative intracellular concentration of substrate (concentration in cells/concentration in medium) computed assuming the functional extracellular space to be the observed low-temperature marker space; ———θ'_{in}, relative intracellular concentration of substrate computed assuming the functional extracellular space to consist of the low-temperature marker space plus the second marker space; - - - - - - - - θ'_{in}/θ_{in}. Note the change in scale at $\theta_{tis} = 1$. Read values of θ_{in} and θ'_{in} at $\theta_{tis} < 1$ and values of θ'_{in}/θ_{in} for all values of θ_{tis} from the left-hand scale; and values of θ_{in} and θ'_{in} for $\theta_{tis} \geq 1$ from the right-hand scale. The figure is based on $S_{in} = 43.0\%$, $S_{ex} = 41.6\%$, and $S_{second} = 7.9\%$ final wet weight of tissue from the penetration of inulin into mouse cerebrum slices incubated in standard HEPES-buffered medium for 60 min plus 10 min preincubation without marker (Table I). (Values from this figure should not be used for calculations as θ_{in}, θ'_{in}, and θ'_{in}/θ_{in} depend on the preparation and the marker.)

extracellular space. The best that can be said from comparing measurements with various markers at various temperatures and the results from other techniques for measuring the extracellular space is that the true extracellular space lies within certain more or less well-defined limits. This may be satisfactory for some purposes.

III. METHOD FOR DETERMINING MARKER SPACE IN BRAIN SLICES

A. Procedure

The author uses the following procedure to determine the marker space in brain slices prepared with a McIlwain tissue chopper (McIlwain and Buddle, 1953). With suitable modifications it can be used to determine *in vitro* marker spaces in other preparations, and the uptake of various other substrates by such preparations.

1. If preincubation is not required, incubate tissue slices, with shaking, at the desired temperature in medium containing radiolabeled marker and unlabeled carrier marker for a period sufficient for equilibration. For 150 mg or less of tissue use 5 ml of medium in a 25-ml stoppered Erlenmeyer flask. If preincubation is required, incubate in 4.5 ml of medium without labeled marker for the preincubation period, then add 0.5 ml of medium containing labeled marker at 10 times the desired final concentration and continue incubation until equilibrium is established. (Twenty to 30 min is required to equilibrate 0.0416-cm-thick mouse cerebrum slices prepared with a tissue chopper. See Section II, A for a discussion of equilibration times.)

2. End the incubation by filtering off slices using a No. 1 Büchner funnel with a 5.5-cm-diameter Whatman No. 54 hardened filter paper. *As soon as the last liquid has passed through the filter, disconnect the vacuum.*

3. Scrape the brain slices from the surface of the filter paper to form a pellet. Freeze the pellet for at least 2 min by covering it completely with dry-ice snow.

4. Weigh the pellet to 0.05 mg.

5. Homogenize the frozen pellet in 2 ml of 5% by weight perchloric acid (0.5 M) in a Potter-Elvehjem tissue homogenizer.

6. Centrifuge the homogenate for 3–5 min at 10,000 g.

7. If inulin is used for the marker substance, heat the clear supernatant for 30 min at 80–90 °C, or allow it to stand at room temperature for 4 hr. (Omit this step with other markers.)

8. Take 0.5 ml of supernatant for liquid scintillation counting.

9. Prepare references by pipetting 100 μl of medium containing labeled marker and carrier into 2 ml of the perchloric acid. If the marker is inulin, heat or let stand at room temperature as in step 7 above. Take 0.5 ml for counting.

B. Notes

1. Unlabeled carrier for inulin and other carbohydrates, at a final concentration of 0.4 mg/ml, is added as a precaution against adsorption on

tissue or glassware, but can be omitted if desired. [The same values are obtained when carrier inulin or sucrose is omitted (S. R. Cohen, unpublished).] Inulin concentrations of up to 1 % (w/v) have been used without affecting brain slices (Varon and McIlwain, 1961). Such concentrations are necessary if inulin is to be determined colorimetrically.

2. It is essential that the inulin contain no appreciable quantity of fructose, sucrose, or low molecular weight oligosaccharides. The quality of radioinulin varies greatly with supplier. It should be tested, and purified if necessary, by semimicro gel filtration chromatography (S. R. Cohen, 1969) or some other suitable method. Thin-layer chromatography on Sephadex G-75, and paper chromatography, which are often used by suppliers to measure radiopurity, will not show low molecular weight fragments in inulin. If the molecular weight is sufficiently high (say, about 5000), moderate variation in molecular weight will not affect the measurements. ^{14}C-carboxyl- and ^{3}H-methoxy-labeled inulin give identical results (Cohen et al., 1970). ^{14}C-hydroxymethylinulin and ^{3}H-inulin, both with molecular weights of 5000 to 5500, are now available.* We have not tested them but they should be as satisfactory as other labeled inulins with the same molecular weight distribution.

3. Media must be heated gently to dissolve the inulin. Once prepared, solutions can be refrigerated for several weeks without precipitation.

4. The author incubates brain slices in a thermostatted bath at a shaking rate of 100 to 110 strokes/min. A reciprocating shaker is used rather than one with swirling ("gyrotary") motion, because oxygenation and mixing of the medium, which occur chiefly at each reversal of direction, may be better. The best shaking rate is somewhat of a problem, although less so in measurements of marker spaces than in other studies. Preliminary studies (S. R. Cohen, unpublished) indicate that the minimum shaking rate for optimum oxygenation may damage tissue upon prolonged incubations.

5. Medium is added to flasks, which are then oxygenated, stoppered, and shaken at the incubation temperature for at least 15 min before tissue is added. Tissue is added with no additional oxygenation. This procedure ensures that tissue is placed in well-oxygenated medium, and eliminates both "dead time" and any artifacts arising from the uncontrolled period of partial anoxia which is present when the medium is oxygenated after adding the tissue.

6. Filtering must be done carefully to remove nonadhering medium without drying the tissue. If nonadherent medium is not removed, the observed inulin space will be high because the specific activity of the medium is greater than that of the tissue. If air is drawn past the tissue after non-

---

* Amersham/Searle Corp., Arlington Heights, Ill. 60005, U.S.A.; the Radio-Chemical Centre, Amersham in the U.K.

adherent medium has been filtered off, the inulin space will be high because the tissue will lose water without losing counts. Whatman No. 50 hardened filter paper can also be used with 0.0416-cm-thick brain slices. Filtration is slower, and this paper is clogged by thinner brain slices.

7. Tissue is frozen to produce a hard pellet that can be handled. Surprisingly, freezing time is not critical. There is little deposition of frost, probably because gaseous carbon dioxide from the dry ice largely prevents water vapor from diffusing to the surface of the pellet. Any frost or solid carbon dioxide on the surface should be chipped off. If this is done properly, frost will not introduce any measurable error.

8. The procedure given is for preparations where the initial weight of tissue cannot be measured or where tissue cannot be recovered completely after incubation, and gives spaces referred to the final wet weight. (These spaces can be converted to spaces based on initial wet weight, dry weight of tissue, DNA content, etc., if desired. See Section III, C.) If the preparation can be weighed before incubation and subsequently recovered completely, as, for example, single first or second cortical slices, it may be weighed before incubation, and formation of a pellet, freezing, and weighing after incubation omitted. Spaces will then be referred to the initial weight of tissue.

9. The contribution of labeled medium adhering to the surface of the slices is small; greater error is introduced by rinsing the tissue with medium that does not contain the labeled marker. (See p. 183). If the same preparation with the same technique for incubating, removing, and weighing the tissue is also being used to measure the *in vitro* uptake of some substrate, no correction is necessary for the contribution of labeled medium adhering to the surfaces of slices when computing the intracellular concentration of substrate because this contribution will be canceled.

10. The supernatants and references must be heated or left standing (step 7) to hydrolyze the inulin to fructose; otherwise inulin may gradually precipitate from the scintillation mixture, reducing the counting efficiency. Inulin precipitates more readily from the references because of their higher concentrations, producing high values for the inulin space. Because this precipitation does not affect the efficiency of the scintillation mixture, it cannot be monitored with an external standard, or with an added internal standard; but it will change the channels ratio. When counting ^{14}C-labeled inulin, one channel should be set for counting ^{3}H. When comparing counts of the same sample made several days apart, precipitation will be indicated by an increase in both the $(^{3}H/^{14}C)$-channels ratio and the count in the ^{3}H-channel, and a decrease in the count in the ^{14}C-channel. Even if there is no change in the counts and in the channel ratio, if the $(^{3}H/^{14}C)$-channels ratio is significantly different for the references than for the tissue supernatants, the results are suspect.

11. If mono- and disaccharides, chloride, sulfate, thiocyanate, or other marker substances that do not precipitate from the scintillation mixture are used, it is not necessary to heat the supernatants and references, or to let them stand.

12. A 100-μl sample of medium is taken to prepare the reference because the slices from one mouse cerebral hemisphere give a pellet containing about 100 mg of water. If the tissue adds an appreciably different quantity of water, the volume taken for the reference should be adjusted to avoid any possible change in counting efficiency from a different quantity of perchloric acid. Omission of tissue or tissue extract from the reference does not affect the counting efficiency (S. R. Cohen, unpublished).

13. Any scintillation mixture that is miscible with the perchloric acid tissue extracts and does not precipitate the marker substance is satisfactory. We use 16 ml per vial of a modified Prockop-Ebert scintillation mixture (Blasberg and Lajtha, 1965) with the composition: 2,5-diphenyloxazole (PPO), 7.5 g; 1,4-bis-2-(5-phenyloxazolyl)-benzene (POPOP), 35 mg; toluene, 1000 ml; and ethylene glycol monomethyl ether (methyl cellosolve), 600 ml.

14. The counting error should be the same or somewhat less than the cumulative random manipulative error. Assuming an error of 1–2% from pipetting, weighing, and handling tissue, etc., activities should be chosen to give a total of 5000 to 10,000 counts above background, which will give a counting error from the random nature of disintegrations of 1.4–1%. For three 10-min counts in a modern, refrigerated, liquid scintillation counter of 0.5 ml of aqueous sample in the modified Prockop-Ebert scintillation mixture, the incubation medium should contain about 0.05 μCi/ml of ^{14}C, or 0.15 μCi/ml of ^{3}H. Suitable channel settings for both single-label and double-label counting of such samples in a Packard Tri-Carb refrigerated liquid scintillation counter are: lower discriminator 150, upper discriminator 1000, gain 20% for ^{14}C; and lower discriminator 50, upper discriminator 300, gain 58% for ^{3}H.

15. Raffinose, sucrose, and unlabeled inulin are determined colorimetrically. A method for inulin is given by Varon and McIlwain (1961), and a method for the fructose formed by the acid hydrolysis of inulin, raffinose, or sucrose, by Kulka (1956). The latter is reported to be reliable, and is widely used [see Law and Phelps, (1966)]. (We have not tested any colorimetric methods.)

C. Computations and Bases for Expressing Marker Spaces

1. Bases

The method of computation given in Section III, C, 3b refers the marker space to the wet weight of tissue after incubation. This basis changes with the extent of swelling; a basis that is independent of swelling is to be preferred. Satisfactory common bases are dry weight of tissue, initial wet weight, and weight of protein. DNA is not suitable because the measured DNA content of brain tissue depends greatly on the method used, and, in addition, the procedures are tedious and difficult. [Compare, for example, Zamenhof *et al.,* (1964); Penn and Suwalski (1969).] Therefore, even if reproducible, consistent DNA assays are obtained, the experimenter cannot have confidence that measurements on different preparations are comparable.

2. Measurement of Fraction of Dry Weight of Tissue

Because slices prepared with a McIlwain tissue chopper and handled as described in the Procedure cannot readily be recovered completely, the initial wet weight and fraction of dry weight after incubation must be measured on parallel preparations. Loss of soluble materials during incubation, which would decrease the observed fraction of dry weight, is negligible (Bourke and Tower, 1966). When tissue is dried, there is some decomposition before the last trace of free water has been driven off. Until tissue drying has been studied in detail, the fraction of dry weight will depend slightly on the procedure with no obvious criterion for choosing among accepted methods. It is best to adopt one procedure that appears to be satisfactory and use it consistently.

The author uses the following method to measure dry weight:

a) Process parallel preparations, with the radioactive label omitted, through to the stage of a frozen tissue pellet (Procedure, steps 1 to 3).

b) Weigh the pellet on a tared planchet to 0.05 mg.

c) Dry the pellet on the planchet in an oven at 100 °C for 24 hr.

d) Cool to room temperature and reweigh on the planchet.

e) Dry for an additional 24 hr, and reweigh to check on the completeness of drying. The two dry weights should be within 0.2 mg of each other.

3. Formulas for Computing Tissue Spaces

The following formulas give tissue spaces in terms of weight, either percentage by weight, or grams per gram of tissue or tissue component. To compute spaces in terms of volume, the density of the liquid in the space is needed. This is usually not known. The common convention is to assume a density of 1, thereby making spaces in terms of weight and spaces in terms of volume the same.

a. Definitions of the Symbols Appearing in This Section and in the Two Following Sections.

A = volume of aliquot of tissue extract taken for counting, in milliliters.

A_R = volume of aliquot of perchloric acid solution of reference taken for counting, in milliliters.

B = volume of perchloric acid used to homogenize tissue pellet, in milliliters.

B_R= volume of perchloric acid used to prepare reference solution, in milliliters.

C = sample counts, or, if different counting times are used for different samples or for sample and reference, sample counts per unit time.

C_R = reference counts, or, if different counting times are used for reference and sample, reference counts per unit time.

D = observed dry weight of tissue after incubation, in percent of final wet weight.

$D°$ = dry weight of tissue, in percent of initial wet weight.

f = dilution factor to convert concentration of labeled substrate in solution used to prepare reference to concentration of labeled substrate in incubation medium.

I = concentration in tissue, in g/g final wet weight of tissue, of indifferent nonvolatile solute used to increase medium tonicity.

L = volume of sample of labeled medium or stock solution added to perchloric acid, to prepare the reference, in milliliters.

m = molecular weight of indifferent nonvolatile solute used to increase medium tonicity.

M = molarity of indifferent nonvolatile solute in incubation medium.

R = equivalent activity of reference, in counts/ml of medium, counting interval.

S = marker space, in percent by weight of final wet weight of tissue.

$S°$ = marker space, in percent by weight of initial wet weight of tissue.

S_I = equivalent tissue space of indifferent nonvolatile solute used to increase medium tonicity, in percent by weight of final wet weight.

V = marker space, in g/g dry weight.

V' = corrected marker space, in g/g dry tissue.

V_w = water content of tissue, in g/g dry weight.

V_w' = corrected water content of tissue, in g/g dry tissue.

V_w^H = water content of tissue at high temperature (usually 37°C), in g/g dry weight.

V_w^L = water content of tissue at low temperature (usually 0°C), in g/g dry weight.

V_1 = "first marker space" = marker space at low temperature (usually 0°), in g/g dry weight.

V_1^H = hypothetical space at high temperature (usually 37°C) corresponding to the "first marker space," in g/g dry weight.

V_2 = "second marker space," in g/g dry weight.

$V_2{}^H$ = "second marker space" at high temperature (usually 37 °C), in g/g dry weight.

$V_2{}^L$ = "second marker space" at low temperature (usually 0 °C), in g/g dry weight.

V_3 = marker space at high temperature (usually 37°C), in g/g dry weight.

$V_3{}^L$ = hypothetical space at low temperature (usually 0°C) corresponding to high-temperature marker space, in g/g dry weight.

w = weight of tissue pellet recovered from incubation, in grams.

$w°$ = initial weight of tissue, in grams.

(In the above, *dry weight* refers to observed dry weight of tissue; *dry tissue* refers to dry weight of tissue minus its content of nonvolatile solute that was added to the medium to increase tonicity.)

b. Marker Space in Percent by Weight of Final Wet Weight. This is given by

$$\text{where} \qquad S = 100C\,[B+(1-0.01D)w]/AwR \qquad (1)$$

$$R = C_R\,[(B_R+L)/A_RL]f \qquad (2)$$

If a sample of the labeled incubation medium is used for preparing the reference, $f = 1$. If the tissue was preincubated without labeled marker, and a stock solution containing label was added subsequently, and if a sample of this stock solution was used to prepare the reference, then f = (volume of stock solution added to the medium) ÷ (total volume of incubation medium after the addition). For the addition of 0.5 ml of labeled stock to 4.5 ml of medium as recommended above, $f = 0.1$.

In Eq. (1), the term $(1-0.01D)w$ is a correction for the water in the tissue pellet, which increases the volume of perchloric acid homogenate. Because the amount of tissue water is small compared to the volume of perchloric acid, this term can be approximated satisfactorily by neglecting the swelling of tissue during incubation, and taking $D \approx D° = 20$, the percentage of dry weight in fresh mature brain tissue. If the volumes recommended in the Procedure are taken, Eqs. (1) and (2) may be further simplified to

$$\text{and} \qquad S = C\,(400+160w)/wR \qquad (3)$$

$$R = 42\,C_R f \qquad (4)$$

c. Marker Space in Grams per Gram Dry Weight. This is given by

$$\text{or} \qquad V = S/D \qquad (5)$$

$$V = S\,(V_w+1)/100 \qquad (6)$$

d. Marker Space in Percent by Weight of Initial Weight. This is given by

$$S^\circ = SD^\circ/D \tag{7}$$

If the weight of the preparation before incubation is known, and if the tissue can be recovered completely after incubation, S° may be computed from

or
$$S^\circ = 100C \, [B + (1 - 0.01D^\circ) \, w^\circ]/AwR, \tag{8}$$
$$S^\circ \approx 100C(B^\circ + 0.8w^\circ)/Aw^\circ R \tag{9}$$

This approximate relation assumes that $D^\circ = 20$.

If the volumes recommended in the Procedure are taken, then Eq. (9) becomes

$$S^\circ = C \, (400 + 160w^\circ)/w^\circ R \tag{10}$$

4. Corrections for the Weight in Dried Tissue of Nonvolatile Solutes from the Medium

The observed dry weight of incubated tissues includes the weight of nonvolatile solutes from the medium that remain after the water has been driven off. No correction for medium solutes is necessary for observed dry weights of tissue incubated in most isotonic media, because the contribution of such solids to the dry weight is small, and is approximately the same as the contribution of nonvolatile solutes in interstitial fluid and cerebrospinal fluid to the dry weight of fresh tissue. The weight of such solids in tissue incubated in highly hypertonic media may be considerable, and obscrved dry weights should be corrected for their content of medium solutes in excess of the amount contributed by isotonic media or extracellular fluids (Cohen and Lajtha, 1970). Because the solutes contributing to the high tonicity frequently enter at least a portion of the intracellular fluid, this correction cannot be made by assuming medium solutes to be restricted to the extracellular space. If the tonicity is increased by adding an indifferent nonvolatile solute to the medium (e.g., mannitol, sorbitol, choline chloride, etc.), the tissue space for that solute should be measured by including a tracer for such solute in the medium and measuring the extent of penetration. The necessary corrections may be computed from the formulas

$$I = MmS_I/100,000 \tag{11}$$
$$V_w' = (100 - D)/(D - 100I) \tag{12}$$
$$V' = S/(D - 100I) \tag{13}$$

Equation (11) assumes implicitly that the equivalent space of the indifferent solute has a density of 1. Any error from this assumption is within the uncertainties of these corrections, even in strongly hypertonic media.

Many workers have observed that the concentration of Na^+ ion, even in good central-nervous-system preparations, is much higher than in the living animal, and often approaches its concentration in the incubation medium. Therefore, if excess NaCl is added to a medium to increase its tonicity, the excess NaCl content of dried, incubated brain tissue should be approximated by assuming a concentration, M, in Eq. (11) equal to the concentration of NaCl in *excess* of that in the corresponding isotonic medium, and a sodium chloride space, S_I, equal to the total tissue water (Cohen and Lajtha, 1970). When dried, tissue that has been incubated in a hypotonic medium contains less nonvolatile solids from the medium than does tissue that has been incubated in the corresponding isotonic medium. The correction to be *added* to the observed dry weight is small and may be ignored. If the medium was made hypotonic by reducing some major component, such as NaCl, the correction may be approximated, if desired, by assuming S_I to be equal to some observed extracellular (marker) space, and considering M to be negative and equal to the difference between the concentration of this component in the hypotonic medium and its concentration in the corresponding isotonic medium.

5. Formulas for Computing the Second Space and Correcting for Changes in Total Tissue Water with Temperature

If the total tissue water after incubation does not depend on the incubation temperature, the second space is given by

$$V_2 = V_2{}^H = V_2{}^L = V_3 - V_1 \tag{14}$$

If the total tissue water after incubation depends on the incubation temperature, the second space will also depend on the temperature, and Eq. (14) cannot be used. Instead, at the high incubation temperature, the second space is given by

where
$$V_2{}^H = V_3 - V_1{}^H \tag{15}$$
$$V_1{}^H = V_1\ (V_w{}^H/V_w{}^L), \tag{16}$$

and at the low incubation temperature, the second space is given by

where
$$V_2{}^L = V_3{}^L - V_1 \tag{17}$$
$$V_3{}^L = V_3\ (V_w{}^L/W_w{}^H) \tag{18}$$

The relations between these various spaces at high and low temperatures are shown by Fig. 4. The above formulas depend on the assumption that the first space, the second space, and the total tissue water change proportionately with temperature; that is, that the ratio of the first space and of the second space to the total tissue water is independent of temperature (Cohen and Lajtha, 1970).

Equations (14) to (18) can be used with spaces that have been corrected (as described in Section III, C, 4) for the weight of nonvolatile solids from the medium that are included in dried tissue to give corrected spaces in g/g dry tissue.

IV. OTHER METHODS

Measuring the uptake of a marker substance is the simplest and most widely used method for determining the extracellular space *in vitro*. Four other methods have been used appreciably, either *in vitro* or *in vivo*. The computation of the extracellular space *in vitro* from steady-state efflux kinetics of a marker, in principle, eliminates errors from the marker entering cells. Marker spaces can be measured more or less successfully in living

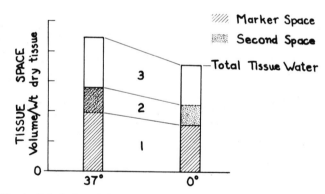

Fig. 4. Calculation of the second marker space. The total tissue water is assumed to be distributed among three compartments: (1) the compartment accessible to marker molecules at 37° and 0°C (the first marker space), (2) the compartment accessible to marker molecules at 37°C but not at 0°C (the second marker space), and (3) the compartment inaccessible to marker molecules at both temperatures. These compartments are assumed to remain proportional to each other at the two temperatures. At 37°C the measured marker space is equal to compartment 1 + compartment 2, both at 37°C; at 0°C the measured marker space is equal to compartment 1 at 0°C. The second space is the difference between the marker spaces at 37° and 0°C corrected for any change in total tissue water. It may be computed for either a tissue temperature of 37°C or one of 0°C. (From Cohen and Lajtha, 1970.)

brain by adopting various sophisticated dodges to circumvent the blood–brain barrier. Although there is little evidence on this point, the interpretation of these spaces may be as complex as the interpretation of marker penetration *in vitro*. The two remaining techniques do not employ markers. Electron microscopy has been used with both *in vivo* and *in vitro* preparations. The observed extracellular space depends on technical factors. The extracellular space can be estimated from the electrical resistance of a tissue, but the value depends on the model assumed for the computation.

A. From Steady-State Efflux Kinetics of a Marker

Analysis of steady-state efflux kinetics of a marker from a tissue preparation is an alternative method that, in favorable cases, should measure the same space as indicated by the uptake of the marker and be free from errors due to penetration into cells. The preparation is incubated with labeled marker until the marker in the extracellular space and in the medium have equilibrated. There may be some penetration of cells, but this is immaterial. The preparation is transferred to fresh medium containing unlabeled marker to extract the labeled marker, and the apparent marker space, S, indicated by the label is measured at various times. The preparation may be rinsed, blotted, or both, before extraction, depending on whether or not the adhering surface film of medium is to be included in the extracellular space. A zero-time marker space, $S°$, is also needed. This is usually measured by analyzing a sample of the preparation (or a parallel preparation) after incubation with the labeled marker, and after any blotting and rinsing that are included in the procedure, but before extraction.

This procedure requires that the exchange of marker from all intracellular compartments which it may have entered be slow compared with the efflux from the extracellular space. Because of this difference in rates, the latter portion of a graph of the apparent marker space, S, as a function of time, t, represents loss of marker from the intracellular compartments. This portion is extrapolated back to zero time to find the intracellular space, S_{in}. The extracellular space, S_{ex}, is found from the zero-time marker space, $S°$, by $S_{ex} = S° - S_{in}$. To a first approximation, the efflux of label from the tissue spaces may be assumed to follow first-order kinetics, giving a two-term exponential decay rate law, $S = S_{ex}\, e^{-k_{ex}t} + S_{in}\, e^{-k_{in}t}$, with $k_{ex} \gg k_{in}$ (Solomon, 1969).* Therefore if S is plotted on a semilogarithmic scale as

---

* The theoretical efflux equation depends on the assumed model. The expression $S = S_{ex}\, e^{-k_{ex}t} + S_{in}\, e^{-k_{in}t}$ is valid if the external and internal compartments are isolated from each other but communicate directly with a sufficient volume of medium to eliminate any reentry of labeled marker, if the resistance to the outflow of marker is restricted to the boundary between the tissue compartment and the medium, and if the size of the com-

a function of time, the portion of the graph representing efflux from the intracellular compartments will be linear or nearly linear, permitting an accurate extrapolation to zero time, as shown by Fig. 5, and the resolution of components to find both compartment sizes and efflux rate constants.

Because the steady-state exchange method compensates for intracellular marker, the experimenter is not restricted to foreign marker substances, such as sucrose, which may alter tissue properties. He can use as marker the ubiquitous physiological ions Na^+ and Cl^-, or even water. It has the disadvantage that many more measurements are needed to determine the extracellular (marker) space of a preparation. Experimental scatter may make the separation of efflux from different compartments, and the extrapolation which this method requires, uncertain. In addition, the tissue must remain stable throughout the total period for loading and extraction, which for

---

partments and the resistances do not change with time. If, instead, all intracellular marker must pass through the extracellular space to leave the tissue, according to the scheme

$$Marker_{in} \xrightarrow{k_{in}} Marker_{ex} \xrightarrow{k_{ex}} Marker_{med}$$

with all other assumptions unchanged, the kinetic expression is again a sum of exponential terms, $S = Ae^{-\lambda_1 t} + Be^{-\lambda_2 t}$, but in this case, A, B, λ_1, and λ_2 are no longer equal to the sizes of the compartments or the rate constants (Huxley, 1960); and in particular

$$S_{ex} = A\,[1 + (B/A)(\lambda_2/\lambda_1)]^2 \,/\, [1 + (B/A)(\lambda_2/\lambda_1)^2]$$

and

$$k_{ex} = \lambda_1[1 + (B/A)\,(\lambda_2/\lambda_1)]^2/[1 + (B/A)\,(\lambda_2/\lambda_1)]$$

If $\lambda_1 \gg \lambda_2$, a necessary condition for good resolution of experimental data, and $A \gg B$, because the intracellular penetration of the marker is comparatively little, the error is small. Assuming $B = 0.3A$ and $\lambda_2 = 0.1\lambda_1$ gives $S_{ex} = 1.06A$ and $k_{ex} = 0.97\lambda_1$. If the difference between λ_1 and λ_2 is less, and if intracellular penetration is greater, the error may be important. Assuming $B = A$ and $\lambda_2 = 0.2\lambda_1$ gives $S_{ex} = 1.38A$ and $k_{ex} = 0.87\lambda_1$. Other models give other rate laws, which are not always expressible as a sum of a few exponential decay terms. If the compartment sizes and the resistance to flow change with time, as with slowly swelling tissue (Fig. 1), the parameters S_{ex}, S_{in}, k_{ex}, and k_{in} become functions of time, and the linear extrapolation to zero time may give incorrect values. Zadunaisky and Curran (1963) assumed as a model of the isolated frog brain an [infinite] cylinder with the extracellular space uniformly distributed, and with the resistance to efflux from this space also uniformly distributed instead of restricted to the surface, and got the expression

$$F = 4\sum_{n=1}^{\infty} \frac{1}{(\mu_n)^2}\, e^{-(\mu_n)^2 Dt/r^2}$$

where F is the fraction of marker remaining in the space, D is the effective diffusion coefficient for the marker, r is the radius of the cylinder, and μ_n are the zeros (roots) of the Bessel function J_0. Because of this dependence of the rate expression on the model and the close fit to the same data that can often be obtained from different models, Zadunaisky and Curran (1963) were able to represent exchange efflux of Na^+ from frog brain by a single exponential term for exit from the "slow compartment" (cells) plus the expression above for exit from the extracellular space, while Bradbury *et al.* (1968) were able to represent exchange efflux of Na^+ from the same preparation by a sum of three exponential decays. In this case the model had little effect on the estimated marker space. Zadunaisky and Curran obtained 24.1% of tissue weight, and Bradbury *et al.*, 23.6% (see Table III).

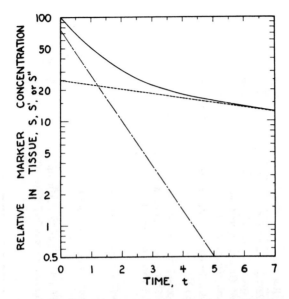

Fig. 5. Graphical resolution of steady-state marker efflux data into components for individual compartments. The efflux data follow the general rate equation $S = S_{ex} e^{-k_{ex}t} + S_{in}e^{-k_{in}t}$, with $k_{ex} > k_{in}$. The relative concentration of labeled marker, S, is plotted semilogarithmically as a function of time, t (——————). The asymptote to the curve at large times (- - - - - - - - - - - -) is extrapolated to zero time to find S_{in}. This line represents the efflux term $S' = S_{in}e^{-k_{in}t}$. Values of S' are subtracted from S, and this difference is plotted (——— - ———). This line, which represents the efflux term $S'' = S - S' = S_{ex}e^{-k_{ex}t}$, is extended to zero time to find S_{ex}. (Alternatively, S_{ex} is found from $S^° - S_{in}$.) The rate constants, k_{ex} and k_{in}, can be found from the slopes of the two straight lines. (In this example $S = 75e^{-t} + 25e^{-0.1t}$.) This process can obviously be extended to resolve efflux data that contain a constant term and several exponential decay terms, $S = S_0 + S_1e^{-k_1t} + S_2e^{-k_2t} + S_3e^{-k_3t} + \ldots$.

brain slices and many other preparations may take at least 2 hr. [One exception is rabbit retina, where the total incubation period was less than 1 hr (Ames and Nesbett, 1966).] There are the usual difficulties of interpretation of the second marker space, and choice of a suitable marker.

There are no published studies of the effect of the second space on exit kinetics. Recent studies by Cohen and Lajtha (1971) show that the effect of temperature on the retention of a marker by brain slices and on the penetration of that marker are not related in any simple way.

Several values for extracellular space measured by exchange kinetics are listed in Table III.

Table III. Extracellular Spaces from Steady-State Efflux of Labeled Marker

Preparation	Marker	Space, % initial wet wt.	Remarks	Reference
Frog brain (*Rana temporia, R. esculenta*)	Na	24.1	Room temperature (20–22°C). Loaded for 30–60 min. Swelling averaged 7% over 1–5 hr. Values presumed to refer to initial wet wt. (Inulin penetration space is 16.2% wet wt. for 40 min incubation.[a])	Zadunaisky and Curran (1963)
Frog brain (*R. pipiens*)	Na Cl	23.6 23.6	Room temperature. Loaded for 60 min. (Marker penetration spaces in Table I.)	Bradbury *et al.* (1968)
Rabbit retina	Na Cl Inulin Mannitol	*60.6* *60.3* *59.1* *62.3*	2.81 ml/g dry wt. 2.80 ml/g dry wt. 2.74 ml/g dry wt. 2.89 ml/g dry wt. Loaded at 37°C extracted at 0°C. Spaces were computed using 21.6% dry wt. for rabbit brain.	Ames and Nesbett (1966)
Cockroach nerve cord (*Periplaneta americana*)	^{3}H as tritiated water	*16.7*	21.6% of tissue water. Space was computed using 25.6% dry wt.	Treherne (1966)
Lobster peripheral nerve (*Homarus americanus*)	^{3}H as tritiated water	*31.4*	35.2% of tissue water. Space was computed using 10.8% dry wt.	Treherne (1966)
Kidney cortex slices	Na Cl 1,3-propane-diol	26.3 18.1 22.2	Loaded for 45 min at 25°C. (Inulin penetration space is 26.7% wet wt.[b])	Kleinzeller and Knotková (1966)

[a] Values in italics were computed from data in the cited reference.
[b] Rosenberg *et al.* (1962).

B. From Marker Spaces *in Vivo*

Attempts have been made for a number of years to measure marker spaces in living brain. Ensuring a steady-state distribution of marker, choosing the correct tissue fluid as the reference, and minimizing marker concentration gradients present grave problems. Early workers injected the marker into the bloodstream, sometimes tying off or removing the kidneys to prevent excretion, a method that had been found acceptable for other soft tissues. After waiting to establish a steady state, the concentration ratio of marker in brain and plasma was measured, and taken as the extracellular space. Because of the blood–brain barrier, this gives very low values; for example, a sulfate space of about 4% (Woodbury *et al.*, 1956; Barlow *et al.*, 1961). Using measured values of 0.12–0.18 in dog (Richmond and Hastings, 1960), 0.13–0.17 in rabbit, or 0.24 in cat (Van Harreveld *et al.*, 1966) for the concentration ratio of sulfate in cerebrospinal fluid and plasma to recompute the extracellular space with the concentration in cerebrospinal fluid as the reference gives a sulfate space of 15–20% (Van Harreveld *et al.*, 1966). Better results are obtained by introducing the marker directly into the cerebrospinal fluid, for example, into the ventricles, the cisterna magna, etc., by a single injection, by repeated injections, or, best, by continuous perfusion. To reduce error from clearance of the marker, it is frequently also injected into the bloodstream. Clearance may also be reduced by saturating the transport systems with a large excess of unlabeled carrier, and by using an inhibitor of the transport system, for example ClO_4^-, when the marker is I^- (Bito *et al.*, 1966). Secretion of cerebrospinal fluid may be suppressed by drugs. Even with these precautions, measurement of the *in vivo* marker space in this way by a single injection, or even by continuous perfusion of marker into the cerebrospinal fluid, is untrustworthy, because equilibration of the marker with the brain tissue is not rapid compared with its clearance from the cerebrospinal fluid or dilution by continuing secretion of cerebrospinal fluid. Woodward *et al.*, (1967) found it required 6 hr of continuous perfusion into the cerebrospinal fluid for the inulin concentration in the cerebral cortex of nephrectomized rats to rise to a steady-state value of 14% of its concentration in perfusate. Ahmed and Van Harreveld (1969) have shown that the iodide space in rabbit brain can be varied from 3 to 22% by changing the experimental conditions.

A method of continuous perfusion of labeled marker into cerebrospinal fluid spaces has recently been described (Rall *et al.*, 1962; Pollay and Davson, 1963; Pollay and Curl, 1967; Curl and Pollay, 1968: Pollay and Kaplan, 1969; Fenstermacher *et al.*, 1970a; Fenstermacher *et al.*, 1970b; Levin *et al.*, 1970). In spite of severe technical difficulties, this method may overcome some limitations of other *in vivo* marker methods and give both reliable marker spaces and indications of penetration into cells. The fluid spaces are perfused until the marker concentration in the space and at the tissue surface has reached a steady state. (The concentration in the bulk of the tissue may still be changing.) The animal is then killed. Brain tissue is removed, frozen, and a series of 0.5- to 1.0-mm-thick slabs parallel to a well-perfused surface are removed and assayed for marker. The marker concentration in the tissue is extrapolated back to the concentration in the surface layer, and the marker space computed as usual as space (in %) = 100 × (marker concentration in tissue)/(marker concentration in medium). The diffusion coefficient and its variation, if any, with perfusion time can also be calculated, and used to decide whether the marker penetrated cells. Spaces determined by this method are listed in Table IV. The values for cat cerebral cortex indicate that the effects of temperature and molecular size on the marker space may not be the same *in vivo* as they are *in vitro*, but more research is needed.

Chapter 7 by Fenstermacher in this volume describes this techinque.

Table IV.   Marker Spaces from *in Vivo* Perfusion

Animal	Region	Perfusion method	Temerpature (°C)	Marker	Space (%)	Reference
Dog	Caudate nucleus	VC	Body (37)	Inulin	19	Fenstermacher *et al.* (1970b)
				Sucrose	19	
				Mannitol	31	
				^{3}H-Water	4	
	Cerebral cortex	SA	38	Inulin	18.8 ± 1.6	Levin *et al.* (1970)
				Sucrose	19.5 ± 1.6	
Cat	Cerebral cortex	SA	37	Inulin	18.4 ± 1.7	Fenstermacher *et al.* (1970a)
				Sucrose	19.8 ± 3.0	
				Mannitol	26.0 ± 3.5	
	Cerebral cortex		15	Inulin	18.4 ± 1.8	Fenstermacher *et al.* (1970a)
				Sucrose	15.3 ± 3.4	
				Mannitol	20.4 ± 1.9	
Rabbit (albino, New Zealand)	Cerebral cortex	SA	38	Inulin	17.6 ± 2.1	Levin *et al.* (1970)
				Sucrose	19.9 ± 2.3	
Rhesus monkey (*Macaca mulatta*)	Cerebral cortex	SA	38	Inulin	18.4 ± 3.0	Levin *et al.* (1970)
				Sucrose	19.6 ± 2.0	

VC = ventriculocisternal perfusion.
SA = subarachnoidal perfusion.

C. By Electron Microscopy

Measurement of extracellular space by electron microscopy has an appealing directness. The space, if any, can be seen and located exactly, and is equal to the average fraction of extracellular space appearing in randomly oriented sections. Most of the classical studies of extracellular space in living brain, for example, those by Horstmann and Meves (1959), have been made by electron microscopy, and show little extracellular space. The observed space depends greatly on the methods used (Karlsson and Schultz, 1965; Schultz and Karlsson, 1965; Torack, 1965; Nevis and Collins, 1967; Van Harreveld and Khattab, 1969; Van Harreveld and Steiner, 1970); some procedures indicate a substantial space. Independent evidence can be adduced to support both the conclusion that there is little extracellular space, and the conclusion that there is appreciable extracellular space in living brain. There is no accepted, independent way to decide which procedures least distort the extracellular space. The common criteria for a satisfactory preparation, such as those given by Palay *et al.* (1962), Sjöstrand (1962), and Karlsson and Schultz (1965), are worthless and have even been used to deny the existence of extracellular space around unmyelinated nerve fibers (Karlsson and Schultz, 1965). After circulatory arrest, cortical asphyxiation, or other insult, and during spreading depression, the electrical resistance of central nervous tissue rises rapidly (Van Harreveld and Ochs, 1956; Ranck, 1964; Van Harreveld, 1966b; Van Harreveld and Khattab, 1967); similar increases occur during fixation by perfusion *in situ,* a commonly used method (Nevis and Collins, 1967; Van Harreveld and Khattab, 1968).* Van Harreveld argues that this increase is due to migration of extracellular fluid into cells (Van Harreveld and Malhotra, 1966; Van Harreveld and Khattab, 1967), and therefore conventional methods of fixation destroy the extracellular space (Van Harreveld, 1966c). To avoid this he rapidly freezes brain tissue *in situ,* a process that is limited to a surface layer 8–15μ thick. The tissue is then either fixed at low temperature (Van Harreveld and Crowell, 1964), or freeze dried and then fixed. With this technique Van Harreveld *et al.* (1965) observed an extracellular space of 18.1 to 25.5% by volume, with a mean of 23.6% in the surface layer of mouse cerebellar cortex, which decreased to less than 6% after asphyxiation for 8 min. Similarly, Bondareff and Pysh (1968) found a mean extracellular space of 21.7% (range, 17.8–26.8%) in the molecular layer of rapidly frozen adult rat cerebral cortex, 20 μ below the pia mater, and a mean extracellular space of 40.5% (range, 35.0 to 48.0%) in the same tissue from 10-day-old rats. For comparison,

---

* Perfusion techniques are described by Palay *et al.* (1962), Sjöstrand (1962), and Karlsson and Schultz (1965.)

Horstmann and Meves (1959) estimated an average extracellular space of 4.6% (range, 2.5–10.6%) in dogfish *(Scylliorhinus canicula)* optic tectum.

Although the values given by Van Harreveld *et al.* (1965) and by Bondareff and Pysh (1968) appear reasonable, especially if one believes that the several lines of investigation make the presence of an appreciable extracellular space in central nervous tissue likely, the spaces may have been distorted, and therefore these values, if accepted, should be considered as, at best, only semiquantitative. In addition, the fraction of extracellular space at the surface of the cerebellar cortex, or the molecular layer of the cerebral cortex, may not be representative of the brain. In regions, such as neuropil, that consist largely of fine fibers, changes in fiber diameter can greatly alter the observed extracellular space (Horstmann and Meves, 1959). Van Harreveld and Khattab (1969) assert that there is no direct relationship between spaces in normal living central nervous tissue and spaces in fixed tissue. In tissues, such as heart muscle, where the existence of extracellular space *in vivo* is not seriously questioned, the spaces shown by electron microscopy are generally smaller than those measured by uptake of markers (Johnson and Simonds, 1962). Until the technical difficulties have been overcome, the chief value of studies of extracellular space in central nervous tissue by electron microscopy is polemical.

The extracellular space has been visualized by introducing or precipitating electron-dense markers, such as ferritin, cupric ferrocyanide, silver iodide, etc., and preparing electron micrographs of the treated tissue. [See, for example, Lasansky and Wald (1962), and Baker (1965).] If the density of marker granules can be related to the concentration of marker, if the marker is fixed in place before any tissue distortion occurs, and if the marker is not adsorbed on cell surfaces before fixation, then electron-dense markers will show both the location and the size of extracellular spaces regardless of distortions caused by tissue preparation. Studies by this method have been only qualitative to date because these conditions have not been established. In some instances they are known to be invalid. Ferritin, for example, sticks to basement membrane in cat visual cortex (Selwood, 1970).

D. From Electrical Resistance of Tissue

Computation of extracellular space from the electrical resistance of tissue is, in principle, a most attractive approach that avoids the ambiguities associated with markers. Van Harreveld (1966d) has published an excellent, brief account of this technique. In simplest terms, this method assumes that because of the high electrical resistance of cell membranes, electric current through tissue is carried by the interstitial fluid, and therefore the conductance (reciprocal of resistance) increases directly with the fraction of extracellular fluid.* The relation between conductance and extracellular fluid is not a simple proportion. As the volume fraction of nonconducting cells increases, not only does the fraction of conducting fluid decrease, but the average path length that the current must traverse also increases, further increasing the resistance, because of the greater number of cells that must be bypassed, and the greater the amount of fluid that is contained in blind pockets where it does not conduct current. The conductance also depends on the shape of the cells, their conductance, if any, and if the tissue is anisotropic, as, for example, a fiber tract or the spinal cord, on the direction of measurement. For any assumed physical model an equation relating the fraction of extracellular space to resistance can be derived. For example, S, the volume fraction of conducting liquid in a suspension of nonconducting spheres, a common model, is related to r, the resistance of the suspension, and $r°$, the resistance of the liquid, by an equation derived by Maxwell, $S = 3(r°/r)/[2+(r°/r)]$.† This relation has been verified for suspensions of sea urchin eggs in sea water containing up to 70% by volume of cells (Cole, 1928). (The maximum volume fraction of close-packed spheres is 74%.) Several other plausible models have also been verified experimentally (Cole et al., 1969). The geometry of nervous tissue is complex, and it is not obvious what tractable physical model provides an acceptable approximation. The extracellular space of any isotropic tissue can be computed from its resistance by the relation $S = (r°/r) L (1-f)+p$, where L is the length factor, that is, the ratio of the length of the physical path taken by the current to the geometrical distance between the two measuring electrodes; f is the shunting factor, that is, the fraction of the current carried by the blood vessels, plus the fraction of the current that passes because of the conductance of the cells; and p is the volume fraction of nonconducting extracellular space contained in blind pockets (Cohen, work in progress). For brain tissue, L is approximately 1.4 to 1.6 from electron micrographs, f is about 0.1 (Ranck, 1963a; Van Harreveld and Ochs, 1956) (assuming that virtually all shunting comes from blood vessels), and p may be arbitrarily assumed to be negligible. The specific resistance of the interstitial fluid in brain is not known, but is probably close to that of cerebrospinal fluid because the concentrations of the two ions, Na^+ and Cl^-, which conduct over 89% of the current, have regional variations in cerebrospinal fluid of less than

---

* Because the reactive component is small at the frequencies used for these measurements (Ranck 1963a; Van Harreveld et al., 1963), conductance and resistance may be taken as numerically equal to admittance and impedance.

† This is a limiting case of the general relation
$$S = 1 - \{[(r°/r) - 1][(r°/r_c) + X]\} / \{[(r°/r_c) - 1][(r°/r) + X]\}$$
where r_c is the specific resistance of the suspended particle (cell), and X is a form factor that depends on the shape of the particle. X is 2 for spheres, and 1 for measurements along the axial direction of parallel cylinders.

2%. If so, $r°$ is 51–62 ohm-cm (Crile *et al.,* 1922), or 55 ohm-cm at body temperature and 85 ohm-cm at 15°C (Fenstermacher *et al.,* 1970).

Typical values for the resistance of neural tissues, and extracellular spaces computed from these values, are listed in Table V. The enormous difference in specific resistance of tissue measured by different reputable investigators, and hence in calculated extracellular space, is striking. The ranges represent measurements on separate animals or groups of animals, not replicate measurements on the same preparation. The published data do not indicate whether these large variations are due to local regional differences, differences in the state of the several preparations, or the inherent inaccuracy of the measurement. Naively, one would assume that the extracellular space varies less than the measured resistances. Uncertainties in the estimates for L, $r°$, and f introduce a relative uncertainty of about 20% in the computed space. This limit to the precision is unimportant in view of the scatter of the data, and the serious disagreement between studies. The data for rabbit cerebral cortex (Van Harreveld *et al.,* 1963) and for conduction along the spinal cord (Ranck and BeMent, 1965) strongly suggest appreciable conduction through cells. Ranck (1963b) finds his measurements for rabbit cortex to be consistent with both an appreciable extracellular space and with the small extracellular spaces reported by most electron microscopists. Earlier, Horstmann and Meves (1959) had pointed out the difficulty of interpreting resistance data by showing that an extracellular space of 8–25% could be calculated from the same conductance data from small changes in the assumed parameters, $r°$, r_c, and X, in the generalized Maxwell equation (footnote, p. 213).

Although resistance measurements support the notion of some, perhaps an appreciable, extracellular space *in vivo,* they give at best only a semi-quantitative estimate of its size. They are invaluable for observing *in vivo* changes, such as the increase in resistance during spreading depression, which may indicate changes in extracellular space (Ranck, 1964; Van Harreveld and Khattab, 1967).

V. CONCLUDING REMARKS

The author should be granted the luxury of expressing a few opinions. Biochemically and physiologically (terms which exclude the phenomenon of "thought"), brain is no more atypical than many other specialized soft tissues. In the absence of firm evidence to the contrary—not the evidence of electron micrographs—it must be considered to have an extracellular space *in vivo* as well as *in vitro.* The indication of various measurements is that in living brain this space lies between 15 and 25% or more conservatively

Table V.   Resistance and Computed Extracellular Space of Central Nervous System Tissues[a]

Animal	Preparation	Temperature (°C)	Specific resistance or impedance (ohm-cm)	Extracellular space (% by vol.)	Conditions	Reference
Rabbit	Cerebral cortex	Body (37)	208±6 (174–249)	35.7 (42.7–29.8)	*In vivo*, 1000 cps (14 aminals)	Van Harreveld et al. (1963)
Rabbit	Subcortical white matter	Body (37)	962±70 (683–1410)	7.7 (10.9–5.3)	*In vivo*, 1000 cps (14 animals)	
Rabbit	Cerebrum (cortex+white)	Body (37)	488±38 (312–804)	15.2 (23.8–9.2)	*In vivo*, 1000 cps (14 animals)	
Rabbit	Cerebral cortex	Body	321±45 230±37	23.1 32.3	*In vivo*, 5 cps *In vivo* 5000 cps	Ranck (1963a)
Cat	Cerebral cortex	36	556±45	13.7	*In vivo*, 0.6–10 msec pulses	Li *et al.* (1968)
Cat	White matter	36	580±53	13.1	*In vivo*, 0.6–10 msec pulses	
Cat	Cerebral cortex	37	527±15 (430–600)	14.1, *15.0*[b] (17.3–12.4)	*In vivo*, 0.6–10 msec pulses (12 animals)	Fenstermacher *et al.* (1970a)
Cat	Cerebral cortex	15	837±9 (800–930)	13.7, *14.7*[b] (14.3–12.3)	*In vivo*, 0.6–10 msec pulses (14 animals)	
Cat	Cervical cord	Body	Longitudinal (138–212) Transverse (1211)	(53.8–35.0)	*In vivo*, 5–10 cps	Ranck and BeMent (1965)
Rabbit	Cerebrum	39	561 (521–621)	14.0[c], 12.6[c]	*In vitro*, fresh tissue, averages of groups of animals	Crile *et al.* (1922)

[a] Except as noted, extracellular spaces were computed from the formula $S = 100 \ (\rho°/\rho) \ L \ (1 - f) + p$ (p. 213), taking $L = 1.5$, $f = 0.1$, $p = 0$, and $\rho° = 52.3$ ohm-cm at 39°C, 55 ohm-cm at 37°C or "body temperature," 56.4 ohm-cm at 36°C, and 85 ohm-cm at 15°C. The indicated uncertainty is the standard deviation of the mean. Values in parentheses show the reported range.

[b] Values in *italics* are given in the citation and were computed from Maxwell's equation for a suspension of nonconducting spheres (p. 213), taking $\rho° = 55$ ohm-cm at 37°C and 85 ohm-cm at 15°C.

[c] Value of 14.0 was computed assuming no conduction through vessels in excised tissue ($f = 0$); value of 12.6 was computed assuming $f = 0.1$.

between 10 and 30% by volume, a range which encompasses the values for most other soft tissues.

In spite of the many unresolved problems of methodology and interpretation—choice of marker, penetration into cells, incomplete equilibration with tissue, interpretation of the second space, changes with time, etc.—marker methods are the only acceptable ones for measuring extracellular space in central nervous tissue, both *in vitro* and *in vivo*. By a proper choice of methodology one can produce any desired value by electron microscopy. Resistance measurements do not allow quite this freedom, but the difficulty of interpretation is such that a wide range of spaces can be computed from any measured tissue resistance.

Until the dependence of the marker space on the marker used and the second marker space phenomenon are both understood, marker spaces in brain and any quantities depending on these spaces must be considered to be *conventionally defined* quantities, completely analogous to the *operationally defined* quantities of the physicist. Section II, C contains some recommendations for suitable conventions. Doubtless as this becomes more widely appreciated, more and better conventions will be proposed. That they are conventional spaces does not mean that marker spaces have no physical meaning. The approximate agreement of measurements made with different markers presumably indicates that they are a rough measure of the true extracellular space. Unfortunately, we cannot at present go from these rough measures to a more accurate determination.

VI. ADDENDUM

Friede and Hu (1971) have recently published a new method for extracellular space *in vitro* employing markers that may penetrate cells. The tissue is equilibrated with media containing at least two different concentrations of a marker, and the marker concentration in the tissue is measured. If the following assumptions hold: (1) the extracellular and intracellular space are independent of the marker concentration, (2) the extracellular concentration of the marker is equal to its concentration in the medium, and (3) the intracellular concentration is independent of the extracellular concentration, then the concentration of marker in the tissue, $[M]_{tis}$, is related to its concentration in the extracellular space, $[M]_{ex}$, and in the intracellular space, $[M]_{in}$, by

$$100 [M]_{tis} = [M]_{ex} S_{ex} + [M]_{in} S_{in}$$

where S_{ex} and S_{in} are the extracellular and intracellular spaces in percent of tissue wet weight. (Any convenient weight concentration units, e.g., molarity, or percent by weight, may be used for marker concentration.) The extracellular space can be calculated (Friede and Hu, 1971) by substituting data from two marker concentrations into this expression and solving the resulting simultaneous equations. The formal solution is

$$S_{ex} = 100 \; ([M]_{tis2} - [M]_{tis1})/([M]_{ex2} - [M]_{ex1})$$

It is preferrable to graph $100 \, [M]_{tis}$ from a series of measurements as a function of $[M]_{ex}$. S_{ex} is the slope of the resulting straight line. It is essential that the assumptions hold. Measurements at two marker concentrations will always give two simultaneous equations with a formal solution, but the calculated space may be meaningless. Although necessary, a linear relation between $[M]_{tis}$ and $[M]_{ex}$ is not a sufficient guarantee. If, for example, the intracellular concentration of a marker is a linear function of its extracellular concentration, that is, if $[M]_{in} = \alpha + \beta \, [M]_{ex}$, then $[M]_{tis}$ will be a linear function of $[M]_{ex}$ given by $100 \, [M]_{tis} = A + B \, [M]_{ex}$ but the slope, B, will now be $B = S_{ex} + \beta$.

As with other marker methods, this can be checked by using several markers. Using Na^+, K^+, and Cl^- as markers in brain from bowfin *(Amia calva)*, a primitive fish, Friede and Hu (1971) found the same extracellular space as that given by sorbitol, 23% at 20°C. (They found a space of 13% with ^3H-methoxyinulin, and a 46% space with ^{14}C-carboxyinulin.) In the preparation they used—the ventricles slit open, but the brain unsliced and otherwise largely intact—swelling is slight, and presumably the intracellular concentrations of these three ions are maintained constant by the normal regulatory processes. Regulation may be much poorer in slices of mammalian brain, which commonly swell extensively during incubation. Obviously, markers like inulin and sorbitol which are not regulated, cannot be used.

This method does not solve the related problems of what the second marker space corresponds to, and which extracellular space, if any, is appropriate for any particular situation.

ACKNOWLEDGMENTS

I wish to thank the following organizations for permission to use copyrighted material: The International Society for Neurochemistry and Pergamon Press for Figs. 1 and 2; and Elsevier Publishing Co. for Fig. 4.

I am indebted to Dr. Miriam Banay-Schwartz for reading the manuscript, and to Miss Candace James for typing.

Finally, I am grateful to the Lord for revealing some of the subtleties of His creation.

REFERENCES

Ahmed, N., and Van Harreveld, A. (1969) *J. Physiol.* **204**, 31–50.
Allen, J. N. (1955) *Arch. Neurol. Psychiat.* **73**, 241–248.
Ames, A., III, and Nesbett, F. B. (1966) *J. Physiol.* **184**, 215–238.
Baker, P. F. (1965) *J. Physiol.* **180**, 439–447.
Barlow, C. F., Domek, N. S., Goldberg, M. A., and Roth L. J. (1961) *Arch. Neurol.* **5**, 102–110.
Barr, L., and Malvin, R. L. (1965) *Amer. J. Physiol.* **208**, 1042–1045.
Becker, N. H., Hirano, A., and Zimmerman, H. M. (1968) *J. Neuropathol. Exp. Neurol.* **27**, 439–452.
Bito, L. Z., Bradbury, M. W. B., and Davson H. (1966) *J. Physiol.* **185**, 323–354.
Blasberg, R., and Lajtha, A. (1965) *Arch. Biochem. Biophys.* **112**, 361–377.
Bondareff, W., and Pysh, J. J. (1968) *Anat. Rec.* **160**, 773–780.
Bourke, R. S., and Tower, D. B., (1966) *J. Neurochem.* **13**, 1071–1097.
Bradbury, M. W. B., Villamil, M., and Kleeman, C. R. (1968) *Amer. J. Physiol.* **214**, 643–651.
Brading, A. F., and Jones, A. W. (1969) *J. Physiol.* **200**, 387–401.
Brightman, M. W. (1965) *Amer. J. Anat.* **117**, 193–220.
Brown, D. A., Stumpf, W. E., and Roth, L. J. (1969) *J. Cell Sci.* **4**, 265–288.
Cohen, S. R. (1969) *Anal. Biochem.* **31**, 539–544.
Cohen, S. R. Blasberg, R., Levi, G, and Lajtha, A. (1968) *J. Neurochem.* **15**, 707–720.
Cohen, S. R., and Lajtha, A. (1970) *Brain Res.* **23**, 77–93.
Cohen, S. R., and Lajtha, A. (1971) *Int. J. Neurosci.* **1**, 251–258.
Cohen, S. R., Stampleman, P. F., and Lajtha, A. (1970) *Brain Res.* **21**, 419–434.
Cole, K. S. (1928) *J. Gen. Physiol.* **12**, 37–54.
Cole, K. S., Li, C.-L. and Bak, A. F. (1969) *Exp. Neurol.* **24**, 459–473.
Crile, G. W., Hosmer, H. R., and Rowland, A. F. (1922) *Amer. J. Physiol.* **60**, 59–106.
Curl, F. D., and Pollay, M. (1968) *Exp. Neurol.* **20**, 558–574.
Farrant, J. L. (1954) *Biochem. Biophys. Acta* **13**, 569–576.
Fenstermacher, J. D., Li, C.-L., and Levin, V. A. (1970a) *Exp. Neurol.* **27**, 101–114.
Fenstermacher, J. D., Ral, D. P., Patlak, C. S., and Levin, V. A. (1970b) in *Capillary Permeability, Alfred Benzon Symposium* II (C. Crone and N. A. Lassen, eds.), Munksgaard, Copenhagen, pp. 483–490.
Friede, R. L., and Hu, K. H. (1971) *J. Physiol.* **218**, 477–493.
Goodford, P. J., and Leach, E. H. (1966) *J. Physiol.* **186**, 1–10.
Horstmann, E., and Meves, H. (1959) *Z. Zellforsch. Mikroskop. Anat.* **49**, 569–604.
Huxley, A. F. (1960) Appendix 2 to A. K. Solomon, Chap. 5, in *Mineral Metabolism,* Vol. IA (C. L. Comar and F. Bronner, eds.) Academic Press, New York, pp. 163–166.
Johnson, J. A., and Simonds, M. A. (1962) *Amer, J. Physiol.* **202**, 589–592.
Karlsson, U., and Schultz, R. L. (1965) *J. Ultrastruct. Res.* **12**, 160–186.
Kleinzeller, A., and Knotková, A. (1966) *Biochem. Biophys. Acta* **126**, 604–605.
Kulka, R. G. (1956) *Biochem. J.* **63**, 542–548.
Lasansky, A., and Wald, F. (1962) *J. Cell Biol.* **15**, 463–479.
Law, R. O., and Phelps, C. F. (1966) *J. Physiol.* **186**, 547–557.
Lehrer, G. M. (1969) in *Autoradiography of Diffusible Substances* (L. J. Roth and W. E. Stumpf, eds.), Academic Press, New York, pp. 191–199.
Levi, G., and Lattes, M. G. (1970) *J. Neurochem.* **17**, 587–596.
Levin, V. A., Fenstermacher, J. D., and Patlak, C. S. (1970) *Amer. J. Physiol.* **219**, 1528–1533.
Li, C.-L., Bak, A. F., and Parker, L. O. (1968) *Exp. Neurol.* **20**, 544–557.
Mcllwain, H., and Buddle, H. L. (1953) *Biochem. J.* **53**, 412–420.
Nevis, A. H., and Collins, G. H. (1967) *Brain Res.* **5**, 57–85.
Nicholls, J. G., and Wolfe, D. E. (1967) *J. Neurophysiol.* **30**, 1547–1592.
Page, E. (1965) in *Advances in Tracer Methodology,* Vol. 2 (S. Rothschild, ed.), Plenum Press, New York, pp. 179–182.

Palay, S. L., McGee-Russell, S. M., Gordon, S., Jr., and Grillo, M. A. (1962) *J. Cell Biol.* **12**, 385–410.

Pappius, H. M. (1965) in *Biology of Neuroglia, Progress in Brain Research,* Vol. 15 (E. D. P. De Robertis and R. Carrea, eds.), Elsevier, Amsterdam, pp. 135–154.

Pappius, H. M., Klatzo, I., and Elliot, K. A. C. (1962) *Can. J. Biochem. Physiol.* **40**, 885–898.

Penn, N. W., and Suwalski, R. (1969) *Biochem. J.* **115**, 563–568.

Phelps, C. F. (1965) *Biochem. J.* **95**, 41–47.

Pollay, M., and Curl, F. (1967) *Amer. J. Physiol.* **213**, 1031–1038.

Pollay, M., and Davson, H. (1963) *Brain* **86**, 137–150.

Pollay, M., and Kaplan, R. J. (1970) *Brain Res.* **17**, 407–416.

Pollay, M., Stevens, A., and Davis, C., Jr. (1968) *Anal. Biochem.* **17**, 192–200.

Rall, D. P., Oppelt, W. W., and Patlak, C. S. (1962) *Life Sci.* **1**, 43–48.

Ranck, J. B., Jr. (1963a) *Exp. Neurol.* **7**, 144–152.

Ranck, J. B., Jr. (1963b) *Exp. Neurol.* **7**, 153–174.

Ranck, J. B., Jr. (1964) *Exp. Neurol.* **9**, 1–16.

Ranck, J. B., Jr., and BeMent, S. L. (1965) *Exp. Neurol.* **11**, 541–463.

Richmond, J. E., and Hastings, A. B. (1960) *Amer. J. Physiol.* **199**, 814–820.

Rosenbaum, J. D., and Lavietes, P. H. (1939) *J. Biol. Chem.* **131**, 663–674.

Rosenberg, L. E., Downing, S. J., and Segal, S. (1962) *Amer. J. Physiol.* **202**, 800–804.

Rosenbluth, J., and Wissig, S. L. (1964) *J. Cell Biol.* **23**, 307–325.

Schultz, R. L., and Karlsson, U. (1965) *J. Ultrastruct. Res.* **12**, 187–206.

Selwood, L. (1970) *Z. Zellforsch. Mikroskop. Anat.* **107**, 6–14.

Sherman, W. R., and Stewart, M. A. (1966) *Biochem. Biophys. Res. Comm.* **22**, 492–497.

Sjöstrand, F. S. (1962) in *The Interpretation of Ultrastructure, Symposium Int. Soc. Cell. Biol.,* Vol. 1, (R. J. Harris, ed.), Academic Press, New York, pp. 47–68.

Solomon, A. K. (1960) Chap. 5 in *Mineral Metabolism,* Vol. IA (C. L. Comar and F. Bronner, eds.), Academic Press, New York, pp. 119–167.

Stewart, M. A., Sherman, W. R., Kurien, M. M., Moonsammy, G. I., and Wigerhof, M. (1967) *J. Neurochem.* **14**, 1057–1066.

Thoft, R. A., and Kinoshita, H. J. (1965) *Exp. Eye Res.* **4**, 287–292.

Torack, R. M. (1965) *Z. Zellforsch. Mikroskop. Anat.* **66**, 352–364.

Treherne, J. E. (1966) *The Neurochemistry of Arthropods,* Cambridge University Press, Cambridge, England, pp. 14–16.

Van Harreveld, A. (1966a) *Brain Tissue Electrolytes,* Butterworths, Washington.

Van Harreveld, A. (1966b) *loc. cit.,* pp. 69–76.

Van Harreveld, A. (1966c) *loc. cit.,* pp. 128–132, 138–140, 161–162.

Van Harreveld, A. (1966d) *loc. cit.,* pp. 50–69.

Van Harreveld, A., Ahmed, N., and Tanner, D. J. (1966) *Amer. J. Physiol.* **210**, 777–780.

Van Harreveld, A. and Crowell, J. (1964) *Anat. Rec.* **149**, 381–385.

Van Harreveld, A., Crowell, J., and Malhotra, S. K. (1965) *J. Cell Biol.* **25**, 117–135.

Van Harreveld, A., and Khattab, F. I. (1967) *J. Neurophysiol.* **30**, 911–929.

Van Harreveld, A., and Khattab, F. I. (1968) *J. Cell Sci.* **3**, 579–594.

Van Harreveld, A., and Khattab, F. I. (1969) *J. Cell Sci.,* **4**, 437–453.

Van Harreveld, A., and Malhotra, S. K. (1966) *J. Cell Sci.,* **1**, 223–228.

Van Harreveld, A., Murphy, T., and Nobel, K. W. (1963) *Amer. J. Physiol.* **205**, 203–207.

Van Harreveld, A., and Ochs, S. (1956) *Amer. J. Physiol.* **187**, 189–192.

Van Harreveld, A., and Steiner, J. (1970) *J. Cell Sci.* **6**, 793–805.

Varon, S., and McIlwain, H. (1961) *J. Neurochem* **8**, 262–275.

Woodbury, D. M., Timiras, P. S., Koch, A., and Ballard, A. (1956) *Fed. Proc.* **15**, 501–502.

Woodward, D. L., Reed, D. J., and Woodbury, D. M. (1967) *Amer. J. Physiol.* **212**, 367–370.

Zadunaisky, J. A., and Curran, P. F. (1963) *Amer. J. Physiol.* **205**, 949–956.

Zamenhof, S., Bursztyn, H., Rich, K., and Zamenhof, P. J. (1964) *J. Neurochem.* **11**, 505–509.

Section III
COMPONENTS OF NEURAL TISSUES

Chapter 9

Ethanolamine Plasmalogens

Lloyd A. Horrocks

Department of Physiological Chemistry
The Ohio State University
Columbus, Ohio

and Grace Y. Sun

Laboratory of Neurochemistry
Cleveland Psychiatric Institute
Cleveland, Ohio

I. INTRODUCTION

The 1-alk-1'-enyl-2-acyl-s*n*-glycero-3-phosphorylethanolamines (ethanolamine plasmalogens) are important components of the central nervous system. Of the total phospholipids in some subcellular fractions, the ethanolamine plasmalogens account for about one-third in the myelin, one-fifth in the microsomes, and one-eighth in the mitochondria. The following procedures are used in our laboratories for determinations of the amount and composition of the ethanolamine plasmalogens. (reviewed by Horrocks, 1972).*

II. LIPID EXTRACTION

The extraction is based on the procedure of Folch *et al.* (1957). The volumes are those used for a single rat brain. Immediately after decapitation and removal of the brain, it is weighed and placed in a Potter-Elvehjem homogenizing tube with 20 ml of chloroform–methanol 2:1 (v/v). The tissue

---

* For an explanation of the nomenclature see *Biochem J.* **105**, 897 (1967) and **112**, 17, (1969).

is thoroughly dispersed at high speed with a Teflon motor-driven pestle, the mixture is transferred to a stoppered calibrated tube with several rinsings, and is diluted to 35 ml with chloroform–methanol 2:1 (v/v). Then 7 ml of 0.1 M NaCl solution is added and the two phases are thoroughly mixed. After standing overnight, the upper phase is aspirated and the lower phase is washed 2 times with 3–5 ml portions of the upper phase solvent (chloroform–methanol– 0.1 M NaCl, 3:48:47 by volume) before filtration through paper. The filtrate is taken to dryness in a rotary evaporator with several additions of 5 ml of absolute ethanol in order to denature the proteolipids. The residue is immediately redissolved in a known amount of chloroform (at least 10 ml/g tissue) and stored at 4°C under nitrogen.

This procedure can be scaled up or down for other amounts of tissue. For the proper separation of the two phases, the amount of water, including that in the tissue, should be one-fifth of the total volume. Aqueous dispersions can be extracted by mixing with 4 volumes of chloroform–methanol 2:1 (v/v). A variety of homogenizers are suitable for the dispersion step. It is also permissible to filter the initial extract, take the filtrate to dryness, and redissolve in 19 volumes of chloroform–methanol 2:1 (v/v) followed by 5 volumes of 0.1 M NaCl. After standing overnight, the two phases are treated as described above.

III. ASSAY OF TOTAL PLASMALOGEN CONTENT

The $1'$, $2'$ double bond in the alkenyl groups is much more reactive than the isolated double bonds in the acyl groups. The iodine addition method (Gottfried and Rapport, 1962) is a quick and simple method for assay of the total alkenyl groups (plasmalogens).

A stock iodine solution is prepared by dissolving about 38 mg iodine in 50 ml of 3% (w/w) aqueous KI. The working reagent is prepared by mixing 1.0 ml of the stock iodine solution with 9.0 ml of 3% KI solution. A lipid sample containing about 0.05 μmoles of plasmalogen is placed in a tube and taken to dryness under a stream of nitrogen. The residue is immediately dissolved in 0.5 ml of methanol with moderate warming (60–70°C for 2–3 min). After the addition of 0.5 ml of the working iodine solution, the mixture is agitated vigorously and left at room temperature for about 10 min. The mixture is diluted with 4.0 ml of ethanol, mixed, and the extinction read against ethanol at 355 nm. Blanks with the iodine reagent must also be carried through the procedure. The content of alkenyl groups is calculated from the difference in extinction between the sample and the blank using a molecular extinction coefficient of 27,500. If the extinction of the sample is less than 0.1, the assay should be done again with a smaller sample. Larger samples can be accommodated if a spectrophotometer is available with a linear range of 0–3 extinction units and if 3.0 ml of the stock iodine solution is diluted with 7.0 ml of 3% KI.

IV. DETERMINATION OF THE PHOSPHOLIPID COMPOSITION INCLUDING THE ALKENYL ACYL AND ALKYL ACYL COMPONENTS

A. Two-Dimensional Thin-Layer Chromatography

A separation-reaction-separation scheme for thin-layer chromatography (TLC) is used in this procedure (Horrocks, 1968). After a separation of phospholipid types by development in the first dimension, the alkenyl groups are cleaved from the plasmalogens by exposure to HCl. The subsequent development in the second dimension further separates the aldehydes, the acid-stable phospholipids, and the lysophospholipids that are derived from the plasmalogens. The acid-stable phospholipids can be subjected to an alkaline hydrolysis to separate the polar components derived from the diacyl type from those of the alkyl acyl type.

Thin-layer plates are coated with a 0.5-mm layer of Silica Gel G suspended in 0.01 M Na$_2$ CO$_3$. The plates are placed in an oven at 110°C for 30 min and stored in a cabinet with dessicant. A sample of the lipid extract that contains between 5 and 15 μg of phosphorus is applied in the lower left corner on a 2-cm line that is 2 cm from each side of the plate. The plate is developed in an unlined tank containing 65 ml of chloroform, 25 ml of methanol, and 4 ml of ammonium hydroxide to a height of 10–13 cm. The plate is then dried for 10 min with a stream of air at ambient temperature from a hair dryer or other suitable source. The plate is then placed face down for 5 min on a Pyrex tray that contains a layer of conc. HCl. The plate is again dried with a stream of air for 10 min, then developed in the second dimension to a height of 10 cm. A mixture of 75 ml of chloroform, 15 ml of methanol, 30 ml of acetone, 15 ml of acetic acid, and 7.5 ml of water gives a better separation of phosphatidic acid, serine phosphoglycerides, inositol phosphoglycerides, and sphingomyelin than does the chloroform–methanol–ammonium hydroxide mixture specified before (Horrocks, 1968). The second-dimensional development will not be successful if the ambient air has a water content that is more than that of air at 22°C and 50% relative humidity.

After the developing solvent has evaporated, the plates are placed face down on another Pyrex tray that contains crystals of iodine. When the spots are stained, the plate is removed and the spots are marked with a sharp pencil point or other stylus. The spots are scraped onto weighing paper with a plas-

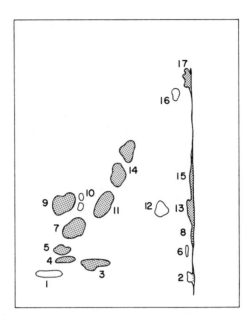

Fig. 1. A diagram of the relative positions of human cerebral lipids after separation-reaction-separation thin layer chromatography. The areas are 1, origin; 2, phosphatidic acids; 3, serine phosphoglycerides; 4, inositol phosphoglycerides; 5, sphingomyelins; 6, unknown; 7, acid-stable choline phosphoglycerides; 8, aldehyde (from choline plasmalogens); 9, acyl GPE (from alkenyl acyl GPE); 10, cerebroside sulfates; 11, acid-stable EPG; 12, unknown; 13, aldehydes (from ethanolamine plasmalogens); 14, cerebrosides; 15, cardiolipin; 16, unknown; 17, cholesterol. The plate was first developed from bottom to top and then from left to right as described in the text.

tic ruler (2.5 × 15 cm). This material can be used for the assay of radioactivity or phosphorus.

Several methods are available for assistance in the identification of the spots. Known mixtures and standards can be spotted on similar plates and on lanes that are exposed to only one developing solvent on the unknown plate. Duplicate plates can be made for use with specific color reactions. For mammalian brain extracts, the aldehydes released from the ethanolomine plasmalogens account for the only large spot at the solvent front of the second dimension. The two remaining spots with the same first-dimension mobility are the acid-stable ethanolamine phosphoglycerides (EPG) and the monoacyl *sn*-glycero-3-phosphoryl ethanolamines (GPE).

B. Assays of Diacyl and Alkyl Acyl GPE

The acid-stable EPG from the preceding separation contains both diacyl GPE and alkyl acyl GPE. The composition of this area can be determined by an alkaline methanolysis followed by phosphorus assays (Panganamala et al., 1971). From 2 to 3 μmoles of phospholipids are applied to a separate TLC plate which is treated as described in Section IV, A. The acid-stable EPG area and a blank of the same size area are scraped into sintered glass filter sticks. The silica gel is eluted three times with 2-ml portions of chloroform–methanol–water 3:6:1 (by volume) into 50-ml Erlenmeyer flasks with a standard taper joint. The eluates are taken to dryness on a rotary vacuum evaporator with additions of absolute ethanol for removal of the water. From 2 to 3 ml of 0.1 M NaOH in methanol is then added to the flask. After 15 min at room temperature, 1 ml of ethyl formate is added and the mixture is again taken to dryness before the addition of 1.0 ml of the upper phase and 2.0 ml of the lower phase that is obtained by mixing 4 volumes of chloroform, 2 volumes of isobutanol, and 3 volumes of water (Dawson, 1960). After thorough shaking, the mixture is poured into a centrifuge tube and centrifuged. Aliquots of 0.25 ml of the upper phase and 0.50 ml of the lower phase are taken for phosphorus assays to determine the relative amounts of diacyl GPE and alkyl acyl GPE. The lower phase sample is taken to dryness with a stream of nitrogen before digestion.

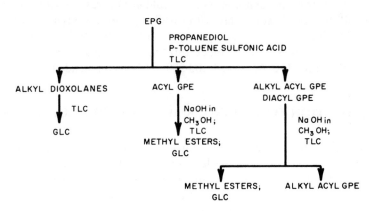

FRACTIONATION OF ETHANOLAMINE PHOSPHOGLYCERIDES FOR GLC

Fig. 2. The reaction sequence for obtaining separate fractions for the determination of the alkenyl and acyl group compositions of the alkenyl acyl glycerophosphoryl ethanolamines and the acyl group composition of the diacyl glycerophosphoryl ethanolamines from a sample of ethanolamine phosphoglycerides.

C. Phosphorus Assays

The procedure of Gottfried (1967) is recommended for the small amounts of phospholipid that are well resolved on TLC plates. The samples and 2.0 ml of $5M$ H_2SO_4 are placed in calibrated tubes (25 × 200 mm) and digested at 250°C. Standards containing 1.0 and 2.0 µg of phosphorus, a reagent blank, and silica gel blanks (from areas of the plate that do not contain phospholipids) are treated in the same manner. All tubes with silica gel should also have three small glass beads. After 15 min, 2 drops of 30% hydrogen peroxide are added to each tube. The tubes are heated for 3 more minutes and removed to a rack. Two drops of a 16% (w/w) Na_2SO_3 solution are added and the tubes are allowed to cool. The contents of each tube are diluted to 20–25 ml with water before the addition of 5 ml of 0.5% ammonium molybdate and 5 ml of 0.025% hydrazine sulfate. Sufficient water is added to each tube to bring the volume to the 35-ml mark. After mixing with a vibrator mixer, the tubes are placed in a boiling water bath for 10 min. The tubes are cooled in an ice bath and, if necessary, the solutions are diluted to 35 ml. Exactly 7.0 ml of n-butanol is added to each tube. The blue color is extracted by thorough mixing with the vibrator mixer. After the upper phase has separated, the mixing is repeated. The extinction of the resulting upper phases is measured with a spectrophotometer at 795 nm against the reagent blank. The extinction of the 1-µg standard should be between 0.19 and 0.21. The butanol extraction step concentrates the molybdenum blue into a small volume and thus permits a large volume during digestion. An acceptable alternate procedure has been described by Rouser et al. (1970).

The tubes from phosphorus assays should not be washed with detergents but should be rinsed thoroughly with distilled water and reserved for these assays. The time for digestion may vary from 5 to 30 min depending on the source of heat that is used. A block tube heater (Hallikainen Instruments, Richmond, Calif., U.S.A. Model 100-300°C) is recommended.

V. ISOLATION OF ETHANOLAMINE PHOSPHOGLYCERIDES

For gas-liquid chromatographic analyses of the acyl and alkenyl group compositions, the most rapid and efficient method for the isolation of lipid classes is preparative thin-layer chromatography. Since some cerebrosides and cerebroside sulfates have mobilities close to those of the EPG, we recommend the following column procedure (adapted from Rouser et al., 1967) for the separation of the phospholipid fraction before thin-layer chromatography.

A 1-cm-diameter glass chromatographic column equipped with a Teflon stopcock is filled with a suspension of 5 g of Unisil silicic acid (Clarkson Chemical Co., Williamsport, Pa.) in 50 ml of chloroform. The Unisil silicic acid column has a high flow rate but the resolution is adequate without regulation. After the chloroform has drained to the top of the silicic acid, the lipid extract from one rat brain is placed on the column. Collection of the eluate is begun. When the extract has drained to the top of the silicic acid, a minimum quantity of chloroform is used to wash any residual extract into the absorbent. The sterols, less polar glycerides, and free fatty acids are eluted with an additional 100 ml of chloroform. All galactolipids are eluted with 50 ml of chloroform–acetone 1:1 (v/v) followed by 50 ml of acetone or by 100 ml of acetone. The phospholipids are eluted with 100 ml of methanol. The methanol eluate is taken to dryness with a rotary vacuum evaporator and immediately made up to 10 ml with chloroform.

From 2 to 4 μmoles of the phospholipid fraction can be applied to each thin-layer plate with a 0.5-mm layer of silica gel G prepared as described in Section IV, A. The sample is applied on a line 2 cm from the bottom across the plate. One lane at the side can be used for an EPG standard or a known mixture. The plate is developed in an unlined tank to a height of 14 cm with a mixture of 65 ml chloroform, 25 ml methanol, and 4 ml water. These conditions give excellent separations of the ethanolamine and choline phosphoglycerides but with some streaking of the serine phosphoglycerides. The latter can be avoided by substituting ammonium hydroxide for the water, but then the EPG and CPG are closer together.

After development, the plate is allowed to dry and then sprayed lightly with a 0.2% solution of 2',7'-dichlorofluorescein in ethanol. The bands are best seen under ultraviolet light. The silica gel containing the EPG is scraped into a tube and thoroughly mixed with 8 ml of chloroform, 4 ml methanol, and 3 ml of water. After the phases have separated, the upper phase is discarded. The lower phase is filtered through a funnel with a paper or sintered glass filter to remove the silica gel and then the filtrate is taken to dryness with a stream of nitrogen. The residue is immediately redissolved in chloroform or used for the preparation of derivatives.

VI. PREPARATION OF DERIVATIVES FOR GAS–LIQUID CHROMATOGRAPHY

The ethanolamine phosphoglycerides from central or peripheral nervous system tissues are a mixture of alkenyl acyl GPE and diacyl GPE with a small amount of alkyl acyl GPE. Since the separation of the intact molecules of the three types is very difficult, a number of approaches have been reported for sequential hydrolyses or separations of derivatives. We have found (Sun and

Horrocks, 1969) that quantitative separations of the alkenyl acyl and the diacyl types can be made by beginning with the reaction described by Rao *et al.* (1967). These procedures can also be used for the corresponding choline compounds (Panganamala *et al.*, 1971).

A sample of EPG containing 5 μmoles or less of alkenyl groups is placed in a culture tube with a Teflon-lined screw cap and taken to dryness with a stream of nitrogen. From 0.5 to 1.0 mg of *p*-toluene sulfonic acid is added as a catalyst. Then 5 ml of a 1 % (w/w) solution of 1,3-propanediol in chloroform is added. The tube is sealed with the screw cap and placed in an 80°C water bath for 1hr. After cooling, additions of 3 ml of chloroform, 4 ml of methanol, and 3 ml of water are made, followed by thorough mixing. After phase separation, the upper phase with excess 1,3-propanediol is removed and discarded. The lower phase is taken to dryness with a stream of nitrogen and redissolved in a small quantity of chloroform for separation of the components by preparative thin-layer chromatography (see Section V). The unreacted diacyl GPE band (typical R_f 0.46) and the monoacyl GPE band (typical R_f 0.30) are scraped into separate stet tubes for the preparation of methyl ester derivatives of the acyl groups. The material at the solvent front is transferred to a sintered glass funnel and eluted with 10 ml of chloroform. The eluate containing the alkyl dioxolanes is applied to another LTC plate that is developed with toluene. A marker lane with an authentic sample of alkyl dioxolanes should be included. The alkyl dioxolane band (typical R_f 0.30) is scraped from the plate and again the alkyl dioxolanes are eluted with chloroform. The eluate is taken to dryness with a stream of nitrogen and redissolved in hexane before analysis by means of gas–liquid chromatography. We have used a 183 cm × 0.317 cm (internal diameter) column with a 10 % polyester packing at 185–200°C for this analysis.

The methyl ester derivatives of the acyl groups are prepared by an alkaline methanolysis (Sun and Horrocks, 1968). The reaction is very rapid and quantitative in the presence of silica gel. The silica gel in each tube is covered with 3 ml of 0.5 M NaOH in methanol for 15 min at room temperature. Then 8 ml of chloroform, 1 ml of methanol, and 3 ml of water are added to each tube and the contents are mixed thoroughly. After separation of the phases, the upper phases are removed and discarded. The lower phases are taken to dryness with a stream of nitrogen. The residues are redissolved in a small amount of chloroform and applied to a TLC plate that is developed with toluene. Separate lanes of the same plate used for isolation of the alkyl dioxolanes can be used. The methyl ester bands (typical R_f 0.60) are also scraped from the plate, eluted with chloroform, and methyl esters are prepared for GLC as described above for the alkyl dioxolanes. The same GLC column can be used for the analysis of the methyl ester mixtures. The origin of the lane used for the TLC of the alkaline methanolysis products from the diacyl GPE band contains any alkyl GPE and alkyl acyl GPE that were present in the latter form in the original sample of the EPG. The alkyl compounds can be eluted for further analysis if desired.

REFERENCES

Dawson, R. M. C. (1960) *Biochem. J.* **75**, 45.
Folch, J., Lees, M., and Sloane-Stanley, G. H. (1957) *J. Biol. Chem.* **226**, 497
Gottfried, E. L. (1967) *J. Lipid Res.* **8**, 321.
Gottfried, E. L., and Rapport, M. M. (1962) *J. Biol. Chem.* **237**, 329.
Horrocks, L. A. (1968) *J. Lipid Res.* **9**, 469.
Horrocks, L. A. (1972) In *Ether Lipids: Chemisty and Biology,* (F. Snyder, ed.) Academic Press, New York, in press.
Panganamala, V., Horrocks, L. A., Geer, J. C., and Cornwell, D. G. (1971) *Chem. Physics Lipids* **6**, 97.
Rao, P. V., Ramachandran, S., and Cornwell, D. G., (1967) *J. Lipid Res.* **8**, 380.
Rouser, G., Kritchevsky, G., Simon, G., and Nelson, G. J. (1967) *Lipids* **2**, 37.
Rouser, G., Fleischer, S., and Yamamoto, A. (1970) *Lipids* **5**, 494.
Sun, G. Y., and Horrocks, L. A. (1969) *J. Lipid Res.* **10**, 153.
Sun, G. Y., and Horrocks, L. A. (1968) *Lipids* **3**, 79.

Chapter 10

Methods for Separation and Determination of Gangliosides

L. S. Wolfe

Donner Laboratory of Experimental Neurochemistry
Montreal Neurological Institute
McGill University
Montreal, Canada

I. INTRODUCTION

Gangliosides constitute a group of glycosylceramides which contain one or more N-acylneuraminic acid residues (5-acetamido- or 5-glycolamido-3, 5-dideoxy-D-*glycero*-D-*galacto*-nonulosonic acids). They were originally isolated by Ernst Klenk in 1939 from cerebral gray matter of the brain as a mixture of different species (Klenk, 1939, 1942). In the past 10 years the resolution, structural chemistry, and metabolism of gangliosides have been intensively studied and have been comprehensively reviewed by a number of authors (Svennerholm, 1964, 1970; Ledeen, 1966, 1970; McCluer, 1968; Roseman, 1968; Wiegandt, 1966, 1971).

The known structures of brain gangliosides together with the generally accepted code names of Svennerholm (1963) are listed in Table I. The carbohydrate sequence galactosyl-N-acetylgalactosaminyl-galactosyl-glucose is the characteristic sequence in all the major brain gangliosides and must be distinguished from the sequence N-acetylgalactosaminyl-galactosyl-galactosyl-glucose present in globoside, the major neutral glycosphingolipid of the erythrocyte membrane. The gangliosides of normal human brain are all N-acetylneuraminic acid derivatives. However, in other species

Table I. Brain Gangliosides

Svennerholm code names	Structure
G_{M3}	N-acetylneuraminyl α2→3 galactosyl β1→4 glucosylceramide
G_{D3}	N-acetylneuraminyl α2→8 N-acetylneuraminyl α2→3 galactosyl β1→4 glucosylceramide

G_{M2}	N-acetylgalactosaminyl β1→4 galactosyl β1→4 glucosylceramide
	            | α2→3
	    N-acetylneuraminyl

G_{M1}	galactosyl β1→3 N-acetylgalactosaminyl β1→4 galactosyl β1→4 glucosylceramide
	            | α→3
	    N-acetylneuraminyl

G_{D1a}	N-acetylneuraminyl α2→3 galactosyl β1→3 N-acetylgalactosaminyl β1→4 galactosyl β1→4 glucosylceramide
	            | α2→3
	    N-acetylneuraminyl

G_{D1b}	galactosyl β1→3 N-acetylgalactosaminyl β1→4 galactosyl β1→4 glucosylceramide
	            | α2→3
	    N-acetylneuraminyl α2→8 N-acetylneuraminyl

G_{T1}	N-acetylneuraminyl α2→3 galactosyl β1→3 N-acetylgalactosaminyl β1→4 galactosyl β1→4 glucosylceramide
	            | α2→3
	    N-acetylneuraminyl α2→8 N-acetylneuraminyl

(ox, horse, dog) N-glycolylneuraminic acid derivatives are present. Although brain gangliosides occur in high concentration in the cerebral cortex (2–3 mg/g fresh tissue weight), it is now clear that gangliosides occur as membrane constituents in many extraneuronal tissues. The principal types in nonneural tissues are hematosides and disialogangliosides. Furthermore, there is an even greater complexity of species than in the central nervous system since N-acetyl and N-glycolylneuraminic acids can occur separately or togehter in the same molecule. A unique feature of brain gangliosides (human, ox) is that almost half of the long chain base is constituted by the homolog of sphingosine, eicosa-4-sphingenine. The predominant fatty acids in brain gangliosides are saturated and stearic acid accounts for 80–90%. On the other hand, lignoceric, nervonic, and behenic acids predominate in many extraneuronal gangliosides.

Evidence strongly supports a neuronal localization of the more complex gangliosides in the central nervous system and particularly in the dendritic and synaptic regions. Gangliosides do occur in lower concentrations in white matter, particularly G_{M1}-ganglioside, but it is uncertain if it is a true myelin constituent or present only on the axolemma.

Ganglioside biosynthesis involves a series of reactions in which sugars are transferred successively by specific glycosyl transferases from their nucleotides to the growing glycolipid acceptor. In brain the glycolipid gly-, cosyl transferases are particulate and appear to be localized in synaptic membranes. Although the overall scheme of ganglioside biosynthesis is fairly well worked out, knowledge of the importance of the several alternate pathways possible in the stepwise buildup of the more complex gangliosides is still very incomplete. Turnover curves do not suggest any precursor-product relationship between the major ganglioside fractions in brain. It has been suggested that multiglycosyl transferase systems are involved in the entire biosynthetic reactions for each ganglioside type. The catabolism of the entire carbohydrate chains of gangliosides proceeds by hydrolytic cleavage of the sialosyl linkages (Ohman *et al.*, 1970) and the terminal glycosyl linkages at the nonreducing end (Gatt, 1969; Shapiro, 1967). These reactions are carried out by a series of glycosyl hydrolases of different substrate specificities and are thought to be localized to the lysosomes. There are several inherited progressive childhood neurological diseases in which there is a primary or secondary deficiency or absence of one or other of the glycosyl hydrolases involved in ganglioside catabolism, leading to excessive storage of gangliosides (Brady, 1969) in neurons.

The physiological function of gangliosides is obscure. Considerable interest at present centers around a possible role in synaptic transmission, in cell surface negative charge and contacts between cells.

II. ISOLATION AND PURIFICATION

Procedures for the extraction of gangliosides from tissues are based on their solubility in organic solvents from which they can subsequently be partitioned into aqueous media essentially by the method described by Folch *et al.* (1957). A mixture of gangliosides is obtained. The procedure outlined below for cerebral cortex is the simplest, most reproducible, and commonly used method. It can be applied to any brain region and as well to extraneural tissues. Highest yields of trisialogangliosides are obtained if the cerebellum is used. An indispensible reference for more details on the extraction and purification of glycolipids is Volume 14 of Methods in Enzymology (Colowick and Kaplan, 1969).

The meninges from fresh cerebral cortex (ox, human) are removed with blunt forceps and the gray matter grossly dissected with curved scissors from the white matter. The weighed tissues are homogenized with 17–20 volumes of chloroform–methanol (2:1, v/v) for 5 min in a mechanical homogenizer (Omnimixer, Lourdes homogenizer, Waring blender) and filtered through a sintered glass Büchner funnel with gentle vacuum or through fat-free filter paper. The residue is reextracted with 10 volumes of chloroform–methanol (1:2, v/v) containing 5% of water and filtered. The filtrates are combined and chloroform added to make a final chloroform–methanol concentration of 2:1. Alternatively, the chloroform–methanol 1:2 filtrate can be evaporated to dryness *in vacuo* in any standard rotatory evaporator and the residue dissolved in the initial 2:1 chloroform–methanol filtrate. The gangliosides are partitioned into an aqueous phase by adding to the 2:1 chloroform–methanol filtrate 1/5 volume of 0.1 M KCl and shaking vigorously. The phases are allowed to separate by standing in a cold room or can be separated more quickly by centrifuging, which efficiently removes microdroplets. The upper phase is removed with care to avoid taking any interfacial material and saved. The lower phase is vigorously shaken again with 1/5 volume of theoretical upper phase containing KCl (chloroform–methanol–0.74% KCl, 3:48:47) and the phases separated as above. The lower phase is again washed with theoretical upper phase containing no salt (chloroform–methanol–water, 3:48:47) and the upper phase collected. Use of pure water causes emulsions but methanol–water is quite satisfactory. The combined upper phases are concentrated to 1/10 volume *in vacuo*. Foaming can be troublesome during this concentration. It can be reduced by using a large volume flask and initially cooling the flask in dry ice–acetone. When the solvents have evaporated off, the addition of pure benzene greatly speeds up the concentration. The concentrate is dialyzed in Visking cellulose tubing for 2 days at 4 °C against a large excess of distilled water changed 2–3 times each day. The dialysis sac contents are freeze dried to obtain a white fluffy powder of the crude mixed gangliosides.

A. Notes on Alternate Procedures

1. Gangliosides can be efficiently extracted from acetone or acetone and ether washed powders which can be prepared and stored in a desiccator in a freezer ($-20°C$) for many months. Fresh brain tissue is homogenized in 20 volumes of cold acetone ($-10°C$) for 5 min and filtered on a Buchner funnel. The residue is homogenized again with 20 volumes of acetone, filtered and finally stirred with 20 volumes of cold diethyl ether (freshly purchased anhydrous ether, analytical grade in tin containers with added antioxidant is quite satisfactory). Alternatively, a 1 to 5 homogenate of brain tissue in distilled water can be poured slowly into 20 volumes of acetone ($-10°C$) with constant stirring in a cold room. The residue obtained after filtration is reextracted with cold acetone and the powder dried in a vacuum desiccator. To extract the lipids from acetone powders, methanol (7–10 ml/g of powder) should be added first and the suspension briefly homogenized. This wets the powder and avoids clumping. Chloroform is then added to bring the chloroform–methanol ratio to 2:1 v/v and the mixture stirred at room temperature for an hour. The procedure from then on is exactly the same as described above for fresh tissue. The author has found that better yields of gangliosides can be obtained from acetone powders if 1 ml of 1 M KCl is added to each gram of acetone powder and the paste then homogenized with 19 volumes of chloroform–methanol (2:1).

2. Dialysis of tissue homogenates or subcellular fractions leads to low extractability of gangliosides due to loss of monovalent cations (Spence and Wolfe, 1967). Therefore, in all dialyzed tissue samples or subcellular fractions obtained by repeated differential or gradient centrifugations, 1 M NaCl or KCl (approximately 1 ml/g wet weight of fraction) should be added before the chloroform–methanol extractions.

3. Small tissue samples are more conveniently extracted in small glass homogenizers with Teflon or glass pestles. For the determination of gangliosides on a microscale (i.e., tissue sections), the tissue is placed in microtubes (6 cm × 5 mm) prepared from standard Pasteur pipets and 0.5 ml of chloroform–methanol–water (16:8:1, v/v/v) added, the tube sealed and heated at 50–55° for 1 hr. The microtubes are opened and the gangliosides partitioned three times into aqueous phases as described above. The phases are separated by centrifuging. All the additions and removals are performed with a 100-µl Hamilton syringe. The combined aqueous phases are transferred to another microtube evaporated to dryness in a vacuum desiccator over NaOH pellets.

4. The crude ganglioside mixture can be prepared by immediate dialysis of the chloroform–methanol extracts of tissues against running tap water in a cold room for 24 hr. The upper phase which appears is removed and the lower phase mixed with an equal volume of methanol and dialyzed again for 24 hr. The combined upper phases of the two dialyses are reduced in volume by evaporation *in vacuo*, dialyzed against distilled water for 24 hr, and lyophilized.

5. Separation of nonlipids and gangliosides from chloroform–methanol extracts can be achieved by Sephadex G-25 chromatography (Siakotos and Rouser, 1965). However, the procedure is quite tedious and does not offer any distinct advantage over aqueous partitioning techniques except perhaps in the complete separation of the relatively less polar gangliosides (e.g., hematosides) which do not completely partition into the aqueous phases.

B. Purification of the Crude Mixed Ganglioside Fractions

1. Mild Alkaline Hydrolysis

Small amounts of contaminating phospholipids can be removed from the crude gangliosides by the mild alkaline hydrolysis procedure of Marinetti (1962). Ceramide linkages in sphingolipids remain intact. The gangliosides are dissolved in methanol (10–20 mg/ml of methanol) and 0.5 N sodium methoxide in methanol added until the pH is approximately 10. The sodium methoxide is freshly prepared by dissolving the appropriate quantity of sodium in methanol placed in an ice bath. The alkaline methanolysis is allowed to proceed at room temperature for 30 min, then cooled in an ice bath and acidified carefully to around pH 2–3.0 (not below!) with 1 N methanolic–HCl. Chloroform is added to make the solution 2:1 v/v of chloroform to methanol and the gangliosides partitioned with 0.1 M KCl and successively with theoretical upper phase–KCl and theoretical upper phase–water as described for the isolation of crude gangliosides. The pooled upper phases are concentrated and dialyzed.

2. Removal of Contaminating Nucleotide Sugars

In vivo or *in vitro* experiments in which the incorporation of radioactive sugars from nucleotide sugars into gangliosides is being investigated, the nucleotide sugars are not readily dialyzable and therefore will contaminate the dialyzed upper phases containing the gangliosides. The nucleotide contamination can be removed by incubation with snake venom phosphodiesterase and *Escherichia coli* alkaline phosphatase. The dialyzed upper phase containing the gangliosides is made 0.1 M with tris-citrate buffer pH 8.5 and 0.03 M with magnesium acetate. *E. coli* alkaline phosphatase and snake venom phosphodiesterase (5 μg of each enzyme to each milliliter of upper phase) is added and the solution incubated at 37°C for 90 min. The mixture is then dialyzed overnight against distilled water. The enzyme protein can be removed by concentration *in vacuo* to dryness with additions of methanol and solution of the gangliosides with chloroform-methanol 2:1, v/v.

3. Barium Salt Precipitation, Formation of Free Acids and Crystallization

The dialyzed gangliosides after mild alkali saponification and removal of nucleotide sugars (if necessary) are passed through a Dowex 50 column (H⁺ form, 200–300 mesh) that has been freshly prepared and thoroughly washed with distilled water until neutral. The ganglioside eluate and water washes from the column are transferred to a beaker on a magnetic stirrer and with continuous monitoring of the pH, saturated barium hydroxide (freshly prepared) is added drop by drop to bring the pH to 9–9.5. Four volumes of absolute ethanol are added and the solution allowed to stand in a cold room (0–4°C) overnight. The precipitate of the barium salts of the gangliosides is collected by centrifuging in the cold and traces of ethanol blown off with a gentle stream of nitrogen or in a vacuum desiccator. The gangliosides are dissolved in a small volume of water (10–15 ml) and passed through another small Dowex 50 (H⁺ form) column. The ganglioside effluent and an equal volume of water wash are collected and immediately lyophilized. For crystallization, to each 100 mg of lyophilized gangliosides 2.0–3.0 ml of boiling methanol is added and the suspension carefully warmed until all the gangliosides have dissolved. The solution is then cooled to −4°C and allowed to stand overnight or longer. The precipitate is collected by filtration through a fine sintered glass funnel and dried in a desiccator *in vacuo*. This material is now a purified mixture of gangliosides.

III. RESOLUTION

A. Column Chromatography

The resolution of mixtures of gangliosides into individual species (G_{M3}, G_{M2}, G_{M1}, G_{D1a}, etc.) by column chromatography on silicic acid is quite laborious and because there is frequently overlap in the elution of the different gangliosides, a second column separation is often needed to obtain reasonably clean fractions. The advantage of the column procedure is that several hundred milligrams of a ganglioside mixture can be fractionated. Final purification can be achieved by preparative thin-layer chromatography using a neutral and ammoniacal system.

The method of Penick *et al.* (1966) has been modified in the author's laboratory and gives reasonably good separations of individual gangliosides. Silica gel H.R. is suspended several times in distilled methanol and the fines removed by suction and then dried at 120°C overnight. A slurry of the silica gel is made in chloroform–methanol–water (65:30:5 by volume). The solvents should be dry since the proportion of water in the solvent mixture is important. The slurry is poured into a column (100 × 2.2 cm); the length to diameter of the column bed should be greater than 20 to 1. The mixed gangliosides dissolved in as small a volume as possible of chloroform–methanol (2:1) are carefully pipetted onto the top of the bed and washed into the column with the same solvent mixture used to prepare the solumn. Eluant reservoirs are attached to the column and the gangliosides eluted first with 500 ml of chloroform–methanol–water (65:30:5), second with a linear gradient of total volume of 1 liter between chloroform–methanol–water (60:37:8) and chloroform–methanol–10% ammonium hydroxide (60:37:8) and finally, with similar gradient of total volume of 1 liter of chloroform–methanol–water (60:40:10) and chloroform–methanol–10% ammonium hydroxide (60:40:10). Fractions of 15 ml are collected in a fraction collector and the flow rate is adjusted to 1.5 ml per minute and regulated by a low positive pressure of nitrogen. The gradient can be achieved simply by connecting two marriotte vessels or similar flasks in series each containing 500 ml of the appropriate solvent mixture. The flask adjacent to the column is mixed by a magnetic stirrer. It takes approximately 30 hr to run the column. The elution is monitored by removing aliquots from the tubes and measuring the *N*-acetylneuraminic acid by the resorcinol method. The resorcinol-positive fractions are evaporated to dryness and tested for homogeneity of ganglioside species by thin-layer chromatography. Homogeneous fractions are pooled and freeze dried. Nonhomogeneous fractions are combined and rechromatographed.

B. Thin-Layer Chromatography on Silica Gel

This technique is the most widely used for the resolution of gangliosides either for analytical or preparative purposes. Both neutral and basic solvent systems have been used (Colowick and Kaplan, 1969; Penick *et al.*, 1966; and Marinetti, 1967).

  (i)   chloroform–methanol–water (60:35:8 by volume)
 (ii)   chloroform–methanol–2.5 N ammonia (60:40:8 by volume)
(iii)   *n*-propanol–water (7:3 by volume)
 (iv)   *n*-propanol–water–conc. NH_4OH (6:2:1 by volume)
  (v)   *n*-butanol–pyridine–water (3:2:1 by volume)

Silica gel G or silica gel H.R. can be used usually on 20 cm × 20 cm thin-layer plates prepared from a slurry of 30 g of silica gel in 60 ml of water. The thickness of the adsorbent can be 250 or 500 μ. After preparation the plates are dried at 110°C for 20–30 min. They can be washed if necessary by a full plate length ascending run with methanol–diethyl ether (4:1 by volume) and redrying the plate. The gangliosides in chloroform–methanol (2:1) are applied preferably with a Hamilton syringe in 1-cm bands.

Because gangliosides are highly polar lipids, their migration rate is slow and the inexperienced worker might find at first that poor separations are obtained. These difficulties can be overcome in a number of ways. The plates can be developed twice, or two successive runs (approx. 7 hr each) can be carried out ascending using plates of double length (20 × 40 cm). The latter technique developed by Ledeen gives good separation of all the major gangliosides (Ledeen, 1966). It may be necessary to slightly modify the proportions of methanol and ammonia (e.g., from 35:8 to 40:9 by volume), but these details must be worked out in individual laboratories since the water content of the solvents and humidity conditions may vary. The descending technique has been described by Korey and Gonatas (1963) in which the solvent is applied to the top of the plate by a filter paper wick. This technique is a little more difficult to set up. The separation of minor gangliosides can be difficult, particularly for the ganglioside G_{D3} which overlaps G_{D1a} in ammoniacal systems and G_{M1} in neutral systems. Thus several solvent systems must be used to identify this ganglioside.

Gangliosides are visualized by spraying with the resorcinol reagent of Svennerholm (1957). It is important to spray the plates evenly but sparsely with a fine spray from a good atomizer. The plate is then covered with a clean glass plate clamped and heated at 130–140°C for 15 to 20 min. If too much reagent is applied, bubbling and breakup of silica gel occurs. Care is necessary on removing the covering plate since strong HCl fumes are given off and the operation should be conducted in a fume hood. The resorcinol reagent is specific for the sialic acid groups in gangliosides. Both gangliosides and nonsialic acid-containing materials can be detected by spraying with 50% concentrated H_2SO_4 and charring in an oven.

Quantification of the N-acetylneuraminic acid in each ganglioside band separated by thin-layer chromatogrpahy can be carried out by the method of Suzuki (1965). Gangliosides are located by a short exposure to iodine vapor and the areas marked with a needle. These areas are scraped off and transferred into centrifuge tubes after all the iodine has sublimated. The N-acetylneuraminic acid is determined directly with the resorcinol reaction without removing the silica gel. The color produced is extracted directly into the butylacetate–butanol (85:15) centrifuged, and the absorbency read at 580 and 450 mμ (see below).

Gangliosides can be resolved on preparative thin-layer plates. The mixed gangliosides are applied as a thin band on 500μ-thick plates of silica gel G. If iodine is used to detect the ganglioside zones after development, it is difficult to be certain when all the iodine has sublimated. If iodine remains, the gangliosides on subsequent freeze drying are brownish in color. The author prefers to air dry the preparative plates after development and spray with bromothymol blue (10 mg/100 ml in 9 N ammonia). The bands are outlined with a needle point and scraped off into medium porosity Gooch crucibles. The bromothymol blue is removed from the gel by two acetone extractions and the gangliosides then extracted with methanol. The methanol is evaporated off, the gangliosides dissolved in water, the solution clarified by centrifuging, and the clear supernatant freeze dried.

IV. ANALYTICAL PROCEDURES

The analysis in detail of the composition of an isolated and purified ganglioside is complex, requiring the setting up of methods for the quantitative determination of sialic acids, hexosamines, neutral hexoses, fatty acids, and sphingosines. For the complete structural determination of the oligosaccharide moiety of a ganglioside, the oligosaccharide must first be cleaved intact from the ceramide part of the molecule and then subjected to a variety of techniques used by carbohydrate chemists to determine sequences, linkages, and their stereoconfigurations. It is beyond the scope of this chapter to give details of these techniques and the investigator should consult the original papers of Kuhn and Wiegandt (1966, 1963a,b). For structural analysis, at least 10–20 mg quantities of the glycolipids are required. These quantities are often unobtainable for ganglioside types present in small quantities in tissues. However, microtechniques are available for compositional analyses and recent advances in mass spectrometry of complex glycolipids indicate that in the near future useful information on structure should be obtainable on samples less than a milligram. However, the determination of the stereoconfiguration of the interglycosidic linkages by NMR spectroscopy still requires 20–50 mg of material.

In this section procedures that have been used successfully for compositional analysis of ganliosides will be mentioned briefly with indications of their particular usefulness and limitations. The reader should consult several excellent books on methods for more extensive accounts (Colowick and Kaplan, 1966, 1969; Marinetti, 1967).

A. Determination of Sialic Acids

Total N-acetylneuraminic acid in gangliosides is usually determined by a reaction based on the Bial's orcinol reaction. The most sensitive method is the resorcinol method of Svennerholm (1957), and the chromogen is extracted into n-butyl acetate-n-butanol (85:15 by volume) as described by Miettinen and Takki-Luukkainen (1959). The absorption is measured at 580 mμ. Aldohexoses have some absorption at this wavelength and in samples in which contamination with hexoses is suspected, a correction can be made by using the formula

$$\text{O.D.}580 = \frac{(\text{O.D.}580 \times R_H - \text{O.D.}450)R_S}{R_S \times R_H - 1}$$

where R_S is the ratio of the O.D. of N-acetylneuraminic acid at 580 mμ and 450 mμ, respectively, and R_H is the ratio of the O.D. of hexose at 450 mμ and 580 mμ, respectively. The resorcinol reagent must be prepared from resorcinol recrystallized from benzene and stored in dark bottles in the refrigerator. It is stable for 2 weeks to a month. The limit of detection is 3–4 μg of N-acetylneuraminic acid. The reagent can be used for spraying thin-layer plates of silica gel for the specific detection of gangliosides. Several concentrations of standards should be run with each assay. Since standard solutions of N-acetylneuraminic acid tend to deteriorate when stored in a refrigerator, a stock solution should be made and divided into small containers and stored in a deep-freeze unit. One container is thawed for the standards in each series of determinations.

Sialic acid can be liberated from gangliosides by mild acid hydrolysis (0.1 N H_2SO_4, 60 min, 80°C), or by purified preparations of *Vibrio cholera* or *Clostridium perfringens* neuraminidases. The free sialic acid can be specifically measured after oxidation with sodium m-periodate and the aldehyde produced reacted with thiobarbituric acid and the red color measured by the procedure of Warren (1959). With the more complex gangliosides there are problems with these methods since it is not possible to quantitatively cleave all the sialic acid by acid or enzymic hydrolysis. The sialic acids liberated by acid or enzymic hydrolyses can be absorbed on Dowex 1 X-8 (formate form, 50–100 mesh) resin columns and eluted with a gradient of formic acid (0.1–1M). N-Acetylneuraminic acid elutes at approximately 0.3 M formic acid. Sialic acids can be chromatographed on paper in an n-butyl acetate–acetic acid–water (3:2:1 by volume) system. The system cleanly separates N-glycolyl and N-acetyl neuraminic acids. The sialic acids are sensitively detected on paper by spraying with a solution of 0.05 M sodium m-periodate in 0.025 M H_2SO_4, after 15 min spraying again with a solution of ethylene glyco-lacetone–conc. sulfuric acid (50:50:0.3 ml), and then after a further

10 min finally spraying with a 6% solution of sodium 2-thiobarbiturate in
1.66% sodium hydroxide. Red spots appear after heating at 100°C for 5 min.
Under UV light a bright red fluorescence is produced.

Hess and Rolde (1964) developed a very sensitive fluorometric method
for ganglioside sialic acid in the nanogram range. It is based on the reaction
of 3,5-diaminobenzoic acid with 2-deoxy sugars to give highly fluorescent
quinaldines. The method outlined by Hess and Rolde must be followed exactly. Recently a reliable method for the analysis of ganglioside sialic acids
by gas-liquid chromatography has been developed by Yu and Ledeen (1970).
As little as 0.3 μg of a sialic acid can be analyzed. This method is particularly
useful for the quantification of N-glycolylneuraminic acids since colorimetric procedures for sialic acids do not differentiate the various types which
may be encountered in gangliosides from different tissue sources.

B. Determination of Hexoses and Hexosamines in Gangliosides

The anthrone reaction has limited value for the determination of total
hexose content of gangliosides since they contain more than one type of
hexose and the different hexoses have different molar extinction coefficients.
Acid hydrolysis to liberate the sugars from gangliosides also poses problems.
The sialic acid is destroyed under the conditions required to liberate free
hexoses and hexosamines and further, in general, stronger hydrolysis conditions are needed to liberate hexosamines than hexoses. Thus there are losses
of free monosaccharides due to their instability in hot acid. Recoveries of
hexoses and hexosamines must be ascertained for the conditions selected.
Usually 4 M HCl with the ganglioside sample in a sealed tube and heated at
100°C for 4–8 hr completely liberates hexoses and hexosamines. If hexosamines are not present, 2 M HCl at 100°C for 1.5–3 hr is sufficient. The HCl
is removed in a vacuum desiccator in the presence of NaOH pellets or in an
all-glass freeze-drying assembly containing NaOH pellets. The hexosamines
can be absorbed on small columns of Dowex 50-X4 (H$^+$ form, 200–400
mesh) (Boas, 1953).

The water eluate and washings contain the neutral hexoses. The hexosamines are eluted with 2 M HCl and the HCl is removed as described
above. A variety of methods are available for analysis of the hexoses and
hexosamines (Colowick and Kaplan; 1966, 1969). Glucose and galactose can
be determined specifically using glucose and galactose oxidases (Glucostat
and Galactostat procedures as outlined in the manual of the Worthington
Biochemical Corp. Freehold, N. J.). Neutral sugars can also be analzyed
by thin-layer chromatographic separation followed by densitometry (Moczar
and Moczar, 1970). Most procedures require 10–20 μg of each sugar. However, a sensitive photodensitometric method developed by Moczar et al.

(1967) has been used by the author for the quantitative determination of 0.1–1 μg of individual hexoses and hexosamines in hydrolyzates of glycolipids and glycoproteins. Total hexosamines may be determined colorimetrically by one or other method based on the Elson-Morgan reaction (Colowick and Kaplan, 1966). Individual hexosamines can be separated on Dowex 50, X-8 (H$^+$ form) by the Gardell procedure (1953). Brain gangliosides contain only N-acetylgalactosamine, but gangliosides from other tissues, particularly erythrocytes, may contain N-acetylglucosamine.

C. Isolation of Sialyloligosaccharides from Gangliosides

The two principal techniques for the cleavage of the oligosaccharide intact from the ceramide moiety of gangliosides take advantage of the fact that the major long chain bases are sphing-4-enine (sphingosine) and eicosasphing-4-enine (eicosasphingosine). The double bond can be oxidized by ozone gas [Wiegandt and Baschang method (1965)] or by osmium tetroxide and sodium metaperiodate [Hakamori method (1966)] the oxidized products hydrolyzed with alkali. The sialyloligosaccharides are released intact through a β-elimination reaction. Unfortunately, either procedure causes considerable degradation of the oligosaccharides and recoveries are low. Our experience favors the Wiegandt and Baschang method and recoveries of sialyloligosaccharides as high as 40% have been achieved. A convenient and cheap ozone generator which has been found very suitable for ganglioside work has been described by Beroza and Bierl (1969). It is simply constructed and very efficient. Gangliosides are dissolved in freshly distilled dry methanol kept ice cold and approximately 5% ozone in oxygen passed through the solution until the solution is yellow to 2% potassium iodide (about 2 min). The ozonolyzed ganglioside is recovered by flash evaporation and dissolved in 10% sodium carbonate (3 mg ganglioside/ml of alkali). This solution is stirred overnight at room temperature and deionized by stirring with Dowex 50 X-8 (H$^+$ form) resin until a final pH of 3.0 is obtained. The crude sialyloligosaccharides are recovered by freeze drying and purified by chromatography on a Dowex-1 X-2 (acetate form) resin column. The sialyloligosaccharides are eluted with a linear gradient between water and 0.8 M pyridine–acetic acid pH. The column is monitored by the resorcinol reaction. The various sialic acid-containing peaks are pooled, concentrated, and analyzed by descending chromatography on Whatman 4 MM paper developed with pyridine–ethylacetate–acetic acid–water (5:5:1:4 by volume). The compounds can be visualized by the thiobarbituric acid reaction outlined above or for reducing oligosaccharides by aniline–diphenylamine–phosphate or other reactions for sugars (Smith, 1960).

D. Analysis of Ganglioside Oligosaccharides by Gas–Liquid Chromatography

The compositional analysis of the sugars in intact gangliosides can be determined readily and conveniently by methanolysis in 0.5–1 M anhydrous methanolic–HCl at 80°C for 18–24 hr. The methyl esters of the fatty acids are partitioned into hexane from aqueous methanol. The methyl glycosides remain in the aqueous methanol. The trimethylsilyl ethers are formed and subjected to gas–liquid chromatography by the methods of Sweeley and Vance (1967). The analysis of the hexosamines by this technique requires the reacetylation of the amino group prior to the formation of the trimethylsilyl derivatives. Deacetylated methyl aminoglycosides do not form trimethylsilyl ethers under the conditions that are used to silylate hexoses (Perry, 1964). The sialic acid residues can be hydrolyzed from the rest of the oligosaccharide under much milder conditions (0.05 M methanolic HCl, 80°C, 1 hr) which does not hydrolyze the acetamido groups. Reacetylation is therefore not necessary prior to formation of the trimethylsilyl derivatives and GLC analysis (Yu and Ledeen, 1970).

The linkages between the constituent sugars of oligosaccharides are usually determined by permethylation of the intact lipid prior to methanolysis. This is followed by gas–liquid chromatographic analysis of the permethylated methyl glycosides. The permethylation is achieved by reaction of the lipid with methyl iodide and silver oxide in anhydrous dimethylformamide (Yamakawa *et al.*, 1963) or methyl iodide and sodium hydride in anhydrous dimethylsulfoxide (Hakamori, 1964). The GLC analysis can be very complex, particularly in the case of high molecular weight glycolipids with a number of different components. Comparison of the retention times of the permethylated sugars with those of known standards is essential to the correct identification of the products and the interpretation of the interglycosidic linkages.

E. Analysis of the Ceramide Part of Gangliosides

The method of Vance and Sweeley (1967) used for the gas–liquid chromatographic analysis of the sugars in gangliosides can also be applied for the analysis of the long chain bases and fatty acids. Following the anhydrous methanolysis of the lipid, the fatty acid methyl esters are extracted with *n*-hexane and analyzed directly by any of a large number of available methods (Colowick and Kaplan, 1969; Marinetti, 1967). The long chain bases partition with the methyl glycosides and can be analyzed as the trimethylsilyl derivatives on the same gas-liquid column as the sugars. The retention times of the bases are considerably longer than those of the trimethylsilyl derivatives of the methyl glycosides. The column temperature must therefore be raised 30–40°C by temperature programming or manually to make the simultaneous determination of the sugars and bases practicable. Unfortunately, under completely anhydrous conditions there is a substantial formation of 3-0 methyl and 5-methoxy-3-deoxy derivatives of sphingenine (Dawson and Sweeley, 1971; Polito et al., 1968). This can be largely overcome by modifying the conditions of hydrolysis according to Gaver and Sweeley (1965). Confirmation of the identity of the long chain bases is achieved by comparison of the retention times of authentic standards or by mass spectrometry (Polito et al., 1968). An excellent detailed review of long chain bases and methods for their determination has recently appeared (Karlsson, 1970).

F. Mass Spectrometry of Gangliosides

Very recently several studies have been done on the feasibility of analyses of intact gangliosides by mass spectrometry (Sweeley and Dawson, 1969; 1971). The results are encouraging and may prove in the future to be an important adjunct to the study of these complex lipids since mass spectrometry can be carried out on 20–100 μg of lipid.

REFERENCES

Beroza, M., and Bierl, B. A. (1969) *Mikrochimica Acta* 4, 720.

Boas, N. F. (1953) *J. Biol. Chem.* 204, 553.

Brady, R. O. (1969) in *Duncan's Disease of Metabolism*, 6th ed. (P K. Bondy, ed.). W. B. Saunders, Philadelphia, p. 357.

Colowick, S. P., and Kaplan, N. O.,eds, (1966) *Methods in Enzymology,* Vol. VIII, *Complex Carbohydrates,* Academic Press, New York.

Colowick, S. P., and Kaplan, N. O., eds. (1959) *Methods in Enzymology,* Vol. XIV, *Lipids,* Academic Press, New York.

Dawson, G., and Sweeley, C. C. (1971) *J. Lipid Res.* 12, 56.

Folch, J., Lees, M., and Sloane-Stanley, G. M. (1957) *J. Biol. Chem.* 226, 497.

Gardell, S. (1953) *Acta Chem. Scand.* 7, 207.

Gatt, S. (1969) in *Methods in Enzymology,* Vol. XIV (J. M. Lowenstein, ed.), Academic Press, New York, p. 134.

Gaver, R. D., and Sweeley, C. C. (1965) *J. Amer. Oil Chem. Soc.* 42, 294.

Hakamori, S. I. (1964) *J. Biochem. (Tokyo)* 55, 205.

Hakamori, S. I. (1966) *J. Lipid Res.* 7, 789.

Hess, H. H., and Rolde, E. (1964) *J. Biol. Chem.* 239, 3215.

Karlsson, K.-A. (1970) *Lipids,* 5, 878.

Klenk, E. (1939) *Z. Physiol. Chem.* 262, 128.

Klenk, E. (1942) *Ibid.,* 273, 76.

Korey, S. R., and Gonatas, J. (1963) *Life Sci.* 2, 296.

Kuhn, R., and Wiegandt, H. (1963a) *Chem. Ber.* 96, 886.

Kuhn, R., and Wiegandt, H. (1963b) *Z. Naturforsch.* 18b, 541.

Ledeen, R. (1966) *J. Amer. Oil Chem. Soc.* 43, 57.

Ledeen, R. (1970) *Chem. Phys. Lipids* 5, 205.

Marinetti, G. V. (1962) *Biochemistry* **1**, 350.

Marinetti, G. V., ed. (1967) *Lipid Chromatographic Analysis,* Vol. 1, Marcel Dekker Inc., New York.

McCluer, R. H. (1968) in *Biochemistry of Glycoproteins and Related Substances* (E. Rossi and E. Stoll, eds.), Karger, New York, p. 203.

Miettinen, T., and Takki-Luukkainen, I. T. (1959) *Acta Chem. Scand.* **13**, 846.

Moczar, E., and Moczar, M. (1970) in *Progress in Thin Layer Chromatography and Related Methods* (A. Niederwieser and G. Pataki, eds.), Ann Arbor-Humphrey Science Publ., Ann Arbor, Mich., p. 169.

Moczar, E., Moczar, M., Schillinger, G., and Robert, L. (1967) *J. Chromatog.* **31**, 561.

Ohman, R., Rosenberg, A., and Svennerholm, L. (1970) *Biochemistry* **9**, 3774.

Penick, R. J., Meisler, M. H., and McCluer, R. H. (1966) *Biochim. Biophys. Acta* **116**, 279.

Perry, M. B. (1964) *Can. J. Biochem.* **42**, 451.

Polito, A. J., Akita, T., and Sweeley, C. C. (1968) *Biochemistry* **7**, 2609.

Roseman, S. (1968) in *Biochemistry of Glycoproteins and Related Substances* (E. Rossi and E. Stoll, eds.), Karger, New York, p. 244.

Shapiro, B. (1967) *Ann. Rev. Biochem.* **36**, 247.

Siakotos, A. N., and Rouser, G. (1965) *J. Amer. Oil Chem. Soc.* **42**, 913.

Smith, I. (1960) *Chromatographic and Electrophoretic Techiniques,* Interscience Publ., New York.

Spence, M. W., and Wolfe, L. S. (1967) *J. Neurochem.* **14**, 585.

Sweeley, C. C., and Vance, D. E. (1967) in *Lipid Chromatographic Analysis* (G.V. Marinetti, ed.), Marcel Dekker, New York, p. 465.

Sweeley, C. C., and Dawson, G. (1969) *Biochem. Biophys. Res. Comm.* **37**, 6.

Suzuki, K. (1965) *J. Neurochem.* **12**, 629.

Svennerholm, L. (1957) *Biochim. Biophys. Acta* **24**, 604.

Svennerholm, L. (1963) *J. Neurochem.* **10**, 613.

Svennerholm, L. (1964) *J. Lipid Res.* **5**, 145.

Svennerholm, L. (1970) in *Handbook of Neurochemistry,* Vol. 3 (A. Lajtha, ed.), Chapter 14. Plenum Press, New York.

Vance, D. E., and Sweeley, C. C. (1967) *J. Lipid Res.* **8**, 621.

Warren, L. (1959) *J. Biol. Chem.* **234**, 1971.

Wiegandt, H. (1966) *Rev. Physiol. Biochem. Exptl. Pharmacol.* **57**, 190.

Wiegandt, H. (1971) *Adv. Lipid Res.* **9**, 249.

Wiegandt, H., and Baschang, G. (1965) *Z. Naturforsch.* **20b**, 164.

Yamakawa, T., Yokoyama, S., and Handa, N. (1963) *J. Biochem. (Tokyo)* **53**, 28.

Yu, R. K., and Ledeen, R. W. (1970) *J Lipid Res.* **11**, 506.

Chapter 11

Mucopolysaccharides and Glycoproteins*

Richard U. Margolis

Department of Pharmacology
New York University School of Medicine
New York, N.Y.

and Renée K. Margolis

Department of Pharmacology
State University of New York
Downstate Medical Center
Brooklyn, N.Y.

I. INTRODUCTION

There have been a number of recent reviews and monographs devoted to various aspects of the isolation, characterization, and analysis of mucopolysaccharides and glycoproteins (Brimacombe and Webber, 1964; Gottschalk, 1972; Neufeld and Ginsburg, 1966; Quintarelli, 1968; Rossi and Stoll, 1968; Hunt, 1970; Balazs, 1970; Roy and Trudinger, 1970; Marshall and Neuberger, 1970). Many of the standard works on carbohydrate chemistry and biochemistry also contain information pertinent to these subjects (Whistler and Wolfrom, 1962–1965; Jeanloz and Balazs, 1965–; Dutton, 1966; Davidson, 1967; Aspinall, 1970; Pigman and Horton, 1970–). The structure, metabolism, and possible functions of mucopolysaccharides and glycoproteins in nervous tissue have recently been reviewed (Margolis, 1969; Brunngraber, 1969).

* Research cited in this review which was carried out in the authors' laboratories was supported by grants from the U.S. Public Health Service (MH-17018 and NS-09348).

The nomenclature and structure of the acid mucopolysaccharides are outlined in Table I, while the glycoproteins can be considered to differ from the acid mucopolysaccharides in the following respects: (1), they do not contain uronic acid; (2) they lack a serially repeating unit; (3) they contain a relatively low number of sugar residues in the heterosaccharide; and (4) they contain several sugars (e.g., fucose, sialic acid, galactose, mannose) which are not major components of the acid mucopolysaccharides. However, the mucopolysaccharides can best be considered as a special subclass of glycoproteins, and both types of compounds have many features in common.

This chapter will concentrate on those techniques which have been used most extensively in our and other laboratories, although a small number of the many alternate methods available will be mentioned where appropriate. Insofar as possible, our aim is to point out the advantages and major limitations of the methods described, as well as any special problems associated with the analysis of mucopolysaccharides and glycoproteins in nervous tissue.

II. EXTRACTION OF MUCOPOLYSACCHARIDES AND GLYCOPROTEINS

Brains are extracted with 20 volumes of chloroform–methanol (2:1, v/v), and the residue thus obtained is reextracted once with the same volume of chloroform–methanol in the reverse ratio (1:2, v/v) to remove remaining traces of gangliosides (Suzuki, 1965). For large-scale brain preparations one can also begin with an acetone powder prepared by homogenizing the brain in a small volume of water and then stirring the homogenate into several volumes of cold acetone (Margolis, 1967). The acetone powder is then extracted with chloroform–methanol as described above.

The lipid-free protein residue is dried *in vacuo* over KOH pellets, suspended at a concentration of 2–3% by weight in 0.2 M boric acid-borax buffer (pH 7.8) containing pronase (0.2–1 mg/ml) and 0.005 M CaCl$_2$ (Narahashi and Yanagita, 1967), and digestion is carried out at 55°C. After 24 hr additional pronase may be added (0.2–1 mg/ml) and the digestion continued for a total of 48–72 hr, although digestion has been reported to be essentially complete after 17 hr (Saigo and Egami, 1970). Since denatured proteins are better substrates for proteolytic enzymes than the native forms, brain protein fractions prepared by other techniques than chloroform-methanol extraction should be denatured by heating for several minutes at 100°C. Digestion with papain instead of pronase has been found by other workers to be equally suitable for the isolation of mucopolysaccharides and glycopeptides from brain (Szabo and Roboz-Einstein, 1962; Brunngraber

Table I. Basic Structures of Acid Mucopolysaccharides

Mucopolysaccharide[a]	Sugars present in disaccharide repeating unit, and linkage	Atypical monosaccharide components[b]
Hyaluronic acid	D-Glucuronic acid (β1→3) N-Acetyl-D-glucosamine (β1→4)	May contain L-arabinose in carbohydrate-protein linkage
Chondroitin	D-Glucuronic acid (β1→3) N-Acetyl-D-galactosamine (β1→4)	
Chondroitin 4-sulfate (Chondroitin sulfate A)	D-Glucuronic acid (β1→3) N-Acetyl-D-galactosamine 4-O-sulfate (β1→4)	
Chondroitin 6-sulfate (Chondroitin sulfate C)	D-Glucuronic acid (β1→3) N-Acetyl-D-galactosamine 6-O-sulfate (β1→4)	
Dermatan sulfate (Chondroitin sulfate B)	L-Iduronic acid (α1→3)[c] N-Acetyl-D-galactosamine 4-O-sulfate (β1→4)	D-Glucuronic acid (β1→3) N-Acetyl-D-glucosamine 6-O-sulfate
Keratan sulfate (Keratosulfate)	D-Galactose and D-galactose 6-O-sulfate (β1→3) N-Acetyl-D-glucosamine 6-O-sulfate (β1→4)	L-Fucose D-Mannose Sialic acid
Heparan sulfate (Heparitin sulfate)	D-Glucuronic acid (α1→4)[d] N-Acetyl-D-glucosamine (α1→4) N-Sulfo-D-glucosamine 6-O-sulfate (α1→4)	L-Iduronic acid N-Acetyl-D-glucosamine 6-O-sulfate N-Sulfo-D-glucosamine
Heparin	D-Glucuronic acid (α1→4)[d] N-Sulfo-D-glucosamine and N-Sulfo-D-glucosamine 6-O-sulfate (α1→4)	L-Iduronic acid[e] D-Glucuronic acid 2-O-sulfate L-Iduronic acid 2-O-sulfate N-Acetyl-D-glucosamine 6-O-sulfate

[a] Older nomenclature in parentheses.
[b] Chondroitin 4-sulfate, chondroitin 6-sulfate, dermatan sulfate, heparin, and heparan sulfate also contain D-galactose and D-xylose in the carbohydrate-peptide linkage (-glucuronosyl-galactosyl-galactosyl-xylosyl-O-serine).
[c] L-iduronic acid is the 5-epimer of D-glucuronic acid, and therefore the iduronosyl group has α-configuration according to the convention of carbohydrate chemistry. Linkage is equatorial, carboxyl group axial.
[d] Linkage details of glucuronidic and glucosaminidic bonds of heparin and heparan sulfate are still incomplete, but all linkages are thought to be α1→4.
[e] Recent evidence indicates that iduronic acid may be the predominant uronic acid in heparin.

et al., 1969). The undigested protein residue can be recovered by centrifugation and retreated with pronase or papain in new buffer. However, this procedure appears to solubilize very little additional material, and is probably not necessary for most studies.

After digestion with pronase or papain, the protease digest is cooled to 4°C, and a portion of the nucleic acids as well as the small amount of protein which remains undigested are precipitated by adding trichloroacetic acid to a concentration of 10%. The solution is then neutralized with NaOH and dialyzed for 1–2 days against running tap water and 1–2 days against two changes of deionized water.

We have found that pronase digestion solubilizes over 95% of the total protein-bound hexose, hexosamine, sialic acid, and uronic acid of brain. Noncarbohydrate-containing proteins are digested primarily to dialyzable amino acids and di-and tripeptides, whereas brain glycoproteins are degraded to glycopeptides of substantially higher molecular weight (3000 to 10,000). This difference is due to the additional bulk of the carbohydrate unit of these glycopeptides, and to the fact that their peptide portion has not been degraded as extensively by the proteolytic enzyme as peptides from other segments of the chain because of steric hindrance from the carbohydrate.

All mucopolysaccharides other than hyaluronic acid have also been shown to be covalently linked to protein at their reducing ends. After dialysis of a protease digest of tissues containing mucopolysaccharides and glycoproteins, the completed oligosaccharide portions are retained, as well as the amino acids located in the immediate vicinity of the carbohydrate-peptide linkage region. The low molecular weight dialyzable glycopeptides (and possibly mucopolysaccharides from pathological tissues and urine) appear to represent various incomplete stages in the stepwise biosynthesis and/or degradation of the complete oligosaccharide chains. The insoluble residue remaining after pronase digestion and dialysis is removed by centrifugation, and the supernatant is made 0.03 to 0.04 M in NaCl. The solution is warmed to 37°C and the acid mucopolysaccharides are precipitated by addition of a slight excess of cetylpyridinium chloride (CPC). For the dialyzed protease digest from a single adult rat brain (1.8 g), 0.2 ml of 10% CPC is usually adequate. For large batches of brain it is convenient to concentrate the dialyzed protease digest so that it contains the mucopolysaccharides and glycopeptides from 4–5 g of brain per ml of 0.04 M NaCl, and after warming to 37°C, 17 ml of 10% CPC are added for each kg of brain. The mucopolysaccharides are allowed to precipitate for 6 to 20 hr at room temperature, centrifuged for 15 min at 2000 rpm, and the supernatant is tested with a few drops of 2% CPC to ensure that sufficient CPC has been added for complete precipitation. The CPC supernatant, containing the glycopeptides derived from brain glycoproteins, is treated at room temperature with excess 2 M KSCN to precipitate free CPC as its insoluble cetylpyridinium thiocyanate. (Since CPC is much less soluble in the cold than at room temperature, solutions containing free CPC should not be refrigerated or dialyzed in the cold in order to avoid its partial precipitation.) After addition of KSCN, the solution is allowed to stand for several hours or overnight at 4°C, centrifuged in the cold, and dialyzed to remove excess KSCN. Excess CPC can also be removed by extraction with an immiscible organic solvent such as amyl alcohol or chloroform (Scott, 1960).

Although keratan sulfate has not been detected in normal brain (Szabo and Roboz-Einstein, 1962; Margolis, 1967; Singh and Bachhawat, 1968; Saigo and Egami, 1970), pathological specimens or other tissues which might contain this mucopolysaccharide should not be treated with excess CPC, since cetylpyridinium complexes of keratan sulfate fractions with low sulfate content redissolve on addition of excess precipitating reagent (Antonopoulos et al., 1961; Cifonelli et al., 1967).

A. Fractionation and Characterization of Mucopolysaccharides

The mucopolysaccharide-CPC complexes are dissolved (with warming if necessary) in a minimum volume of 2.5 M NaCl–methanol (2:1, v/v), and the sodium salts of the mucopolysaccharides are precipitated by the slow addition (with stirring) of 60% ethanol followed by 90% ethanol, in the volume ratios of 6:10:25 (methanolic NaCl:60% ethanol:90% ethanol). The precipitate is allowed to remain for at least 12 hr at 4°C, washed sucessively with ethanol and ether, and dried in vacuo over paraffin and P_2O_5.

The mucopolysaccharides can be separated into sulfated (chondroitin sulfate and heparan sulfate) and nonsulfated (hyaluronic acid) fractions by selective precipitation with CPC utilizing the principle of "critical electrolyte concentration" described by Scott (1960). If the mucopolysaccharides (or their CPC-complexes) are dissolved in 0.3 M NaCl, the sulfated compounds can be precipitated with CPC, while hyaluronic acid remains in the supernatant. When present in relatively high concentration, hyaluronic acid can be quantitatively precipitated from the CPC supernatant by dilution to 0.1 M NaCl. At lower concentrations it can be recovered from the dialyzed supernatant (after removal of excess CPC with KSCN) either by lyophilization, or by concentrating the solution and precipitating the hyaluronic acid from 0.1 M NaCl with 3 volumes of ethanol.

It has been shown that in the brains of all species examined, hyaluronic acid, chondroitin 4- and 6-sulfate, and heparan sulfate account for greater than 95% of the acid mucopolysaccharide present (Szabo and Roboz-Einstein, 1962; Margolis, 1967; Singh and Bachhawat, 1968; Saigo and

Egami, 1970). We have found that for metabolic and other studies, hyaluronic acid can be most easily isolated by CPC fractionation as described above. Heparan sulfate can then be isolated by gel filtration or paper chromatography after digestion of the chondroitin sulfates in the sulfated mucopolysaccharide fraction to lower molecular weight disaccharides, using chondroitinase AC or ABC, as described in Section IV,A.

When mucopolysaccharides are isolated from tissues such as brain, where they are present in relatively low concentration, the initial preparation obtained by CPC precipitation usually contains appreciable amounts of nucleic acids, since these polyanions are also precipitated with CPC. Nucleic acids represent a significant source of interference in many of the colorimetric carbohydrate determinations used for the analysis of mucopolysaccharides, including those for uronic acid, N-sulfated hexosamine, and sialic acid.

It is often quite difficult to completely remove nucleic acids from mucopolysaccharides isolated from brain, although the degree of contamination appears to vary somewhat among different species. A considerable portion of the nucleic acids are removed with the undigested protein after treatment of the pronase digest with trichloroacetic acid. Most of the remainder can be precipitated by repeated treatment of a more concentrated solution of the crude mucopolysaccharides (10–15 mg/ml) with 10% trichloroacetic acid at 4°C. Any nucleic acid remaining after these treatments can then be removed by one or more treatments with pancreatic ribonuclease (0.05 M phosphate buffer, pH 7.0, 5 hr at 37°C) followed by digestion in the same buffer for 12 hr after the addition of pancreatic deoxyribonuclease and $MgCl_2$ (0.005 M). In both cases an enzyme-to-substrate ratio of 1:10 is used. After dialysis, the mucopolysaccharides can be reprecipitated with CPC from 0.04 M NaCl.

Hyaluronic acid, heparan sulfate, and chondroitin sulfate can also be partially fractionated by elution from Dowex 1-X2 (200–400 mesh) in the chloride form (Schiller et al., 1961; Pearce et al., 1968). Hyaluronic acid is eluted with 0.5 M NaCl (Schiller et al., 1961), and when this procedure was used for the purification of hyaluronic acid from bovine (Margolis, 1967) and other brains, much of the accompanying nucleic acid was also removed.

Two fractions of heparan sulfate have been found in rat brain. A minor component is eluted from Dowex 1 with 1.0 M NaCl, while the major fraction is eluted between 1.1 and 1.5 M NaCl (Fig. 1). Most of the chondroitin sulfate is eluted as a single peak between 1.3 and 1.7 M NaCl, although there is appreciable overlap between the heparan sulfate and chondroitin sulfate fractions (Fig. 2). Because of its inability to achieve a clean separation between heparan sulfate and chondroitin sulfate, anion-exchange

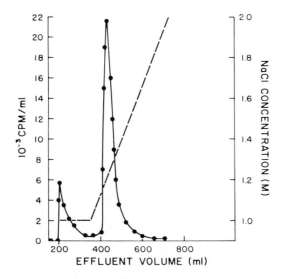

Fig. 1. ³⁵S-Labeled heparan sulfate was isolated by gel
filtration on Sephadex G-25 after digestion of the sulfated
mucopolysaccharides from rat brain with chondroitinase
ABC. Figure shows the elution of two fractions of labeled
heparan sulfate from Dowex 1 (Cl⁻) with 1.0 *M* NaCl
followed by a linear gradient of NaCl.

chromatography alone has only a limited usefulness for the fractionation
of mucopolysaccharides from brain. Other anion-exchange materials such
as DEAE-Sephadex (Schmidt, 1962) and ECTEOLA-cellulose (Antonopoulos *et al.,* 1967; Fransson and Anseth, 1967; Stefanovich and Gore, 1967)
have also been used for the column chromatographic fractionation of
mucopolysaccharides, but are reported to have no significant advantages
over Dowex 1 (Pearce *et al.,* 1968). The method of Scott (1960) for the
fractional precipitation of various polyanions with long-chain aliphatic
ammonium compounds has also been adapted for the determination of
mucopolysaccharides from tissues on a microgram scale (Antonopoulos
et al., 1964; Svejcar and Robertson, 1967; Dorner *et al.,* 1968). This method,
which is based on the stepwise elution of the CPC-mucopolysaccharide
complexes from a cellulose column with a set of specific eluants, has also
been successfully scaled down for such applications as the microchemical
analysis of mucopolysaccharides in histological layers of nasal septum
cartilage (Szirmai *et al.,* 1967). However, since this method distinguishes
mucopolysaccharides not strictly by their chemical nature, but also to some

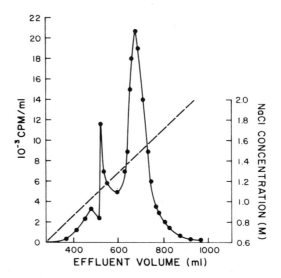

Fig. 2. Gradient elution of sulfated mucopolysaccharides from rat brain on Dowex 1 (Cl⁻). The first two peaks contain predominantly glucosamine, and represent the two fractions of heparan sulfate shown in Fig. 1. The third peak, containing predominantly galactosamine, is removed by digestion with chondroitinase ABC and represents chondroitin sulfate (90% chondroitin 4-sulfate).

extent by their molecular size (Laurent and Scott, 1964), it is necessary to characterize the fractions from each new tissue under investigation. For this reason such fractionation methods cannot be used routinely without prior testing with material from the same organ, species, etc., and in sufficient quantity so that the identity and homogeneity of the isolated fractions can be determined unequivocally on the basis of other criteria such as chemical and enzymic analyses. These limitations also apply to Dowex 1 column chromatography and to cellulose acetate electrophoresis, which are affected by the degree of sulfation of the mucopolysaccharides, as well as to the analysis of pathological samples using techniques devised on the basis of experiments with normal tissue.

Although mucopolysaccharides prepared by these methods will be polydisperse, the identity and homogeneity of the fractions can be evaluated on the basis of their carbohydrate composition and electrophoretic behavior. The presence of nucleic acids can be determined by measuring the absorption at 260 (and 280) mμ. The percent composition, in terms of hexosamine (including the differential determination of glucosamine and galactosamine), uronic acid, neutral sugars, amino acids, sulfate and N-sulfate can be determined by the methods described in Section III.

Because the mucopolysaccharides are highly charged and asymmetric molecules, molecular weights calculated from gel filtration experiments on columns calibrated with protein markers are greatly in error. However, it is possible to obtain accurate molecular weight data by gel filtration using a Sephadex G-200 column calibrated with mucopolysaccharides of known molecular weights (Constantopoulos et al., 1969). Number average molecular weights can be calculated from intrinsic viscosity measurements (Mathews, 1956; Laurent et al., 1960), and relatively simple techniques have recently been described for estimation of the molecular weights of acid mucopolysaccharides by polyacrylamide gel electrophoresis (Mathews and Decker, 1971; Hilborn and Anastassiadis, 1971).

Cellulose acetate strip electrophoresis is also often helpful in identifying acid mucopolysaccharides and evaluating their homogeneity (Mathews, 1961). The mucopolysaccharide in a 0.5–2% solution is spotted once on a prewetted strip of cellulose acetate. Electrophoresis is carried out for 80 min at 100 V or for 45 min at 170 V, using either pyridine-formic acid buffer, pH 3.0, or 0.05 M phosphate buffer, pH 7.0. Strips are stained by spraying with 1% aqueous acridine orange containing 0.2% of a detergent such as "Tergitol" (Carbon and Carbide Chemicals, New York), and then washed for 3–5 min in running tap water.

It is usually possible to obtain a good separation of hyaluronic acid, chondroitin sulfate, heparan sulfate, and heparin. Methods have also been described for the electrophoretic separation of isomeric chondroitin sulfates on cellulose acetate strips (Seno et al., 1970), and for mucopolysaccharide electrophoresis on acrylamide (Hilborn and Anastassiadis, 1969), starch (Brookhart, 1965), and agarose (Horner, 1967) gels.

One should note, however, that the migration distances of the mucopolysaccharides in any particular sample are greatly influenced by such factors as molecular size and degree of sulfation (see, for example, Cifonelli, 1970). Therefore, one cannot rely solely on electrophoresis for the identification of mucopolysaccharides, since the reference compounds may not be comparable to the sample being examined.

B. Fractionation and Characterization of Glycopeptides and Glycoproteins

Any discussion of the fractionation or structural analysis of glycopeptides (or their oligosaccharide side chains) derived from glycoproteins by proteolytic enzyme treatment must consider the various types of heterogeneity which are characteristic of these substances. It is now well recognized that glycoproteins cannot be conceived merely in terms of a protein core to which is linked a carbohydrate side chain of rigorously defined structure. Rather, there appears to be considerable heterogeneity not only in terms of the carbohydrate components themselves (hexoses, hexosamines, sialic acid), but also with respect to the groups attached to the various components (e.g., sulfate, acetyl, and glycolyl residues). Various terms have been used to describe the different types of heterogeneity encountered in studies of mucopolysaccharides and glycoproteins (cf. Huang *et al.,* 1970). The acid mucopolysaccharides are usually described as being *polydisperse,* meaning that although the molecules have essentially the same polymeric covalent structure (i.e., the same disaccharide repeating units), they differ in molecular size. However, even in this relatively simple case the situation is complicated by the existence of hybrid molecules as exemplified by dermatan sulfate, in which both iduronic and glucuronic acids are present in different segments of the molecule (Fransson and Havsmark, 1970). Glycoproteins and glycopeptides are usually described as being *microheterogeneous,* which implies that all molecules in a preparation have the same primary backbone structure, but differ from each other in substitutions of small monomer residues or chemical groups on the primary chain. It is also evident that the dispersion of a biopolymer may be categorized in more than one way, depending on the parameter that is used for reference.

Thus, because the biosynthesis of the glycoproteins and mucopolysaccharides is not controlled by a particular template as in the case of the proteins and nucleic acids (where the natural error in the copying process is estimated to be extremely small), but rather by much less specific glycosyl transferases, one cannot expect to obtain a product in which all of the molecules have identical primary, covalent structures (i.e., are monodisperse). These facts have an important bearing on the limits to any attempt to purify glycoproteins or glycopeptides for structural or metabolic studies, since one is working with a population of molecules whose structure and composition can often be defined only in statistical terms. In attempting to purify these substances to an ever more elusive "homogeneity," one often merely obtains innumerable fractions and subfractions, none of which contains enough material for useful structural or metabolic studies. The situation has been well summarized by Jeanloz (1968), who states that "methods of purification, in order to obtain side-chains possessing a definite structure, have found limited success, and it is questionable, in the case of glycoproteins containing up to seven carbohydrate components, whether side-chains with definite structure and molecular weight exist in preponderant proportion."

For the reasons discussed above it is clear why the few attempts to purify and characterize brain glycoproteins and glycopeptides have met with only limited success. Some degree of fractionation of glycopeptides prepared from brain glycoproteins has been achieved by gel filtration and column electrophoresis on formalated cellulose (Di Benedetta *et al.*, 1969). Glycopeptides from other sources have also been partially resolved by ion exchange or charcoal-Celite column chromatography (Spiro, 1966).

Glycopeptides prepared by proteolytic enzyme digestion of glycoproteins contain a peptide fragment of variable size attached to the carbohydrate chains. In many cases oligosaccharide chains of quite different structures are located close to one another on the original protein core, and are subsequently recovered together, attached to the same peptide. This is because of steric and other factors which limit the extent of proteolytic digestion, as discussed earlier. In all glycopeptides, however, the properties of the amino acids in the peptide fragment may influence the separation of such glycopeptides by ion-exchange chromatography or electrophoresis, and the added bulk of the residual peptide may also affect their behavior on gel filtration columns. For these reasons it is often desirable to remove the peptide portion when possible. This can be achieved by alkali treatment of glycopeptides containing *O*-glycosidic linkages of *N*-acetylgalactosamine to serine and threonine, although it has no effect on *N*-acetylglucosaminylasparagine linkages. This technique has been used for structural studies of the alkali-labile oligosaccharides in rat and rabbit brain glycoproteins, where approximately 10% of the carbohydrate is attached to protein by *O*-glycosidic linkages (Margolis and Margolis 1971). Although alkali and alkaline-borohydride treatment can also yield considerable information concerning the carbohydrate structure and the carbohydrate-peptide linkages of such glycopeptides, a detailed discussion of these techniques is beyond the scope of this review.

Some attempts have also been made to purify and characterize native glycoproteins from brain by chromatography on calcium hydroxylapatite (Brunngraber *et al.*, 1969). However, this approach is hindered by the fact that most of the brain glycoproteins appear to be membrane bound (Dekirmenjian and Brunngraber, 1969), and are therefore difficult to extract and purify without considerable degradation.

III. ANALYTICAL METHODS

A. Hexosamines

Hexosamines are usually determined spectrophotometrically by one of the numerous manual or automated modifications of the original Elson-Morgan method. This involves their reaction with an alkaline solution of 2,4-pentanedione, followed by treatment with an acid solution of *p*-dimethylaminobenzaldehyde to yield a colored product. Prior to colorimetric determination, the hexosamines must be liberated by acid hydrolysis. We have found the manual technique described by Swann and Balazs (1966) to be one of the most reliable forms of the Elson-Morgan reaction. For the mucopolysaccharides found in brain (hyaluronic acid, chondroitin 4- and 6-sulfate, and heparan sulfate), optimum hydrolysis conditions are 6 N HCl for 3 hr at 100°C, and give an average destruction of 5–7% with glucosamine and galactosamine standards. No hydrolysis technique gives complete recovery of hexosamine from mucopolysaccharides or glycoproteins, since in all cases a point is reached at which liberation of additional hexosamine occurs at approximately the same rate as destruction. It is important to avoid conditions (such as dilute acid) under which cleavage of the acetamido bond precedes that of the glycosidic bond, since these lead to the formation of highly acid-resistant glycosides of the deacetylated hexosamines (Moggridge and Neuberger, 1938). Since NaCl in moderate quantities depresses color formation in most of the published procedures, it is necessary to remove under vacuum the HCl used for hydrolysis before performing the Elson-Morgan reaction. A convenient procedure for evaporating a large number of samples is described by Swann and Balazs (1966).

Maximum release of hexosamine from brain glycoproteins occurs after hydrolysis at 100°C for 2 hr in 6 N HCl or for 8 hr in 4 N HCl. Under the latter conditions there is less than 5% destruction of hexosamine or hexosaminitol standards. However, the determination of total hexosamine in glycoproteins or glycopeptides is considerably more susceptible to interference than the analysis of mucopolysaccharides, since neutral sugars in the presence of amino acids can also form colored products which absorb at the same wavelength used for measuring the Elson-Morgan chromogen (530 mμ). For this reason it is advisable when studying glycoprotein hydrolyzates to separate the hexosamines from the neutral sugars and some of the amino acids and peptides using a short column of Dowex 50 (Boas, 1953; Spiro, 1966). Although this step will usually remove interfering substances unless they are present in much greater concentrations than the hexosamines, condensation products of amino acids may still cause interference in the analysis of certain samples (Chotiner et al., 1968).

We have found that the differential determination of glucosamine and galactosamine is most conveniently accomplished using the 15-cm column intended for analysis of the basic amino acids on a Beckman amino acid analyzer (Spackman et al., 1958; Walborg et al., 1963). If the pH of the eluting buffer is decreased from 5.28 to 5.20 a single quantitation of as little as 0.003 μmole of glucosamine and galactosamine can be completed in less than 40 min, after which the column is regenerated with NaOH to remove the basic amino acids. The accelerated systems devised for amino acid determinations in protein hydrolyzates are not usually satisfactory for the analysis of glycoproteins, since hexosamines usually appear after the neutral and acidic amino acids, and may not be resolved from phenylalanine. Spiro (1966) has described buffer modifications for the differential determination of amino acids, glucosamine, and galactosamine using the Technicon single-column amino acid analyzer.

Although glucosamine and galactosamine are the only amino sugars which have been detected so far as structural components of glycoproteins or mucopolysaccharides, many other amino sugars occur in nature or are formed chemically by procedures such as periodate oxidation of glyco-peptides and oligosaccharides. These other amino sugars can usually be resolved by modifications of buffers and programming on an amino acid analyzer (Heyns et al., 1966; Lüderitz et al., 1968; Yaguchi and Perry, 1970; Steele et al., 1970). In preliminary studies we have found that approximately 1.5% of the total hexosamine in rabbit brain glycopeptides appeared at the same elution volume as mannosamine when analyzed on the amino acid analyzer using the pH 5.06 citrate-borate buffer of Bella and Kim (1970). All of this material appears to be a component of the alkali-stable glycopeptide fraction. However, since no peak corresponding to mannosamine was detected in hydrolyzates of rat brain glycopeptides, further study will be required to confirm the presence of this small amount of mannosamine in rabbit brain glycoproteins, and to evaluate its possible significance.

The amino acid analyzer also provides a convenient method for the separation from hexosamines and the quantitation of glucosaminitol and galactosaminitol obtained after reduction of oligosaccharides derived from glycoproteins, or produced by alkaline-borohydride cleavage of O-glycosidic carbohydrate-peptide linkages in glycoproteins (Weber and Winzler, 1969; Bella and Kim, 1970).

Several colorimetric procedures have been described for the differential determination of glucosamine, galactosamine, and other amino sugars (Radhakrishnamurthy and Berenson, 1964; Risse and Lüderitz, 1964; Swann and Balazs, 1966; Glowacka et al., 1967; Ludowieg and Benmaman, 1968). However, these methods are often quite sensitive to interference by compounds other than hexosamines, and there is one report of inconsistent results when applied to glycopeptides from brain glycoproteins (Brunngraber et al., 1970).

Simplified column chromatographic procedures for the separation and analysis of glucosamine and galactosamine, such as the widely used Dowex 50 method described by Gardell (1953), are a great improvement over most differential colorimetric assays. However, the Gardell column does not always eliminate interfering amino acids, and improvements have been proposed (Kelleher and Smith, 1968).

Gas chromatographic methods for the determination of hexosamines have also been described (Perry, 1964; Karkkainen *et al.,* 1965; Radhakrishnamurthy *et al.,* 1966).

B. *N*-Acetylhexosamines

N-Acetylhexosamines are conveniently determined by the Morgan-Elson reaction as modified by Reissig *at al.* (1955). In this method the sample is boiled briefly with potassium tetraborate, and then treated at 37°C with an acid solution of *p*-dimethylaminobenzaldehyde to form a red-violet color which is measured spectrophotometrically. The structural features required in an amino sugar derivative for a positive Morgan-Elson reaction are a 2-acylamido group, a free reducing group, and a free hydroxyl group at C-4. Alkali-labile substituents at C-1 or C-4, such as *O*-acetyl groups, are eliminated in the first stage of the determination, and such derivatives thus give a positive reaction. The modification described by Reissig *et al*, reduces interference from such factors as minor variations in the pH of the sample, the presence of sugars plus amino acids, and magnesium ions. It is also more sensitive and less time-consuming than previous versions of the Morgan-Elson reaction.

The determination of *N*-acetylhexosamine reducing groups is often useful in following the course of mucopolysaccharide digestion with enzymes such as testicular hyaluronidase, or for the assay of hyaluronidase activity in crude tissue extracts where turbidimetric and other methods are not satisfactory (Mathews, 1966). An enzymic method for the quantitative differential determination of chondroitin 4-sulfate and chondroitin 6-sulfate in a mixture of the two mucopolysaccharides has also been described by Mathews and Inouye (1961), and is based on the lack of reactivity of *N*-acetylgalactosamine 4-sulfate in the Morgan-Elson reaction.

Further details on the chemistry and reactions of the hexosamines and *N*-acetylhexosamines can be found in the review by Horton (1969).

C. *N*-Sulfated Hexosamine

Heparin and heparan sulfate contain variable amounts of *N*-sulfate in addition to *O*-sulfate groups (Brimacombe and Webber, 1964). One of the major differences between these two mucopolysaccharides, whose structures are still not well established, is that heparin usually has a considerably higher molar ratio of *N*-sulfate and a lower ratio of *N*-acetyl groups to total glucosamine. Nitrous acid treatment of heparin and heparan sulfate results in the deamination of *N*-sulfated D-glucosamine residues, and the formation of reducing terminal 2,5-anhydromannose groups which can be determined colorimetrically (Lagunoff and Warren, 1962; Cifonelli, 1968). The procedure of Lagunoff and Warren is a convenient method for the direct assay of N-sulfated hexosamine in purified samples of heparin and heparan sulfate, but there is considerable interference by 2-deoxyribose when DNA is present. The specific hydrolysis with dilute HCl (0.04 N, 90 min, 100°C) of sulfoamino bonds in [35S]-labeled heparan sulfate provides a simple method for determining the extent of labeling of N-sulfate and O-sulfate groups in heparan sulfate isolated from brain after chondroitinase digestion of the sulfated mucopolysaccharides (Margolis and Margolis, 1972). Inorganic sulfate radioactivity can be measured after its separation from the N-desulfated heparan sulfate by gel filtration or paper chromatography.

D. Uronic Acids

Uronic acids can be conveniently determined in mucopolysaccharide samples by conversion to a furfural-type chromogen after heating with strong acid. A reliable and widely used method is the modification by Bitter and Muir (1962) of Dische's carbazole reaction. This modification, which involves the use of borate in concentrated sulfuric acid, has the advantages of increased sensitivity, greater stability of the color formed, greater reproducibility, reduction of interference by chloride ion and oxidants, and the immediate development of maximum color. The greatest source of interference in the analysis of mucopolysaccharides isolated from brain is the frequent presence of contaminating nucleic acids in partially purified preparations. Large amounts of neutral sugars can also lead to the formation of an anomalous yellow color in the absence of uronic acid, but the extent of this reaction can be evaluated by measuring the ratio of the absorbancy at 350 mμ as compared to that at 430 mμ (Mathews and Cifonelli, 1965).

The dependence of the carbazole reaction on factors such as temperature, borate concentration, etc., has been extensively investigated, and various methods have been proposed for the differential determination of several uronic acids in a mixture, or in the presence of neutral sugar (Gauthier and Kenyon, 1966; Dische and Rothschild, 1967; Galambos, 1967; Knutson and Jeanes, 1968). Other colorimetric methods which have been employed for the determination of uronic acid include the orcinol, napthoresorcinol, and anthrone procedures. These three methods often give marked interference from neutral sugar or protein, but like the original procedure of Dische (1947), they may provide tentative evidence for the presence of iduronic acid in the analysis of samples containing dermatan sulfate. All of the colorimetric methods can be used directly on polymeric material, since "hydrolysis" takes place during the reaction with acid.

There are many problems involved in the isolation and identification of uronic acids from mucopolysaccharides. Because they are very labile to acid and alkali, techniques such as direct acid hydrolysis are often not feasible because the rates of destruction of uronic acid and the liberation of hexosamine are roughly parallel (Wolfrom and Karabinos, 1945; Brimacombe and Webber, 1964). Iduronic acid, although the characteristic constituent of dermatan sulfate, is also present in significant amounts in heparin and heparan sulfate (Cifonelli and Dorfman, 1962; Wolfrom *et al.*, 1969), and may constitute the major uronic acid in heparin (Perlin and Sanderson, 1970). However, it has been reported that deaminative cleavage of the $(1\rightarrow4)$ glycosidic linkage between D-glucosamine and D-glucuronic acid may result in the concomitant epimerization of D-glucuronic acid to L-iduronic acid (Yamauchi *et al.*, 1968; Carter *et al.*, 1969).

Although samples may be hydrolyzed directly in acid (Fransson *et al.*, 1968), the resin hydrolysis procedure described by Jeffrey and Rienits (1967) may give more quantitative recoveries. The isolated uronic acids may then be separated by paper chromatography (Marsh, 1966) or electrophoresis (St. Cyr, 1970). Since glucuronic and iduronic acids lactonize under conditions used for hydrolysis, these may show two spots. Methods have also been described for the separation of uronic acids and uronic acid-containing oligosaccharides by manual or automated ion-exchange chromatography (Dziewiatkowski, 1962; Johnson and Samuelson, 1966; Fransson *et al.*, 1968).

Analysis of the sulfated mucopolysaccharides of brain by chondroitinase AC and ABC digestion (Section III, A), and by ion-exchange chromatography of the uronic acids according to the method of Fransson *et al.* (1968), has revealed that only traces of dermatan sulfate are present in rat, rabbit, and bovine brain. We have found that iduronic acid comprised 2–5% of the total uronic acid isolated from brain mucopolysaccharides. However, it is known that dermatan sulfate accumulates in brain in certain pathological conditions such as Hurler's syndrome. The uronic acid composition of normal brain mucopolysaccharides would also appear to warrant further investigation since there has been a preliminary report of the presence of a novel galacturonic acid-containing mucopolysaccharide in rabbit and human brain (Stary *et al.*, 1964).

E. Sulfate

The sulfate content of mucopolysaccharides or glycoproteins can be quantitatively determined as inorganic sulfate after hydrolysis in 1 N HCl for 4 hr at 100°C. Spencer (1960) has described ultramicro modifications of the benzidine and barium chloranilate methods for the determination of inorganic sulfate. We have found the barium chloranilate method to be less tedious and more suitable for routine use, although it is known to be sensitive to variations in the ionic concentration of the sample (Sutherland, 1966), and thus requires careful neutralization of the hydrolyzate. Other modifications of the benzidine method have also been described (Muir, 1958; Antono-poulos, 1962).

The turbidimetric method of Dodgson and Price (1962) has been widely used for the determination of ester sulfate in mucopolysaccharides. Although it has the advantages of speed and simplicity, this method is not suitable for partial hydrolyzates of mucopolysaccharides (such as would occur in mea-suring the rate of acid hydrolysis of ester sulfate in a sulfated polysaccharide) because undegraded polysaccharides will also produce turbidity and thus cause interference, particularly in the initial stages of the hydrolysis. Turbidi-metric methods are also susceptible to interference by ultraviolet-absorbing materials formed during hydrolysis of the sample (Dodgson and Price, 1961). Most of these limitations have been overcome by the modification of Kawai et al. (1969) in which undegraded mucopolysaccharides are removed by precipitation with cetylpyridinium chloride, although certain samples of keratan sulfate may not precipitate under the recommended conditions.

Inorganic sulfate can also be determined on a micro scale after preci-pitation as the salt of 4-amino-4'-chlorobiphenyl (Jones and Lethan, 1956), by flame photometry (Barker et al., 1968), or by gas chromatography (Srini-vasan et al., 1970).

F. Total Neutral Sugar

The phenol-sulfuric acid reaction described by Dubois et al. (1956) provides one of the most rapid and convenient methods for the determination of simple sugars and their derivatives. In this procedure, 1 ml of 5% phenol is added to 1 ml of sample containing 10–80 μg of sugar. Five milliliters of concentrated sulfuric acid are then added rapidly directly onto the surface of the water layer. Rapid addition of acid is necessary since the heat required for color development is provided by the exothermic reaction of sulfuric acid and water.

Hexoses, pentoses, methylpentoses, uronic acids, disaccharides, and oligo-and polysaccharides (including their methylated derivatives possessing a free or potentially free reducing group) produce an orange-yellow color with an absorption maximum at 480–490 mμ. For the sugars present in glycoproteins, the absorption is read at 490 mμ after the samples have stood for 30 min at room temperature, and the color remains stable for up to 3 hr. Since the extinction coefficients vary among the different sugars (xylose> mannose > galactose > fucose), standard solutions with approximately the same composition as the sample should be used for greatest accuracy in the measurement of total sugar in a mixed sample. Amino sugars and sialic acids do not react, and although the method is especially useful for the analysis of glycoproteins, insofar as it is largely unaffected by the presence of protein, it is advisable to include an internal standard when the assay is used for the determination of small amounts of carbohydrate in the presence of a large excess of protein. α- and β-keto acids and aliphatic aldehydes and ketones also give a yellow color with the phenol-sulfuric acid reagent (Montgomery, 1961). Although these substances would not constitute a common source of interference in the carbohydrate analysis of glycoproteins, when ketones are used as solvents, as in chromatographic systems, it is necessary to remove them completely before proceeding with quantitative carbohydrate determinations by the phenol-sulfuric acid method.

Another possible source of interference is borate, which, because of its well-known ability to form anionic complexes with polyhydroxy compounds, has been used extensively for the separation of carbohydrates by paper electrophoresis or column chromatography. The absorbance of solutions containing hexoses is reduced slightly, and that of pentoses is lowered significantly, by the presence of borate in solutions tested by the phenol-sulfuric acid procedure (Lin and Pomeranz, 1968).

The anthrone method (Hodge and Hofreiter, 1962) has also been widely used for the determination of reducing sugars and carbohydrates. However, in addition to being more tedious than the phenol-sulfuric acid method, it requires the use of an expensive and relatively unstable reagent, and is affected by certain salts, oxidizing agents, acids, solvents, preservatives, amino acids, and proteins.

G. Methylpentoses

Fucose is the only methylpentose whose presence in glycoproteins has been firmly established, although rhamnose and various 3-O-methyl-6-methylpentoses are known to occur in the cardiac glycosides and other biological materials. Methylpentoses can be estimated after conversion to furfural derivatives and other degradation products, which are then reacted with a mercapto-containing compound. They are usually determined by the cysteine-sulfuric acid procedure of Dische and Shettles (1948), which involves heating the sample for 10 min at 100°C with sulfuric acid, and, after cooling, adding cysteine hydrochloride to give a yellow-green color. The optical density is read at 400 and 430 mμ after allowing the solution to stand for several hours at room temperature, and the difference between these values is compared with that given by standard fucose solutions. Hexoses, pentoses, and hexuronic acids do not interfere. We have found it advantageous to use the modification introduced by Gibbons (1955), who has substituted thioglycolic acid for cysteine hydrochloride, and has shown that the values obtained are little affected by the presence of large amounts of other sugars, hexosamines, or amino acids, including tryptophan. Moreover, the accuracy is improved, and thioglycolic acid produces a more rapid development of color which then remains stable for at least 3 hr. Prior hydrolysis of the sample is not required as a separate step in the analysis of glycoprotein-bound fucose.

Free fucose can also be measured enzymically using L-fucose dehydrogenase prepared from pork liver or *Pseudomonas* (Finch *et al.*, 1969).

H. Hexoses

Galactose, mannose, and glucose can be differentially determined in mixtures with each other and with methylpentose by the so-called primary and secondary cysteine-sulfuric acid reactions of Dische (Dische *et al.*, 1949; Dische, 1955). Modifications have recently been described which increase the sensitivity and make the reactions better reproducible (Dische and Danilchenko, 1967). The major source of interference is from pentoses in contaminating nucleic acids or nucleotides, but this can be partially corrected for by the use of appropriate internal standards. The reactions can be carried out using either unhydrolyzed samples or HCl hydrolyzates of polysaccharides.

The enzymic determination of galactose using D-galactose dehydrogenase offers a more sensitive and specific method for the measurement of galactose in brain glycoproteins (Margolis and Margolis, 1970a). Samples are hydrolyzed for 3 hr in 1 N HCl at 100°C and neutralized with NaOH. Neutralized sample (0.2 ml) containing 0.03 to 0.3 μmole of D-galactose is assayed after the addition of Tris buffer, NAD, and D-galactose dehydrogenase. Correspondingly smaller sample volumes can be used if semimicro or micro cells are employed. The amount of galactose present is calculated from the extent of NAD reduction as measured at 340 mμ. There is no interference by amino acids or by any of the other sugars present in brain glycoproteins.

Galactose can also be measured enzymically using galactose oxidase, although this is not as specific as D-galactose dehydrogenase insofar as D-galactosamine is also oxidized. Therefore, galactosamine must be either removed by passing the sample through a short column of Dowex 50, or measured separately by another method (such as ion exchange chromatography) and the appropriate correction applied to the galactose assay.

There is unfortunately no sensitive and specific colorimetric or spectrophotometric method available for the determination of mannose. Mannose can be determined by difference after measurement of total neutral sugar by the phenol-sulfuric acid reaction, and galactose and fucose with D-galactose dehydrogenase and the thioglycolic-sulfuric acid reaction, respectively. We have found this procedure to be more accurate, sensitive, and convenient than the differential determination of galactose and mannose using the primary and secondary cysteine reactions.

Finch *et al.* (1969) have described an enzymic microassay for mannose which involves its phosphorylation to mannose-6-phosphate by hexokinase and ATP, followed by a measurement of ADP formation using pyruvate kinase and lactic dehydrogenase. The extent of NADH oxidation is measured spectrophotometrically and corresponds to the amount of mannose originally present in the sample. However, the method is not specific for D-mannose since both D-glucosamine and D-glucose are also phosphorylated by hexokinase. This difficulty can be overcome by removing D-glucosamine on a short cation-exchange column prior to assay, and by measuring D-glucose, if present, with a specific assay (see below) and applying the appropriate correction for glucose to the mannose assay.

The most sensitive and specific method for mannose determination is gas chromatography (cf. Section III, K).

Glucose is not a well-established constituent of any animal glycoproteins except collagen, and the small amounts reported by some investigators as occurring in brain glycoproteins may be derived from connective tissue in the meninges or brain vasculature. By means of a spectrophotometric assay for glucose using yeast hexokinase and glucose-6-phosphate dehydrogenase (Slein, 1965), we have found that less than 0.3% of the carbohydrate in glycopeptides prepared from rat and rabbit brain glycoproteins can be accounted for as glucose. In studying sugars which may be present in very low concentration in glycoproteins, it is also important to avoid such steps as dialysis, gel filtration on Sephadex, and chromatography on cellulose columns, since these procedures may lead to contamination with extraneous carbohydrate.

I. Sialic Acids

The most sensitive and specific of the commonly used methods for the determination of sialic acid is the thiobarbituric acid assay of Warren (1959). In this colorimetric assay, the sialic acids are oxidized with sodium periodate in concentrated phosphoric acid, the periodate oxidation product is coupled with thiobarbituric acid, and the resulting pink chromophore is extracted into cyclohexanone. The mechanism of the reaction has been studied by Paerels and Schut (1965). Since the method measures only unbound sialic acid, it can be used for the differential determination of both free and bound sialic acid in samples assayed before and after mild acid hydrolysis. Glycosidically bound sialic acid can be released from brain glycopeptides by hydrolysis for 1 hr in 0.1 N H_2SO_4 at 80°C. Values must be corrected for destruction during hydrolysis (approximately 10%) under these conditions. The thiobarbituric acid method allows the measurement of approximately 5 μg of sialic acid.

The most important interfering substance found in biological materials is 2-deoxyribose, although suitable methods for correcting for the presence of this sugar have been described (Warren, 1959). It has also been reported that small amounts of ferrous salts decrease the color yield significantly (Hartree and Brown, 1970).

An alternative method for the colorimetric determination of *total* sialic acid is the resorcinol method of Svennerholm (1957), as modified by Miettinen and Takki-Luukkainen (1959). Although this method is less sensitive (requiring approximately 10 μg of sialic acid) and less specific than the thiobarbituric acid assay, it has recently been further modified by introducing a periodate oxidation step prior to heating with the resorcinol reagent (Jourdian *et al.,* 1971). With this modification it is also possible to determine total, free, or bound sialic acid. The periodate-resorcinol method is reported to be more sensitive than the resorcinol procedure, is not affected by lipids, amino acids, or sugars, and can be used to detect free or glycosidically-bound sialic acids on paper chromatograms.

A sensitive fluorometric method which can measure 0.3 μg or less of sialic acid has also been described (Hess and Rolde, 1964).

Yu and Ledeen (1970) have described a gas chromatographic method for the assay of lipid-bound sialic acid. This method also appears to be adaptable for the determination of sialic acid in glycopeptides and glycoproteins. It has the advantages of high sensitivity (0.3 μg) and the capacity to simultaneously determine both N-acetylneuraminic acid and N-glycolylneuraminic acid. O-Acetyl-N-glycolylneuraminic acid could be detected but not quantified, due to partial removal of the highly labile O-acetyl group during methanolysis. Although rat and rabbit brain glycoproteins contain only N-acetylneuraminic acid (Yu and Margolis, unpublished results), it is possible that there are species differences in the sialic acid composition of brain glycoproteins similar to those reported for the gangliosides (Yu and Ledeen, 1970). The gas chromatographic method may also be advantageous for the analysis of sialic acids in crude or only partially purified samples, since these often yield false chromogens in colorimetric procedures.

J. Column Chromatographic Separation of Neutral Sugars

Most neutral sugars form anionic complexes in alkaline borate buffers, and are therefore amenable to separation by ion-exchange chromatography.

A number of chromatographic systems have been described for the automated analysis of neutral mono- and oligosaccharides using alkaline borate buffers (Ohms *et al.*, 1967; Kesler, 1967; Jolley and Freeman, 1968; Lee *et al.*, 1969), and Technicon Instruments Co manufactures an automated chromatographic system based on this principle. However, since alkaline rearrangement and other degradative reactions have been reported to occur during the chromatography of saccharides at elevated temperatures in alkaline borate buffers, Walborg and co-workers have described procedures for their elution at neutral pH utilizing boric acid–glycerol or boric acid–2,3-butanediol buffers (Walborg and Lantz, 1968; Walborg *et al.*, 1969). This latter system has also been automated, employing the Hitachi Perkin-Elmer liquid chromatograph (Walborg and Kondo, 1970). These methods are capable of quantitating a variety of mono- and oligosaccharides with a precision of approximately $\pm 5\%$, and absolute recoveries of 90 to 100% have been reported for monosaccharides eluted from anion exchangers with either alkaline or neutral borate buffers at elevated temperatures. Although such automated chromatographic systems have found limited use up to now in the analysis of the carbohydrate components of glycoproteins, they offer a sensitive and specific method which will undoubtedly be more widely employed in the future.

Other systems have been described for the partition chromatography of sugars on strongly basic anion exchangers in the sulfate form, or cation exchangers in the lithium form, using water–ethanol mixtures for elution (Larsson *et al.*, 1966; Jonsson and Samuelson, 1967; Martinsson and Samuelson, 1970).

K. Gas Chromatographic Methods

Gas chromatography provides a very sensitive and specific method for the determination of neutral sugars and hexosamines in glycoproteins and mucopolysaccharides. A great number of procedures have been described using different derivatives and operating conditions. The *O*-trimethylsilyl ethers of the carbohydrates (Sweely *et al.*, 1966) have been employed in many published procedures. Clamp *et al.* (1967) have described a method for the simultaneous estimation in glycopeptides and glycoproteins of fucose, mannose, galactose, *N*-acetylglucosamine, and *N*-acetylneuraminic acid as trimethylsilyl ethers of their methyl glycosides, after methanolysis and re-*N*-acetylation. In their study, methanolysis was found to be preferable to aqueous acid hydrolysis of the oligosaccharides in these biological materials. Methods have also been described which give resolution of eleven alditol acetates of the neutral monosaccharides commonly found in glycoproteins and mucopolysaccharides (Lehnhardt and Winzler, 1968).

Procedures employing the trimethylsilyl ethers have the advantage that preparation of the derivatives is simple, and standard reference compounds are commercially available. On the other hand, the trimethylsilyl derivatives of most samples of a single sugar will show two or more peaks due to the presence of various isomeric forms. This does not usually constitute a serious disadvantage, although it may complicate the interpretation of chromatograms in which unknown sugars are present.

L. Paper Chromatography and Electrophoresis

In Table II the relative migration distances are given for a number of sugars which have been reported to be present in brain mucopolysaccharides or glycoproteins. These are presented mainly to indicate the separation which can be expected for any particular combination of sugars, as an aid in the selection of appropriate solvent systems. Other useful solvents and tables of R_f values are given in monographs on paper chromatography (Smith, 1969; Sherma and Zweig, 1971).

For paper chromatographic identification of their component sugars, glycopeptides or oligosaccharides can be hydrolyzed for 3 hr in 1 N HCl at 100°C, and the hydrolyzate neutralized with Dowex 3 (CO^{2-}_3). Sialic acid is destroyed under these conditions, but can usually be quantitatively released

Table II. Relative Migration Distances on Paper of Sugars Found in Glycoproteins and Mucopolysaccharides

	$R_{galactose}$				
	A	B	C	D	E
Galactose 6-sulfate	0.44	0.40	0.67	0.53	0.53
N-Acetylglucosamine 6-sulfate	0.65	—	0.98	—	0.63
N-Acetylgalactosamine 6-sulfate	0.63	—	0.96	—	0.69
Galactosamine	0.71	0.36	0.84	0.68	0.80
Glucosamine	0.73	0.48	0.84	0.79	0.86
Glucose	1.11	1.17	—	1.15	1.05
Mannose	1.36	1.32	1.14	1.31	1.21
Arabinose	1.32	1.51	1.24	1.26	1.21
Xylose	1.48	1.78	—	1.49	1.32
Fucose	1.63	1.71	1.41	1.47	1.57
Rhamnose	1.89	—	1.51	1.78	1.79

Solvent systems:
A. propanol–ethyl acetate–water (7:1:2), 20 hr.
B. ethyl acetate–pyridine–water (8:2:1), 17 hr.
C. ethyl acetate–acetic acid–water (6:3:2), 15 hr.
D. ethyl acetate–pyridine–butanol–butyric acid–water (10:10:5:1:5), 22 hr.
E. butanol–acetic acid–water (50:12:25), 15 hr.

by milder acid hydrolysis (0.1 N H$_2$SO$_4$, 1 hr, 80°C) or by neuraminidase, and then separated from the remaining glycopeptide by gel filtration on Sephadex G-15, or by adsorption on and elution from a short column of Dowex 1 (Spiro, 1966). Silver carbonate has also been utilized for neutralization, but in our experience has not been found to be as satisfactory as Dowex 3 since it often gives rise to multiple spots from standard sugars in certain solvent systems. It should also be noted that solvent systems containing pyridine are extremely sensitive to salt in the sample, leading to streaking of the chromatogram. Hydrolysis in 2 N trifluoroacetic acid for 2 hr at 120°C also gives good yields of monosaccharides from glycopeptides, and has the advantage that the acid can be easily removed by evaporation under vacuum.

The most sensitive and generally useful detection reagent for sugars is alkaline silver nitrate (Trevelyan *et al.,* 1950). The paper is rapidly pulled through a saturated solution of silver nitrate in acetone, air-dried, and then sprayed in a fume hood with 0.5 N ethanolic NaOH (prepared by diluting saturated aqueous NaOH with ethanol). After fixing with 5% sodium thiosulfate (Anet and Reynolds, 1954), reducing sugars and glycols give dense brown or black spots of silver on a gray or white background. The sensitivity is approximately 1 µg for hexoses and methylpentoses, 2 µg for pentoses, hexosamines, and glucuronic acid, 4 µg for N-acetylhexosamines, and 5 µg for glucuronolactone (Mes and Kamm, 1968).

The aniline hydrogen phthalate spray of Wilson (1959) is also useful but often less sensitive than alkaline silver nitrate. The dried chromatogram is sprayed with the reagent (1.66 g *o*-phthalic acid, 0.9 ml aniline, 48 ml *n*-butanol, 48 ml ethyl ether, 4 ml water), and then heated at 105°C for 5–10 min to develop the spots. Hexoses, methylpentoses, uronic acids, and hexosamines give brown or orange-brown spots, while pentoses give red spots. One to two micrograms of hexose, pentose, glucuronic acid, or hexosamine can be detected. Methylpentoses, glucuronolactone, and acetylhexosamines require larger amounts (Mes and Kamm, 1968). If the paper contains borate buffer, this should first be volatilized as trimethyl borate by spraying the paper twice with methanol containing 7% acetic acid, followed each time by heating for 15 min at 60°C (Spiro and Spiro, 1965). This also greatly increases the sensitivity of the alkaline silver nitrate procedure with borate-impregnated paper. The aniline hydrogen phthalate method has also been used for the quantitative determination of sugars after elution of the stained spots from the chromatogram (Wilson, 1959). Mes and Kamm (1968) have reported on the relative sensitivity of a large number of other reagents for the detection and differentiation of sugars and sugar derivatives found in glycoproteins after their separation by paper chromatography.

Sugars can also be separated by high voltage paper electrophoresis using 0.05 M borate buffer (pH 9.2) or 0.05 N acetic acid–pyridine buffer (pH 6.0). Relative migration distances and other buffer systems are described by Zweig and Whitaker (1967).

IV. ENZYMIC ANALYSIS OF MUCOPOLYSACCHARIDES AND GLYCOPROTEINS

A. Bacterial Chondroitinases and Chondrosulfatases

The recent purification and characterization by Yamagata and co-workers (1968) of a series of bacterial chondroitinases and chondrosulfatases marked a significant advance in the methods available for the analysis of sulfated mucopolysaccharides. Two chondroitinases have been purified to apparent homogeneity and their properties described. "Chondroitinase ABC," purified from extracts of *Proteus vulagris,* degrades chondroitin 4-sulfate (CS-A), chondroitin 6-sulfate (CS-C), and dermatan sulfate (CS-B) by an elimination reaction to yield the corresponding $\triangle$4,5-unsaturated disaccharide 4- and 6- sulfates (Fig. 3). The unsaturated disaccharides formed from chondroitin 4-sulfate and dermatan sulfate are identical due to the conversion of C-5 of the uronosyl group to the same symmetrical $-CH=C<$ grouping. Although chondroitinase ABC also degrades hyaluronic acid and chondroitin at a slower rate than the three chondroitin sulfates, it does not attack keratan sulfate, heparin, or heparan sulfate. Another type of chondroitinase, "chondroitinase AC," has been purified from extracts of *Flavobacterium heparinum,* and carries out essentially the same reactions as chondroitinase ABC except that it has no measurable ac-tivity with dermatan sulfate (chondroitin sulfate B).

Two sulfatases, "chondro-4-sulfatase" and "chondro-6-sulfatase," also occur in the crude extract of *Proteus vulgaris,* and have been separated from the accompanying chondroitinase ABC and from each other. These chondrosulfatases catalyze the hydrolytic desulfation of the $\triangle$ 4,5-unsaturated disaccharide sulfates obtained as products of chondroitinase digestion.

Chondro-4-sulfatase catalyzes the conversion of $\triangle$4,5-unsaturated disaccharide 4-sulfate (i.e., the product of chondroitinase ABC degradation of chondroitin 4-sulfate or dermatan sulfate) and its saturated analog (*N*-acetylchondrosine-4-sulfate) to the corresponding nonsulfated disaccharides and inorganic sulfate. It does not attack $\triangle$4,5-unsaturated disaccharide 6-sulfate (obtained by chondroitinase digestion of chondroitin 6-sulfate) or its saturated analog (*N*-acetylchondrosine 6-sulfate).

In contrast, chondro-6-sulfatase carries out the desulfation of the disaccharide 6-sulfates and *N*-acetylgalactosamine 4,6-disulfate at position 6, but it does not attack the disaccharide 4-sulfate isomers.

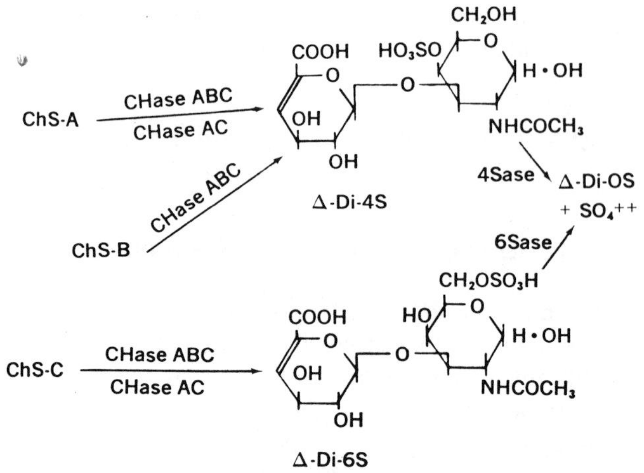

Fig. 3. Activities and end products of chondroitinase AC and ABC, and chondro-4-sulfatase and 6-sulfatase.

The chondrosulfatases do not desulfate polymer chondroitin sulfates or dermatan sulfate, hexa-, penta-, tetra-, or trisaccharides derived from these mucopolysaccharides by digestion with testicular hyaluronidase, or N-acetylgalactosamine 4- and 6-sulfates.

The sulfated and unsulfated disaccharide products of chondroitinase and chondrosulfatase digestions can be easily separated by paper chromatography, and Saito *et al.* (1968) have described methods utilizing these enzymes for the differential measurement of microgram quantities of chondroitin 4- and 6-sulfates and dermatan sulfate in mixtures containing these and other mucopolysaccharides. The unsaturated disaccharides can be detected on paper chromatograms and measured spectrophotometrically by virtue of their absorbancy in the region of 230 mμ. However, the presence of nucleic acids in preparations of brain mucopolysaccharides may require preliminary separation of the disaccharides from undigested high molecular weight material by procedures such as gel filtration. This also provides a convenient method for the isolation of heparan sulfate from brain. Chondroitinase digestion can also be used for the study of "oversulfated" and "undersulfated" chondroitin sulfates by analysis of the resulting disaccharides (Suzuki *et al.*, 1968; Saigo and Egami, 1970).

The chondroitinases and chondrosulfatases as well as certain reference disaccharides are produced commercially by Seikagaku Kogyo Co, Tokyo, Japan, and are distributed in the Western hemisphere by Miles Laboratories, Kankakee, Illinois.

B. Testicular Hyaluronidase

A number of enzymes are known which depolymerize hyaluronic acid, and often other mucopolysaccharides as well. These are known collectively as hyaluronidases, and have been reviewed by several authors (Gibian, 1959; Gibian, 1966; Mathews, 1966; Linker, 1966; Meyer, 1971). The best-characterized enzyme of this group is the endo-β-hexosaminidase produced by sperm and isolated from mammalian testis (testicular hyaluronidase, hyaluronate glycanohydrolase (EC 3.2.1.35)). This enzyme hydrolyzes β-(1→4)-hexosaminidoglucuronic acid bonds of hyaluronic acid to yield at first relatively high molecular weight oligosaccharides, and later a tetrasaccharide as the main (approximately 80–90%) end product. Disaccharides are produced in only small amounts after exhaustive digestion with a large excess of enzyme. The speed of the reaction decreases rapidly with the decrease in chain length of the substrate. In addition to digesting hyaluronic acid, this enzyme also degrades chondroitin 4- and 6- sulfates and chondroitin, but at a considerably slower rate. The degradation leads to sulfated oligosaccharides, and, after exhaustive digestion, to tetrasaccharides and disaccharides. Testicular hyaluronidase has no effect on heparin, heparan sulfate, or keratan sulfate. However, dermatan sulfate, which has been shown to be a hybrid molecule containing both iduronosyl and glucuronosyl linkages, is partially degraded by testicular hyaluronidase (Fransson and Havsmark, 1970).

This enzyme also has transglycosylase activity, as evidenced by the formation of higher oligosaccharides from hexasaccharides (Weissmann, 1955), and of hybrid tetrasaccharides and hexasaccharides from a substrate containing both hyaluronic acid and chondroitin sulfate (Hoffman et al., 1956).

Digestion of mucopolysaccharides with testicular hyaluronidase is usually carried out for 12–24 hr at 37°C in 0.1 M sodium acetate buffer at pH 5.0 containing 0.15 M NaCl. The extent of digestion of a mucopolysaccharide by testicular hyaluronidase can be quantitatively determined using the acid albumin turbidimetric procedure described by Mathews (1966) for the assay of hyaluronidase. When this method is used to determine the extent of digestion of a mucopolysaccharide, excess enzyme (600–700 N.F. units/ml) is added to a dilution of mucopolysaccharide (approximately 1 mg/ml) which gives an absorbance (at 600 mμ) of 0.5 to 0.7 when mixed with acid albumin before digestion. Control and unknown solutions are incubated for 2 hr at 38–40°C. Thunell (1967) has also described a considerably more elaborate microprocedure for studying the depolymerization of mucopolysaccharides by testicular hyaluronidase. The method is based on the increased solubility in salt solutions of the mucopolysaccharide-cetylpyridinium complex which occurs on depolymerization of the mucopolysaccharide. The solubility changes are followed with the aid of the CPC-cellulose microcolumn technique. Oligosaccharides resulting from the digestion of mucopolysaccharides with testicular hyaluronidase can also be fractionated by gel filtration (Flodin *et al.,* 1964) or paper chromatography.

Testicular hyaluronidase is inhibited by sulfated mucopolysaccharides (especially those which are not substrates for the enzyme), as well as by other polyanions and nonspecific protein inhibitors found in tissues and body fluids (for reviews see Mathews and Dorfman, 1955; Gibian, 1959; Bernfeld, 1966).

It should be noted that even very highly purified preparations of testicular hyaluronidase (16,000 NF units/mg) contain significant amounts of contaminating ribonuclease and deoxyribonuclease activity (Margolis and Margolis, 1970b). Considerable amounts of other hydrolytic enzyme contaminants (e.g., acid and alkaline phosphatases, sulfatase, esterases, lipase, β-galactosidase, and β-glucuronidase) have also been found in less highly purified preparations of testicular hyaluronidase (Chauncey *et al.,* 1953). For this reason it is essential to perform appropriate control experiments in physiological and histochemical studies in which conclusions are based on the presumed ability of testicular hyaluronidase to remove only certain mucopolysaccharides. The use of leech hyaluronidase or one of the bacterial mucopolysaccharidases would probably be preferable for such purposes (Margolis and Margolis, 1970b).

C. Other Mucopolysaccharidases

In addition to the chondroitinases and chondrosulfatases described earlier, hyaluronidases (hyaluronate lyases, EC 4.2.99.1) have also been isolated from various other microorganisms, including streptococci, clostridia, pneumococci, staphylococci, and *Escherichia.* These enzymes are all endo-β-hexosaminidases, and in this respect they resemble testicular hyaluronidase. However, like the previously described chondroitinases from adapted strains of *Proteus vulgaris* and *Flavobacterium heparinum,* the bacterial hyaluronidases form $\triangle$4,5-unsaturated uronides by the elimination of water, rather than the saturated oligosaccharides produced by testicular hyaluronidase digestion. Bacterial mucopolysaccharidases are also usually more specific than chondroitinase AC and ABC, in that they digest only *unsulfated* mucopolysaccharides (i.e., hyaluronic acid and chondroitin). Since chondroitin has not been detected in tissues other than cornea, these bacterial hyaluronidases can, for most purposes, be considered as specific enzymes for the digestion of hyaluronic acid. The hyaluronidase from *Streptococcus mitis* or *hemolyticus* has been most commonly used. Digestion can be carried out in 0.1 M phosphate–0.15 M NaCl buffer, pH 5.2, for 12–24 hr at 37°C.

No transglycosylation has been observed with the bacterial hyaluronidases, and the end products are△4,5-unsaturated disaccharides. Also, in contrast to testicular hyaluronidase, the chain length of the substrate has no marked influence on the speed of reaction. Unfortunately, all of the bacterial hyaluronidases are fairly crude, and attempted purification has been difficult.

Ohya and Kaneko (1970) have recently described a novel hyaluronidase from a strain of *Streptomyces*. This enzyme is absolutely specific for hyhyaluronic acid, and does not degrade chondroitin or other mucopolysaccharides. The end products are tetrasaccharides and hexasaccharides, with △4,5-unsaturated glucuronic acid residues at the nonreducing ends.

An endo-β-glucuronidase present in leech heads (salivary glands) also has an absolute specificity for hyaluronic acid and higher oligosaccharides obtained from hyaluronic acid by other types of hyaluronidase. The major end product is a tetrasaccharide with glucuronic acid as the reducing end group (Linker *et al.,* 1960). Leech hyaluronidase has been partially purified and characterized by Yuki and Fishman (1963).

A hyaluronidase which has a selective activity toward hyaluronic acid and chondroitin 4-sulfate has been isolated from tadpole tail fin (Silbert and DeLuca, 1970), and provides a possible means of obtaining chondroitin 6-sulfate free from chondroitin 4-sulfate.

Heparin and heparan sulfate are resistant to the various hyaluronidases, but they are both degraded by enzymes from adapted strains of *Flavobacterium heparinum* (Linker, 1966; Gibian, 1966; Linker and Hovingh, 1968; Dietrich, 1969). Crude "heparinase" has been fractionated by Linker and Hovingh (1965) into an eliminase which produces unsaturated disaccharides and an α-glucuronidase which further degrades the disaccharides to monosaccharide units. The crude eliminase obtained from heparin-induced flavobacteria has recently been further purified, and fractionated into a heparanase acting on heparan sulfates and related compounds, and a heparinase acting mainly on heparin (Hovingh and Linker, 1970).

A multienzyme system present in the liver of a marine mollusk *(Charonia lampas)* is capable of degrading keratan sulfate to yield galactose, *N*-acetylglucosamine, and inorganic sulfate, but no oligosaccharides or sulfated sugars (Nishida-Fukuda and Egami, 1970). The authors concluded that degradation of keratan sulfate resulted from the concerted action of β-galactosidase, β-*N*-acetylglucosaminidase, and a keratosulfatase, which was partially purified and characterized. The keratosulfatase apparently first removes the sulfate, after which the exo-glycosidases hydrolyze the glycosidic bonds in the desulfated carbohydrate moiety.

It was also found that purified β-galactosidase (but not β-*N*-acetylglucosaminidase) released approximately 6% of the total galactose in a preparation of shark cartilage keratan sulfate (Nishida-Fukuda and Egami,

1970). The combined action of β-galactosidase and β-N-acetylglucosamini-
dase released a further amount of reducing material, and in the presence of
the two glycosidases and keratosulfatase, keratan sulfate is almost completely
degraded. This indicates the presence at the nonreducing end of some
galactose and N-acetylglucosamine residues which are not sulfated, and
probably also explains the finding by Öckerman (1970) of enzyme activity
in a number of rat and human tissues, including brain, which liberates
1–4% of the total galactose in various preparations of keratan sulfate.
Since the galactose liberated was in inverse proportion to the chain length
of the keratan sulfate, it would appear that the enzyme activity measured
by Öckerman was β-galactosidase rather than a specific keratan sulfate
degrading anzyme.

   Enzymes with a substrate specificity similar to that of testicular hyaluronidase have been isolated from many tissues, including liver (Aronson
and Davidson, 1967), serum (De Salegui et al., 1967; Bowness and Tan,
1968), skin (Cashman et al., 1969), and brain (Margolis, unpublished results).
Tissue hyaluronidase activity appears to be of lysosomal origin, and to differ
from the testicular enzyme in having a considerably lower pH optimum
(usually less than pH 4). The cellular degradation of mucopolysaccharides
and glycoproteins has recently been reviewed by Davidson (1970).

D. Glycosidases Acting on Glycopeptides and Glycoproteins

   The sequential treatment of glycopeptides or glycoproteins with purified
glycosidases is a widely used procedure for structural studies of these complex
carbohydrates. Because of their usually high specificity and because they
generally release monosaccharides only from the terminal, nonreducing ends
of oligosaccharide chains, the glycosidases may give less ambiguous data
than those obtained by other techniques such as graded acid hydrolysis.
They may also give information concerning the anomeric configuration of
the bond which is split. Certain applications of glycosidases in structural
studies of glycoproteins have been reviewed by Spiro (1966) and by Marshall
and Neuberger (1970). These enzymes may also be employed for the release
of specific sugars in metabolic studies using labeled glycopeptides or glycoproteins. Because of these several advantages, it is unfortunate that with
few exceptions (e.g., bacterial and viral neuraminidases, and β-galactosidase
from E. coli) these enzymes are not available commercially at the present
time. Table III lists references for the purification and properties of a number
of glycosidases which may be useful for structural or metabolic studies of
glycoproteins. However, it should be noted that full interpretation of data
derived from the use of these enzymes must await further understanding of
their specificities, of the nature of the residual oligosaccharide obtained

Table III.   Isolation and Properties of Glycosidases Acting on
Glycopeptides and Glycoproteins

Enzyme	Source	Reference
Neuraminidase	Influenza virus	Rafelson *et al.* (1966)
	Clostridium perfringens	Cassidy *et al.* (1966);
		Balke and Drzeniek (1969);
		Kraemer (1968)
	Vibrio cholerae	Ada and French (1959)
α-Galactosidase	Coffee bean	Courtois and Petek (1966)
	Phaseolus vulgaris	Agrawal and Bahl (1968)
	Aspergillus niger	Pazur and Kleppe (1962); Spiro (1967)
β-Galactosidase	*E. coli*	Hu *et al.* (1959);
		Spiro (1962); Marchesi *et al.* (1969)
	Diplococcus pneumoniae	Hughes and Jeanloz (1964a)
	Jack bean	Li and Li (1968)
	P. vulgaris	Agrawal and Bahl (1968)
	A. niger	Bahl and Agrawal (1969)
	Rat epididymis	Levvy and Conchie (1966)
α-Mannosidase	Jack bean	Li and Li (1968);
		Snaith and Levvy (1968)
	Rat epididymis	Snaith and Levvy (1969)
	Charonia lampas	Muramatsu (1967);
		Muramatsu and Egami (1967)
	Hog kidney	Okumura and Yamashina (1970)
α-L-Fucosidase	Abalone liver	Tanaka *et al.* (1968)
	C. perfringens	Aminoff and Furukawa (1970)
β-Xylosidase	*C. lampas*	Fukuda *et al.* (1969)
β-*N*-Acetyl-hexosaminidase	*D. pneumoniae*	Hughes and Jeanloz (1964b)
	Jack bean	Li and Li (1970)
	A. niger	Bahl and Agrawal (1969)
	P. vulgaris	Bahl and Agrawal (1968); Agrawal and Bahl (1968)
	Boar epididymis	Levvy and Conchie (1966)
α-*N*-Acetyl-galactosaminidase	Bovine and pig liver	Weissmann and Hinrichsen (1969)

after enzyme treatment, and of the problem of microheterogeneity discussed
earlier.

REFERENCES

Ada, G. L., and French, E. L. (1959) *Nature* **183,** 1740.
Agrawal, K. M. L., and Bahl, O. P. (1968) *J. Biol. Chem.* **243,** 103.
Aminoff, D., and Furukawa, K. (1970) *J. Biol. Chem.* **245,** 1659.
Anet, E. F. L. J., and Reynolds, T. M. (1954) *Nature* **174,** 930.

Antonopoulos, C. A. (1962) *Acta Chem. Scand.* **16,** 1521.
Antonopoulos, C. A., Borelius, E., Gardell, S., Hannström, B., and Scott, J. E. (1961) *Biochem. Biophys. Acta* **54,** 213.
Antonopoulos, C. A., Fransson, L.-Å., Heinegard, D., and Gardell, S. (1967) *Biochim. Biophys. Acta* **148,** 158.
Antonopoulos, C. A., Gardell, S., Szirmai, J. A., and De Tyssonsk, E. R. (1964) *Biochim. Biophys. Acta* **83,** 1.
Aronson, Jr., N. N., and Davidson, E. A. (1967) *J. Biol. Chem.* **242,** 437, 441.
Aspinall, G. O. (1970) *Polysaccharides,* Pergamon Press, Oxford.
Bahl, O. P., and Agrawal, K. M. L. (1968) *J. Biol. Chem.* **243,** 98.
Bahl, O. P., and Agrawal, K. M. L. (1969) *J. Biol. Chem.* **244,** 2970.
Balazs, E. A. (ed.) (1970) *Chemistry and Molecular Biology of the Intercellular Matrix,* 3 vols, Academic Press, New York.
Balke, E., and Drzeniek, R. (1969) *Z. Naturforsch.* **24b,** 599.
Barker, S. A., Kennedy, J. F., Somers, P. J., and Stacey, M. .1968) *Carbohyd. Res.* **7,** 361.
Bella, Jr., A. M., and Kim, Y. S. (1970) *J. Chromat.* **51,** 314.
Bernfeld, P. (1966) in *The Amino Sugars,* Vol. IIB (E. A. Balazs and R. W. Jeanloz, eds.), Academic Press, New York, p. 213.
Bitter, T., and Muir, H. M. (1962) *Anal. Biochem.* **4,** 330.
Boas, N. F., Jr. (1953) *J. Biol. Chem.* **204,** 553.
Bowness, J. M., and Tan, Y. H. (1968) *Biochim. Biophys. Acta* **151,** 288.
Brimacombe, J. S., and Webber, J. M. (1964) *Mucopolysaccharides-Chemical Structure, Distribution and Isolation.* Elsevier Publishing Co., Amsterdam.
Brimacombe, J. S., and Webber, J. M. (1964) *Mucopolysaccharides.* Elsevier, Amsterdam, p. 104.
Brookhart, J. H. (1965) *J. Chromat.* **20,** 191.
Brunngraber, E. G. (1969) in *Handbook of Neurochemistry,* Vol. 1 (A. Lajtha, ed.), Plenum Press, New York, p. 223.
Brunngraber, E. G., Aguilar, V., and Aro, A. (1969) *Arch. Biochem. Biophys.* **129,** 131.
Brunngraber, E. G., Brown, B. D., and Aguilar, V. (1969) *J. Neurochem.* **16,** 1059.
Brunngraber, E. G., Aro, A., and Brown, B. D. (1970) *Clinica Chim. Acta* **29,** 333.
Carter, H. E., Kisic, A., Koob, J. L., and Martin, J. A. (1969) *Biochemistry* **8,** 389.
Cashman, D. C., Laryea, J. U., and Weissmann, B. (1969) *Arch. Biochem. Biophys.* **135,** 387.
Cassidy, J. T., Jourdian, G. W., and Roseman. S. (1966) in *Methods in Enzymology,* Vol. 8 (E. F. Neufeld and V. Ginsburg, eds.), Academic Press, New York, p. 680.
Chauncey, H., Lionetti, F., and Lisanti, V. (1953) *Science* **118,** 219.
Chotiner, G., Smith, J. G., Jr., and Davidson, E. A. (1968) *Anal. Biochem.* **26,** 146.
Cifonelli, J. A. (1968) *Carbohyd. Res.* **8,** 233.
Cifonelli, J. A. (1970) in *Chemistry and Molecular Biology of the Intercellular Matrix,* Vol. 2 (E. A. Balazs, ed.), Academic Press, New York, p. 961.
Cifonelli, J. A., and Dorfman, A. (1962) *Biochem. Biophys. Res. Commun.* **7,** 41.
Cifonelli, J. A., Saunders, A., and Gross, J. L. (1967) *Carbohyd. Res.* **3,** 478.
Clamp, J. R., Dawson, G., and Hough, L. (1967) *Biochim. Biophys. Acta* **148,** 342.
Constantopoulos, G., Dekaban, A. S., and Carroll, W. R. (1969) *Anal. Biochem.* **31,** 59.
Courtois, J. E., and Petek, F. (1966) in *Methods in Enzymology,* Vol. 8 (E. F. Neufeld and V. Ginsburg, eds.), Academic Press, New York.
Crumpton, M. J. (1959) *Biochem. J.* **72,** 479.
Davidson, E. A. (1967) *Carbohydrate Chemistry,* Holt, Rinehart and Winston, Inc., New York.
Davidson, E. A. (1970) in *Metabolic Conjugation and Metabolic Hydrolysis,* Vol. 1 (W. H. Fishman, ed.), Academic Press, New York, p. 327.
Dekirmenjian, H., and Brunngraber, E. G. (1969) *Biochim. Biophys. Acta* **177,** 1.
De Salegui, M., Plonska, H., and Pigman, W. (1967) *Arch. Biochem. Biophys.* **121,** 548.
Di Benedetta, C., Brunngraber, E. G., Whitney, G., Brown, B. D., and Aro, A. (1969). *Arch. Biochem. Biophys.* **131,** 404.
Dietrich, C. P. (1969) *Biochemistry* **8,** 2089.

Dische, Z. (1947) *J. Biol. Chem.* **167**. 189.
Dische, Z. (1955) in *Methods of Biochemical Analysis,* Vol. 2 (D. Glick, ed.), Interscience, New York, p. 313.
Dische, Z., and Danilchenko, A. (1967) *Anal. Biochem.* **21**, 119.
Dische, Z., and Rothschild, C. (1967) *Anal. Biochem.* **21**, 125.
Dische, Z., and Shettles, L. B. (1948) *J. Biol. Chem.* **175**, 595.
Dische, Z., Shettles, L. B., and Osnos, M. (1949) *Arch. Biochem.* **22**, 169.
Dodgson, K. S., and Price, R. G. (1962) *Biochem. J.* **84**, 106.
Dorner, R. W., Antonopoulos, C.A., and Gardell, S. (1968) *Biochim. Biophys. Acta* **158**, 336.
Dubois, M., Gilles, K. A., Hamilton, J. K., Rebers, P. A., and Smith, F. (1956) *Anal. Chem.* **28**, 350.
Dutton, G. H. (1966) *Glucuronic Acid: Free and Combined. Chemistry, Biochemistry, Pharmacology, and Medicine,* Academic Press, New York.
Dziewiatkowski, D. (1962) *Biochim. Biophys. Acta* **56**, 167.
Finch, P. R., Yuen, R., Schachter, H., and Moscarello, M. A. (1969) *Anal. Biochem.* **31**, 296.
Flodin, P., Gregory, J. D., and Rodén, L. (1964) *Anal. Biochem.* **8**, 424.
Fransson, L.-Å., and Anseth, A. (1967) *Exptl. Eye Res.* **6**, 107.
Fransson, L.-Å. and Havsmark, B. (1970) *J. Biol. Chem.* **245**, 4770.
Fransson, L.-Å., Rodén, L., and Spach, M. (1968) *Anal. Biochem.* **21**, 317.
Fukuda, M., Muramatsu, T., and Egami, F. (1969) *J. Biochem. (Tokyo),* **65**, 191.
Galambos, J. T. (1967) *Anal. Biochem.* **19**, 119, 133.
Gardell, S. (1953) *Acta Chem. Scand.* **7**, 207.
Gauthier, P. B., and Kenyon, A. J. (1966) *Biochim. Biophys. Acta* **130**, 551.
Gibbons, M. N. (1955) *Analyst* **80**, 268.
Gibian, H. (1959) *Mucopolysaccharide und Mucopolysaccharidasen,* Franz Deuticke, Vienna.
Gibian, H. (1966) in *The Amino Sugars,* Vol. IIB (E. A. Balazs and R. W. Jeanloz, eds.), Academic Press, New York, p. 181.
Glowacka, D., Kopacz-Jodczyk, T., and Popowicz, J. (1967) *Anal. Biochem.* **19**, 1.
Gottschalk, A. (ed.) (1972) *Glycoproteins—Their Composition, Structure and Function,* 2 vols., 2nd ed. Elsevier Publishing Co., Amsterdam.
Hartree, E. F., and Brown, C. R. (1970) *Analyt. Biochem.* **35**, 259.
Hess, H. H., and Rolde, E. (1964) *J. Biol. Chem.* **239**, 3215.
Heyns, K., Müller, G., and Kiessling, G. (1966) *Hoppe-Seyler's Z. Physiol. Chem.* **346**, 108.
Hilborn, J. C., and Anastassiadis, P. A. (1969) *Anal. Biochem.* **31**, 51.
Hilborn, J. C., and Anastassiadis, P. A. (1971) *Anal. Biochem.* **39**, 88.
Hodge, J. E., and Hofreiter, B. T. (1962) in *Methods in Carbohydrate Chemistry,* Vol. 1 (R. L. Whistler and M. L. Wolfrom, eds.), Academic Press, New York. p. 380.
Hoffman, P., Meyer, K., and Linker, A. (1956) *J. Biol. Chem.* **219**, 653.
Horner, A. A. (1967) *Can. J. Biochem.* **45**, 1009, 1015.
Horton, D. (1969) in *The Amino Sugars,* Vol. IA (R. W. Jeanloz, ed.), Academic Press, New York, p. 1.
Hovingh, P., and Linker, A. (1970) *J. Biol. Chem.* **245**, 6170.
Hu, A. S. L., Wolfe, R. G., and Reithel, F. J. (1959) *Arch. Biochem. Biophys.* **81**, 500.
Huang, C.-C., Mayer, H. E., Jr., and Montgomery, R. (1970) *Carbohyd. Res.* **13**, 127.
Hughes, R. C., and Jeanloz, R. W. (1964a) *Biochemistry* **3**, 1535.
Hughes, R. C., and Jeanloz, R. W. (1964b) *Biochemistry* **3**, 1543.
Hunt, S. (1970) *Polysaccharide-Protein Complexes in Invertebrates,* Academic Press, London.
Jeanloz, R. W. (1968) in *Biochemistry of Glycoproteins and Related Substances,* Part II (E. Rossi and E. Stoll, eds.), S. Karger, Basel, p. 94.
Jeanloz, R. W., and Balazs, E. A. (eds.) (1965-) *The Amino Sugars,* Academic Press, New York.
Jeffrey, P. L., and Rienits, K. G. (1967) *Biochim. Biophys. Acta* **141**, 179.
Johnson, S., and Samuelson, O. (1966) *Analytica Chim. Acta* **36**, 1.
Jolley, R. L., and Freeman, M. L. (1968) *Clin. Chem.* **14**, 538.

Jones, A. S., and Letham, D. S. (1956) *Analyst* **81,** 15.
Jonsson, P., and Samuelson, O. (1967) *J. Chromat.* **26,** 194.
Jourdian, G. W., Dean, L., and Roseman, S. (1971) *J. Biol. Chem.* **246,** 430.
Kärkkäinen, J., Lehtonen, A., and Nikkari, T. (1965) *J. Chromat.* **20,** 457.
Kawai, Y., Seno, N., and Anno, K. (1969) *Anal. Biochem.* **32,** 314.
Kelleher, P. C., and Smith C. J. (1968) *J. Chromat.* **34,** 7.
Kesler, R. B. (1967) *Anal. Chem.* **39,** 1416.
Knutson, C. A., and Jeanes, A. (1968) *Anal. Biochem.* **24,** 470, 482.
Kraemer, P. M. (1968) *Biochim. Biophys. Acta* **167,** 205.
Lagunoff, D., and Warren, G. (1962) *Arch. Biochem. Biophys.* **99,** 396.
Larsson, L.-I., Ramnäs, O., and Samuelson, O. (1966) *Anal. Chim. Acta* **34,** 394.
Laurent, T. C., Ryan, M., and Pietruszkiewicz, A. (1960) *Biochim. Biophys. Acta* **42,** 476.
Laurent, T. C., and Scott, J. E. (1964) *Nature* **202,** 661.
Lee, Y. C., McKelvy, J. F., and Lang, D. (1969) *Anal. Biochem.* **27,** 567.
Lehnhardt, W. F., and Winzler, R. J. (1968) *J. Chromat.* **34,** 471.
Levvy, G. A., and Conchie, J. (1966) in *Methods in Enzymology,* Vol. 8 (E. F. Neufeld and V. Ginsburg, ed.), Academic Press, New York, p. 571.
Li, Y.-T., and Li, S.-C. (1968) *J. Biol. Chem.* **243,** 3994.
Li, S.-C., and Li, Y.-T. (1970) *J. Biol. Chem.* **245,** 5153.
Lin, F. M., and Pomeranz, Y. (1968) *Anal. Biochem.* **24,** 128.
Linker, A. (1966) in *Methods in Enzymology,* Vol. 8 (E. F. Neufeld and V. Ginsburg, eds.), Academic Press, New York, p. 650.
Linker, A., and Hovingh, P. (1965) *J. Biol. Chem.* **240,** 3724.
Linker, A., and Hovingh, P. (1968) *Biochim. Biophys. Acta* **165,** 89.
Linker, A., Meyer, K., and Hoffman, P. (1960) *J. Biol. Chem.* **235,** 924.
Lüderitz, O., Gmeiner, J., Kickhofen, B., Mayer, H., Westphal, O., and Wheat, R. W. (1968) *J. Bact.* **95,** 490.
Ludowieg, J. J., and Benmaman, J. D. (1968) *Carbohyd. Res.* **8,** 185.
Marchesi, S. L., Steers, E., and Shifrin, S. (1969) *Biochim. Biophys. Acta,* **181,** 20.
Margolis, R. U. (1967) *Biochim. Biophys. Acta* **141,** 91.
Margolis, R. U. (1969) in *Handbook of Neurochemistry,* Vol. 1 (A. Lajtha, ed.), Plenum Press, New York, p. 245.
Margolis, R. K., and Margolis, R. U. (1970a) *Biochemistry* **9,** 4389.
Margolis, R. U., and Margolis, R. K. (1970b) *Anal. Biochem.* **35,** 77.
Margolis, R. U., and Margolis, R. K. (1971) *Abstracts, Third International Meeting of the International Society for Neurochemistry,* Akadémiai Kiadó, Budapest, p. 276.
Margolis, R. U., and Margolis, R. K. (1972) *Biochim. Biophys, Acta* **264,** 426.
Marsh, C. A. (1966) in *Glucuronic Acid: Free and Combined. Chemistry, Biochemistry, Pharmacology, and Medicine* (G. H. Dutton, ed.), Academic Press, New York. p. 3.
Marshall, R. D., and Neuberger, A. (1970) *Adv. Carbohyd. Chem. Biochem.* **25,** 407.
Martinsson, E., and Samuelson, O. (1970) *J. Chromat.* **50,** 429.
Mathews, M. B. (1956) *Arch. Biochem. Biophys.* **61,** 367.
Mathews, M. B. (1961) *Biochim. Biophys. Acta* **48,** 402.
Mathews, M. B. (1966) in *Methods in Enzymology,* Vol. 8 (E. F. Neufeld and V. Ginsburg, eds.), Academic Press, New York, p. 654.
Mathews, M. B., and Cifonelli, J. A. (1965) *J. Biol. Chem.* **240,** 4140.
Mathews, M. B., and Decker, L. (1971) *Biochim. Biophys. Acta* **244,** 30.
Mathews, M. B., and Dorfman, A. (1955) *Physiol. Rev.* **35,** 381.
Mathews, M. B., and Inouye, M. (1961) *Biochim. Biophys. Acta* **53,** 509.
Mes, J., and Kamm, L. (1968) *J. Chromat.* **38,** 120.
Meyer, K. (1971) in *The Enzymes,* 3rd ed., Vol. 5 (P. D. Boyer, ed.), Academic Press, New York, p. 307.
Miettinen, T., and Takki-Luukkainen, I.-T. (1959) *Acta Chem. Scand.* **13,** 856.
Moggridge, R. C. G., and Neuberger, A. (1938) *J. Chem. Soc.,* p. 745.
Montgomery, R. (1961) *Biochim. Biophys. Acta* **48,** 591.
Muir, H. (1958) *Biochem. J.* **69,** 195.

Muramatsu, T. (1967) *J. Biochem. (Tokyo)* **62**, 487.
Muramatsu, T., and Egami, F. (1967) *J. Biochem. (Tokyo)* **62**, 700.
Narahashi, Y., and Yanagita, M. (1967) *J. Biochem. (Tokyo)* **62**, 633.
Neufeld, E. F., and Ginsburg, V. (eds.) (1966) *"Complex Carbohydrates,"* in *Methods in Enzymology,* Vol. 8 (S. P. Colowick and N. O. Kaplan, eds.), Academic Press, New York.
Nishida-Fukuda, M., and Egami, F. (1970) *Biochem. J.* **119**, 39.
Öckerman, P. A. (1970) *Carbohyd. Res.* **12**, 429.
Ohms, J. I., Zec, J., Benson, J. V., and Patterson, J. A. (1967) *Anal. Biochem.* **20**, 51.
Ohya, T., and Kaneko, Y. (1970) *Biochim. Biophys. Acta* **198**, 607.
Okumura, T., and Yamashina, I. (1970) *J. Biochem. (Tokyo)* **68**, 561.
Paerels, G. B., and Schut, J. (1965) *Biochem. J.* **96**, 787.
Pazur, J. H., and Kleppe, K. (1962) *J. Biol. Chem.* **237**, 1002.
Pearce, R. H., Mathieson, J. M., and Grimmer. B. J. (1968) *Anal. Biochem.* **24**, 141.
Pearson, C. H. (1963) *Biochem. J.* **88**, 540.
Perlin, A. S., and Sanderson, G. R. (1970) *Carbohyd. Res.* **12**, 183.
Perry, M. B. (1964) *Can. J. Biochem.* **42**, 451.
Pigman, W., and Horton, D. (eds.) (1970-) *The Carbohydrates—Chemistry and Biochemistry,* 2nd ed., Academic Press, New York.
Quintarelli, G. (ed.) (1968) *The Chemical Physiology of Mucopolysaccharides,* Little, Brown and Co., Boston.
Radhakrishnamurthy, B., and Berenson, G. S. (1964) *Clinica Chim. Acta* **10**, 562.
Radhakrishnamurthy, B., Dalferes, E. R..Jr., and Berenson, G. S.(1966) *Anal. Biochem.* **17**, 545.
Rafelson, M. E., Gold, S., and Priede, I. (1966) in *Methods in Enzymology,* Vol. 8 (E. F. Neufeld and V. Ginsburg, eds.), Academic Press, New York, p. 677.
Reissig, J. L., Strominger, J. L., and Leloir, L. F. (1955) *J. Biol. Chem.* **217**, 959.
Risse, H. J., and Lüderitz, O. (1964) *Biochem. Z.* **341**, 1.
Rossi, E., and Stoll, E. (eds.) (1968) *Biochemistry of Glycoproteins and Related Substances,* S. Karger, Basel.
Roy, A. B., and Trudinger, P. A. (1970) *The Biochemistry of Inorganic Compounds of Sulphur,* Cambridge University Press, Cambridge.
Saigo, K., and Egami, F. (1970) *J. Neurochem.* **17**, 633.
Saito, H., Yamagata, T., and Suzuki, S. (1968) *J. Biol. Chem.* **243**, 1536.
Schiller, S., Slover, G. A., and Dorfman, A. (1961) *J. Biol. Chem.* **236**, 983.
Schmidt, M. (1962) *Biochim. Biophys. Acta* **63**, 346.
Scott, J. E. (1960) in *Methods of Biochemical Analysis,* Vol. 8 (D. Glick, ed.), Interscience, New York, p. 145.
Seno, N., Anno, K., Kondo, K., Nagase, S., and Saito, S. (1970) *Anal. Biochem.* **37**, 197.
Sherma, J., and Zweig, G. (1971) in *Paper Chromatography and Electrophoresis,* Vol. 2 (G. Zweig and J. R. Whitaker, eds.), Academic Press, New York.
Silbert, J. E., and DeLuca, S. (1970) *J. Biol. Chem.* **245**, 1506.
Singh, M., and Bachhawat, B. K. (1968) *J. Neurochem.* **15**, 249.
Slein, M. W. (1965) in *Methods of Enzymatic Analysis* (H. U. Bergmeyer, ed.), Academic Press, New York, p. 117.
Smith, I. (ed.) (1969) *Chromatographic and Electrophoretic Techniques,* Vol. 1, 2nd ed., Wiley/Interscience, New York.
Snaith, S.M., and Levvy, G.A. (1968) *Biochem. J.* **110**, 663.
Snaith, S.M., and Levvy, G.A. (1969) *Biochem. J.* **114**, 25.
Spackman, D.H., Stein, W.H., and Moore, S. (1958) *Anal. Chem.* **30**, 1190.
Spencer, B. (1960) *Biochem. J.* **75**, 435.
Spiro, R.G. (1962) *J. Biol. Chem.* **237**, 646.
Spiro, R.G. (1966) in *Methods in Enzymology,* Vol. 8 (E. F. Neufeld and V. Ginsburg, eds.), Academic Press, New York, pp. 3–52.
Spiro, R. G. (1967) *J. Biol. Chem.* **242**, 4813.
Spiro, R. G., and Spiro, M. J. (1965) *J. Biol. Chem.* **240**, 997.

Srinivasan, S. R., Radhakrishnamurthy, B., Dalferes, Jr., E. R., and Berenson, G. S. (1970) *Anal. Biochem.* **35,** 398.

St. Cyr, M. J. (1970) *J. Chromat.* **47,** 284.

Stary, Z., Wardi, A., and Turner, D. (1964) *Biochim. Biophys. Acta* **83,** 242.

Steele, R. S., Brendel, K., Scheer, E., and Wheat, R. W. (1970) *Anal. Biochem.* **34,** 206.

Stefanovich, V., and Gore, I. (1967) *J. Chromat.* **31,** 473.

Sutherland, I. T. (1966) *Clinica Chim. Acta* **14,** 554.

Suzuki, K. (1965) *J. Neurochem.* **12,** 629.

Suzuki, S., Saito, H., Yamagata, T., Anno, K., Seno, N., Kawai, Y. and Furuhashi, T. (1968) *J. Biol. Chem.* **243,** 1543.

Svejcar, J., and Robertson, W. van B. (1967) *Anal. Biochem.* **18,** 333.

Svennerholm, L. (1957) *Biochim. Biophys. Acta* **24,** 604.

Swann, D. A., and Balazs, E. A. (1966) *Biochim. Biophys. Acta* **130,** 112.

Sweeley, C. C., Wells, W. W., and Bently, R. (1966) in *Methods in Enzymology.* Vol. 8, (E. F. Neufeld and V. Ginsburg, eds.), Academic Press, New York, p. 95.

Szabo, M. M., and Roboz-Einstein, E. (1962) *Arch. Biochem. Biophys.* **98,** 406.

Szirmai, J. A., Van Boven-De Tyssonsk, E., and Gardell, S. (1967) *Biochim. Biophys. Acta* **136,** 331.

Tanaka, K., Nakano, T., Noguchi, S., and Pigman, W. (1968) *Arch Biochem. Biophys.* **126,** 624.

Thunell, S. (1967) *Ark. Kemi* **27,** 33.

Trevelyan, W. E., Proctor, D. P., and Harrison, J. S. (1950) *Nature* **166,** 444.

Walborg, E. F., Cobb, III, B. F., Adams-Mayne, M., and Ward, D. N. (1963) *Anal. Biochem.* **6,** 367.

Walborg, E. F., and Kondo, L. E. (1970) *Anal. Biochem.* **37,** 320.

Walborg, E. F., and Lantz, R. S. (1968) *Anal. Biochem.* **22,** 123.

Walborg, E. F., Ray, D. B., and Öhrberg, L. E. (1969) *Anal. Biochem.* **29,** 433.

Warren, L. (1959) *J. Biol. Chem.* **234,** 1971.

Weber, P., and Winzler, R. J. (1969) *Arch Biochem. Biophys.* **129,** 534.

Weissmann, B. (1955) *J. Biol. Chem.* **216,** 783.

Weissmann, B., and Hinrichsen, D. F. (1969) *Biochemistry* **8,** 2034.

Whistler, R. L., and Wolfrom, M. L., eds. (1962–1965) *Methods in Carbohydrate Chemistry,* Academic Press, New York.

Wilson, C. M. (1959) *Anal. Chem.* **31,** 1199.

Wolfrom, M. L., Honda, S., and Wang, P. Y. (1969) *Carbohyd. Res.*.**10,** 259.

Wolfrom, M. L., and Karabinos, J. V. (1945) *J. Am. Chem. Soc.* **67,** 679.

Yaguchi, M., and Perry, M. B. (1970) *Can. J. Biochem.* **48,** 386.

Yamagata, T., Saito, H., Habuchi, O., and Suzuki, S. (1968) *J. Biol. Chem.* **243,** 1523.

Yamauchi, F., Kosaki, M., and Yosizawa, Z. (1968) *Biochim. Biophys. Res. Commun.* **33,** 721.

Yu, R. K., and Ledeen, R. W. (1970) *J. Lipid Res.* **11,** 506.

Yuki, H., and Fishman, W. H. (1963) *J. Biol. Chem.* **238,** 1877.

Zweig, G., and Whitaker, J. R. (1967) *Paper Chromatography and Electrophoresis,* Vol. 1, Academic Press, New York.

Section IV
BIOLOGICALLY ACTIVE AMINES

Chapter 12

Assay of Biogenic Amines and Their Deaminating Enzymes in Animal Tissues*

Solomon H. Snyder
and Kenneth M. Taylor

Department of Pharmacology and Experimental Therapeutics
and
Department of Psychiatry
The Johns Hopkins University School of Medicine
Baltimore, Maryland

I. INTRODUCTION

The biogenic amines, dopamine, norepinephrine, serotonin, and histamine have in recent years played an important role as suspected neurotransmitters in neurochemical investigations of brain functions. Much of this interest can be ascribed to the development of highly sensitive and specific spectrophotofluorometric and isotopic procedures for estimating tissue concentrations of these amines, their metabolism *in vivo,* and the activity of their synthetic and catabolic enzymes. This chapter describes techniques used in this laboratory for measuring endogenous concentrations of dopamine, norepinephrine, serotonin, and histamine in animal tissues. The catecholamines and serotonin are estimated by spectrophotofluorometry, while tissue histamine is assayed by a procedure in which the specific enzymic methylation of tissue histamine reflects its endogenous content. Fluorometric and radiometric methods for the assay of monoamine oxidase and diamine oxidase activities are also described.

* Supported by USPHS grants 1-R01-NB-07275, 1-P01-GM-16492, and MH-18501. Solomon H. Snyder is a recipient of NIMH Research Scientist Development Award, K3-MH-33128.

II. SPECTROPHOTOFLUOROMETRIC ASSAY OF CATECHOLAMINES AND RELATED COMPOUNDS

During the past 10 years chemical assay has tended to replace biological assay for catecholamine estimation, due to increased sensitivity, specificity, and the ability to assay biologically inactive compounds. For the routine chemical assay of minute amounts of catecholamines and metabolites, only fluorometric methods appear at present to be sensitive enough, although recent radioisotopic and double isotopic labeling techniques have great potential (Engelman *et al.*, 1968; Saelens *et al.*, 1967).

Biological extracts containing catecholamines and/or their metabolites must be purified and concentrated before the appropriate estimation technique can be applied. This is achieved after homogenization and precipitation of proteins with either acid, alcohol, trichloracetic acid, or perchloric acid (Von Euler, 1959), by absorption onto alumina, ion-exchange chromatography or by solvent extraction. Paper, thin-layer, and gas chromatography (Von Euler, 1961; Häggendal, 1966) have been used for separation as well as identification but generally require prior purification and concentration of the tissue extract.

The main solvent extraction method is that of Shore and Olin (1958) in which the catecholamines are extracted with butanol. Anton and Sayre (1964) have employed ether to extract metanephrine and normetanephrine from urine, tissue, and plasma samples.

All catecholamines are adsorbed by alumina at pH 8.4 and can be removed by elution with dilute acid. Due to the inability of alumina to separate catecholamines, the ion-exchange method has tended to become the purification and concentration technique of choice, because of separation of amines by differential elution. Strong ion-exchange resins are superior to weaker resins in being able to cope with extracts of high ionic strength.

There have been a wide variety of methods published for the fluorometric estimation of catecholamines and related compounds in biological materials (Von Euler, 1959; Häggendal, 1966) and an even greater number of unpublished variations on these methods. Many of them are based on the production of a fluorescent indole derivative ("lutin") by means of oxidation and subsequent rearrangement. This technique has been applied to a wider range of compounds than, for example, the ethylenediamine condensation which is applicable only to compounds having a catechol grouping. Iodine is the most suitable oxidant as it has been shown to react efficiently with a wide range of compounds (Carlsson and Lindquist, 1962; Carlsson and Waldeck, 1958).

The establishment of conditions for maximal fluorescence and their use has resulted in an increased sensitivity in estimating the pure amines in solution. Of more significance, it has provided increased sensitivity, consistency, and reproducibility when applied to the detection and measurement of these compounds in biological extracts.

The following method describes how catecholamines and amine metabolites can be determined in tissue samples. Basically the method involves separation of the amines using a column of Dowex-50W cation-exchange resin followed by fluorometric determination using the trihydroxyindole method (Laverty and Taylor, 1968; Taylor and Laverty, 1969).

A. Materials

1. Reagents

Freshly distilled deionized water is used in all cases.

1.2 N HCl   (3.6 % v/w hydrochloric acid)
2 N HCl   (6 % v/w hydrochloric acid)
3 N HCl   (9 % v/w hydrochloric acid)
5 N K_2CO_3 (34.5 % v/w potassium carbonate)
1 M sodium acetate, pH 6.5; 20 g NaOH + 30 ml glacial acetic acid
to 500 ml with water. The pH is adjusted to 6.5

2. Ion-Exchange Resin

Dowex-50W–X8 cation exchange resin 200–400 mesh. (H^+ form). Biorad Laboratories.

3. Catecholamines and Related Compounds

l-Norepinephrine bitratrate (NE), dopamine (3,4-dihydroxyphenethylamine) hydrochloride (DA), and metanephrine hydrochloride [L. Light & Co.]; *l*-epinephrine, tyramine hydrochloride (TA), and tyrosine (TS) [Koch-Light]; DL-normetanephrine hydrochloride (NM), DL-dihydroxyphenylalanine (dopa), 3-methoxytyramine (4-hydroxy-3-methoxyphenethylamine) hydrochloride (3MT), DL-octopamine hydrochloride (OA), 3,4-dimethoxyphenethylamine hydrochloride (DMP), and α-methylnorepinephrine (3,4-dihydroxynorephedrine) hydrochloride (mNA) [Calbiochem]; α-methyltyrosine (mTS) and α-methyldihydroxy-phenylalanine (mdopa) [Merck, Sharp and Dohme]. Amine solutions are made up in approximately 0.01 N HCl; the quantities are expressed in terms of the base.

4. Buffers

The following standard buffer solutions are used:

Phosphate: 1/15 M monopotassium phosphate + 1/15 M disodium phosphate.

Borate: 0.1 M boric acid in 0.1 M KCl + 0.1 N NaOH.

Carbonate: 0.2 M anhydrous sodium carbonate + 0.2 M sodium bicarbonate.

Citrate-phosphate: 0.1 M citric acid + 0.2 M disodium phosphate.

B. Procedure

1. Tissue Samples

The rate of postmortem loss of catecholamines is very rapid. Therefore, after decapitation the tissue required is rapidly removed, enclosed in aluminum foil, chilled in dry ice, and weighed. When extraction is not carried out immediately, tissues are stored in a deep freeze at − 14°C.

2. Extraction

The tissue is ground in a glass homogenizer with 2 ml 0.01 N HCl, 20 mg of ascorbic acid and 10 mg of EDTA. Two additional 2-ml portions of 0.01 N HCl are used to wash the homogenate into a 10 × 1.5-cm polypropylene centrifuge tube. Care must be taken to keep the extract at 0°C during the homogenization. For recovery experiments, pure amine samples are now added. Three milliliter of 1.2 N HClO₄ are now added to precipitate proteins. After mixing and centrifugation (7000 $g \times 5$ min) the supernatant fluid is poured off into a 10 × 2.5-cm cellulose nitrate centrifuge tube, and the pH adjusted to 4.0 (maximum stability of catecholamines) with 5 N K₂CO₃. A second centrifugation (7000 $g \times 5$ min) is now carried out to remove precipitated potassium perchlorate and the supernatant is poured carefully onto the ion-exchange column.

3. Separation

A 0.4 × 3.5 cm Dowex-50W cation-exchange resin column is prepared by the method of Juorio et al. (1966). The resin is washed with 20 ml of 2 N hydrochloric acid followed by 10 ml of water. It is then converted to the acetate form by 20 ml of 1 M sodium acetate solution (pH 6.5) followed by a 10-ml wash with water. The column is now ready for the passage of the tissue extract.

The tissue extract is now applied carefully to the column. When all of the extract has passed through the column, the reservoir and column are carefully washed with 10–15 ml of water. Elution of the cation-exchange column with increasing concentrations of hydrochloric acid separates catecholamines and their amine metabolites in the following order.

6 ml 1.2 N HCl norepinephrine (NE), epinephrine

6 ml 2 N HCl dopamine (DA), normetanephrine (NM), metanephrine (M)

6 ml 3 N HCl 3-methoxytyramine (3MT)

Normetanephrine and metanephrine occur in the same fraction as dopamine but there is no cross interference in the fluorometric methods for these compounds. Epinephrine is eluted in the norepinephrine fraction but again these compounds can be measured separately by the differential fluorometric methods described later. The recoveries of pure solutions of catecholamines and metabolites added to the chromatography system as carrier substances are indicated in Table I. The recovery of NE $-^3$H, DA $-^3$H, and NH $-^3$H is also given in Table I.

Overlap of acids and amines into adjacent fractions was determined and was found to be less than 5 % of applied pure compound for all the above catecholamines and metabolites. For the extraction of amines in blood samples, 10 ml of whole blood are centrifuged (8000 g × 10 min) and the plasma removed. Samples of plasma (0.5–1.0 ml) are diluted to 3 ml with water, and 1 ml of 30% tricholracetic acid is added (internal standards added at this stage). The mixture after shaking is centrifuged for 10 min at 1000 g. The supernatant fluid is removed for separation as specified above.

4. Estimation

The acid eluate containing the required amine is adjusted to the specific oxidation pH (Table II) with 5 N K$_2$CO$_3$, using a pH meter and the volume of K$_2$CO$_3$ required is recorded. A sample of this pH-adjusted eluate is taken and estimated by the appropriate fluorometric method. Internal standard and blank estimation are also performed using an equal sample volume.

In outline, the general fluorometric method is as follows:

1. 0.1–0.5 ml sample containing the compound to be measured is made up to 1.1 ml with the appropriate buffer.
2. Iodine (0.05 ml) is added; after all additions the mixture is shaken vigorously.
3. After 3 min alkaline sulfite solution in appropriate volume is added.

Table I. The Recovery of Added Catecholamines and Metabolites from Pure Solutions and Tissue Samples Using the Separation Technique and Fluorimetric or Radioisotopic Analysis

Catecholamine or metabolite	Mean percentage recovery ± S.E.M. (number of determinations)			
	From pure solution		From tissue sample	
	Fluorimetric	Radioisotopic	Fluorimetric	Radioisotopic
NA	95±2(12)	90±1(4)	88±2(12)	84±1(4)
DA	80±2(12)	84±2(4)	69±3(12)	72±2(4)
NM	80±3(12)	76±2(4)	74±3(12)	74±2(4)
3MT	85±6(12)		78±3(12)	

4. After 1 or 5 min the appropriate volume of glacial acetic acid is added.
5. After the appropriate time, with heating if necessary, the sample is read in the fluorometer at the appropriate wavelength maxima.
6. Samples with added internal standard, and completely reversed blanks are run in parallel with the unknown sample

The specific volumes of reagents in the above method and the values of the various parameters that produce maximal fluorescence and the sensitivity obtained using pure amine solutions are shown in Table II.

5. Oxidation

0.05 ml of an iodine solution (added to 1.1 ml buffered solution containing the compound being tested) gives maximal or near-maximal fluorescence with all compounds. A 3-min oxidation time is satisfactory for all compounds; small changes in these two parameters have little effect on the amount of fluorescence produced.

Oxidation pH, however, has a significant influence on the amount of fluorescence produced by any compound. The choice of buffer also affects the fluorescence production; for instance, borate buffer gives a greater fluorescence than phosphate-citrate, phosphate, or bicarbonate in the pH 8–9 range.

6. Tautomerization

In many methods for catecholamines, ascorbic acid has been used as an antioxidant and stabilizer in the alkaline tautomerization stage. The other common method is to use sulfite or some similar reducing agent as an antioxidant, with ascorbic acid, BAL, or thiopropionic acid as a stabilizer. In the present method, acidification of the final fluorescent solution stabilizes the product without any additional reducing agent. Sulfite can thus be used as an antioxidant.

Peak fluorescence is obtained when the sulfite and alkali are added together; so for all compounds an alkaline sulfite solution is used. As shown in Table II, most compounds require 0.4 or 0.5 ml of solution for maximal fluorescence except for DA, dopa and 3MT, which only require 0.25 ml. Small changes in alkaline sulfite volume from these optimal values do not affect the fluorescence greatly. All compounds require 5 min exposure to the alkaline conditions for tautomerization except l-epinephrine and metanephrine hydrochloride which require only 1 min. Small changes in time interval from the maximal time do not affect the results greatly.

Oxidation and tautomerization give maximal results under these conditions when carried out at room temperature (18–20°C).

Table II. Structure—Reactivity Relationships for T.H.I. Reaction

Amine	Structure					Oxidation				Tautom.		Acid		Develop.		Wavelengths			Sens
	ring	ring	β-C	α-C	N	Buffer Type	pH	I₂ soln. (ml)	Time (min)	SO₃ and OH (mml)	Time (in)	HAc (ml)	Final pH	Time (min)	Temp (°C)	Excit. λ (mλ)	Emiss. λ (mλ)	Minor λ (mλ)	Twice blank (ng)
NA	OH	OH	OH	H	H	PO₄	6.5	0.05	3	0.5	5	0.14	4.8	25	20	380	480	285	0.5
A	OH	OH	OH	H	CH₃	CIT	4.0	0.05	3	0.5	1	0.1	5.0	0	20	410	500	290	2
NM	OH	OCH₃	OH	H	H	BO₃	8.6	0.05	3	0.5	5	0.3	4.2	25	20	380	475	290	4
M	OH	OCH₃	OH	H	CH₃	BO₃	9.1	0.05	3	0.5	1	0.1	5.6	0	20	410	490	295	3
DA	OH	OH	H	H	H	PO₄	7.0	0.05	3	0.25	5	0.1	4.4	40	100	320	375		2
Dopa	OH	OH	H	COOH	H	CIT	5.4	0.05	3	0.25	5	0.05	5.7	40	100	330	380		4
3MT	OH	OCH₃	H	H	H	BO₃	8.8	0.05	3	0.25	5	0.25	4.5	40	100	320	375		8
OA	OH	H	OH	H	H	CO₃	9.0	0.05	3	0.4	5	0.2	4.7	30	100	375	475	285	200
TA	OH	H	H	H	H	CO₃	9.9	0.05	3	0.4	5	0.15	4.5	40	100	320	375		200
TS	OH	H	H	COOH	H	CO₃	10.6	0.05	3	0.4	5	0.1	5.0	40	100	330	380		50
mNA	OH	OH	OH	CH₃	H	PO₄	6.5	0.05	3	0.5	5	0.1	5.0	20	20	385	485	290	20
mdopa	OH	OH	H	CH₃ COOH	H	CIT	5.4	0.05	3	0.25	5	0.15	4.7	30	100	320	400		25
mTS	OH	H	H	CH^a COOH	H	CO₃	10.6	0.05	3	0.4	5	0.1	5.0	20	100	320	390		500
DMP	OCH	OCH₃	H	H	H	No reaction													

ᵃ CH₃ and COOH on α—C (noH)

7. Final Solution

Acidification of the alkaline reaction mixture using glacial acetic acid results in increased fluorescence with all compounds. The amount of glacial acetic acid and the resulting final pH for maximal fluorescence are given in Table II. Changes in the final pH affects the final fluorescence appreciably; glacial acetic acid is used in preference to other acids because of the buffering action of acetate in the required pH range.

Contrary to published reports (Carlsson and Waldeck, 1958, 1964), no fluorescence is obtained with DA and other phenethylamine derivatives unless the final solution is heated. The rate of production of fluorescence by other compounds is also increased by heating, but often at the expense of reduced stability and consistency. The temperature and time of heating for maximal fluorescence, consistent with reproducible results, are shown in Table II. The fluorescence is stable for at least 60 min at room temperature once maximal fluorescent conditions have been achieved.

8. Blanks

With solutions of pure compound, all forms of blank give similar readings. However, for tissue samples, a completely reversed blank is preferable, since with other types of blank any "chrome" derivatives formed by atmospheric oxidation would be converted to the fluorescent "lutin," yielding a false blank. However, no blank as yet devised can be regarded as completely satisfactory.

9. Comparison of Acidification and Alkaline Ascorbic Acid for Stabilization

If the oxidized reaction mixture remains alkaline, no fluorescence is observed unless ascorbic acid is present. After acidification, however, in the absence of ascorbic acid, the fluorescent derivatives are stable for at least 100 min, whether exposed or protected from visible or UV light. Addition of ascorbic acid to an acid system reduces fluorescence, increases blank values, and abolishes the secondary activation peak at approximately 290 $m\mu$ (Table II).

Alternation of acid and alkaline conditions shows that the fluorescent "lutin" product is present in both cases, but that the required ionic form for fluorescence is slower to develop in alkaline solution than in acid solution. This change in ionic form is accompanied by a hypochromic wavelength shift, small in the case of norepinephrine and other phenethanolamine derivatives (from 390/505 $m\mu$ in alkali to 380/480 $m\mu$ in acid for NE) but larger in the case of phenethylamine derivatives (380/460 $m\mu$ in alkali to 320/375 $m\mu$ in acid for DA), and an increase in fluorescent intensity in the acid form.

10. Structure-Reactivity Relationships

The use of a wide range of compounds with a standard type of reaction enables the structural requirements for reactivity to be determined. These are:

1. A phenethylamine nucleus.
2. The amino group can be primary or secondary; secondary amines are tautomerized more readily to the final "lutin" form.
3. A *meta, para* catechol grouping yields highest fluorescence; a *para* hydroxy is essential for the reaction.
4. β-Hydroxylation of the side chain increases the ease of formation of final fluorescent product; phenethylamine derivatives require heat for fluorescence development. β-Hydroxylation also determines the degree of wavelength shift on acidification.
5. Methoxyl groups on the *m*-position decrease the fluorescence; methylation of the *p*-hydroxy group eliminates the reaction completely, suggesting that demethylation does not occur during the reaction.
6. A methyl group on the α-carbon atom of the side chain decreases the fluorescence of the final indole product. A carboxyl group has little effect on the fluorescence but has a slight effect on the final wavelenghts. Compounds having both methyl and carboxyl groups on the α-carbon must lose one grouping, presumably the carboxyl, in order form a hydroxyindole compound, the postulated end product of this oxidative rearrangement.

11. Specificity of Reaction

The use of different oxidation pH values, different treatments of the final solution, and different wavelength maxima permits some compounds to be measured accurately in the presence of others. However, cross interference may occur. In particular NE, *l*-epinephrine and NM; *l*-epinephrine and metanephrine hydrochloride; DA, dopa, and 3MT; NA, and NM, metanephrine hydrochloride with OA; TS and TA; ethylamine derivatives with the corresponding α-methyl compound; all these combinations cause interference to an appreciable extent. Hence chemical separation is required to deal with some mixtures of compounds. It is possible to reduce the interference between epinephrine and NE to very low levels without losing sensitivity by oxidizing at pH 3.5, at which the fluorescence from NE is very small while the *l*-epinephrine fluorescence is still appreciable. This enables a differential assay of *l*-epinephrine and NE in mixtures to be carried out.

Recoveries of added standard estimated on rat brain tissue are shown in Table III. Also shown is the sensitivity for the complete method, i.e., the amount of each amine required in the original tissue extract to give a sample

Table III. Recoveries of Catecholamines and Metabolites Added to
Brain Homogenates and Sensitivity of the Method for Multiple
Extraction of Amines from a Single Sample

Compound	Amount (μg) added to homogenate	Recovery, mean $\pm$ S.E.M. (No. of observations)	Sensitivity, μg/total homogenate
NA	0.5	86$\pm$4(6)	0.025
A	0.5	77$\pm$4(4)	0.08
DA	0.5	78$\pm$9(6)	0.25
NM	0.5	70$\pm$6(6)	0.25
3MT	1.0	78$\pm$6(6)	0.4

Table IV. Endogenous Catecholamine Levels in Various Regions
of the Brain of the Rat[a]

Brain region	Weight (g)	Amine concentration (μg/g)			
		NA	NM	DA	3MT
Whole brain	1.75$\pm$0.06	0.38$\pm$0.02	0.05$\pm$0.01	0.46$\pm$0.05	0.04$\pm$0.01
Brainstem	0.25$\pm$0.01	0.44$\pm$0.01	0.05[b]	0.08$\pm$0.01	ND[c]
Cerebellum	0.23$\pm$0.04	0.26$\pm$0.02	0.03[b]	0.03[b]	ND
Cortex	0.53$\pm$0.02	0.22$\pm$0.01	0.04$\pm$0.01	0.04[b]	ND
Corpus striatum	0.24$\pm$0.03	0.28$\pm$0.01	0.03[b]	3.08$\pm$0.07	0.39$\pm$0.13
Thalamus-hypothalamus-midbrain	0.50$\pm$0.03	0.58$\pm$0.02	0.07$\pm$0.01	0.13$\pm$0.01	ND

[a] Sprague-Dawley male rats (180–200 g) were used. Brain regions were dissected by the method of Taylor and Laverty (1969). Each value is the mean $\pm$ S.E.M. of eight determinations.
[b] Metabolite detectable but not consistently measurable.
[c] ND = Metabolite not detectable.

reading of twice blank value. This value not only depends on the sensitivity of the oxidation reaction but also includes the volume factor introduced by the separation of the compounds. When only specific amines are present, conditions can be chosen, e.g., by alumina absorption rather than Dowex, to reduce the sample volume and so increase the sensitivity value.

The concentrations of catecholamines and metabolites in regions of the rat brain, determined by the above procedure are shown in Table IV. In regions where dopamine, normetanephrine, and 3-methoxytyramine are not consistently measurable, a more accurate concentration can be obtained by pooling brain tissue samples.

C. Discussion

The method described represents a collection into a single comprehensive technique of many of the variations already applied by other workers to the determination of individual catecholamines or related compounds. By employing a standardized technique using as many standardized reagents as possible, the method becomes one that may be readily adopted for routine variety of compounds, and the elucidation of factors controlling the amount of fluorescence produced by a compound after formation of a hydroxyindole derivative has also produced an increase in the sensitivity of the method when applied to many compounds.

III. SPECTROPHOTOFLUOROMETRIC ASSAY OF TISSUE SEROTONIN BY THE NINHYDRIN PROCEDURE

The first chemical method for the estimation of tissue serotonin (5-hydroxytryptamine) which was specific, relatively sensitive, and suitable for general use by neurochemists was the method of Bogdanski et al. (1956). This procedure measures the native fluorescence of serotonin in acid soultion, which is specific for 5-hydroxyindoles. However, this technique could not accurately measure less than 0.3 μg of tissue serotonin. The present method depends on the formation of an intensely fluorescent product when serotonin is heated with ninhydrin (Snyder et al., 1965). It is based on the ninhydrin-serotonin complex described earlier by Jepson and Stevens (1953) and Vanable (1963). The present assay is highly specific and about 8 times as sensitive as that of Bogdanski et al. (1954), so that as little as 10 mμg of tissue serotonin can be reliably measured.

A. Procedure

The method involves extraction of serotonin into l-butanol from a salt-saturated solution at pH 10. Serotonin is then returned to an aqueous solution, pH 7.0, by the addition of heptane and reacted with ninhydrin to yeild a fluorescent product.

Tissues are homogenized in 8 ml of ice-cold 0.4 N perchloric acid in a motor-driven glass homogenizer. Homogenates are centrifuged at 900 g for 10 min. A 4-ml aliquot of the supernatant fluid is adjusted to pH 10.0 with sodium hydroxide solutions and a glass electrode and then transferred to a 40-ml glass-stoppered centrifuge tube containing 0.5 ml of 0.5 N borate buffer at pH 10, 1.5 g sodium chloride, and 15 ml l-butanol. Tubes are shaken for 10 min, centrifuged, and the aqueous phase removed by aspiration. The organic phase is then shaken for 3 min with 2 ml of 0.1 M borate buffer (pH 10), previously saturated with sodium chloride, and centrifuged. Ten milliliters of the organic phase are transferred to a 40-ml glass-stoppered centrifuge tube containing 1.4 ml of 0.05 M phosphate buffer, pH 7.0, and 15 ml of *n*-heptane. After shaking for 2 min, the tube is centrifuged and the organic phase carefully aspirated.

A 1.2-ml aliquot of the aqueous phase is transferred to a small tube containing 0.1 ml of 0.1 M ninhydrin solution and the tubes heated for 30 min at 75°C. One hour after heating, the solution is transferred to a quartz cuvette and the fluorescence measured at 490 mμ after activation at 385 mμ (uncorrected). The activation and fluorescent spectra are essentially the same as described by Banable (1963). The fluorescence increases about 10% in the first 20 min after heating but is then stable for at least 6 hr. A small reagent blank is obtained by carrying 4 ml of 0.4 N perchloric acid through the above procedure. The fluorescence intensity is proportional to serotonin concentration over the range 0.005–0.5 μg/ml. Serotonin added to tissues is recovered to the extent of 90–100% after correcting for 85% extraction.

1. Fluorescence of a Variety of Compounds After Reacting with Ninhydrin

The capacity of a number of biologically occurring substances and indole derivatives to form fluorescent compounds when heated with ninhydrin at pH 7.0, as described above, but without prior butanol extraction appears in Table V. The fluorescence is highly specific for serotonin. The fluorescence of bufotenin is about 2% and that of 5-hydroxytryptophan about 1% of an equal concentration of serotonin, while other compounds tested produce negligible fluorescence. When tested at 0.1 M concentrations, leucine and methionine give appreciable fluorescence but with a fluorescent peak at 450 mμ and an activation peak at 380 mμ. Tyrosine at 0.1 M concentrations produces fluorescence with an activation peak at 400 mμ and fluorescent peak at

Table V. Relative Fluorescence of Serotonin and Other Compounds after Heating with Ninhydrin[a]

Compound	Units
Serotonin	850
Bufotenin	20
5-Hydroxytryptophan	10
5-Hydroxyindoleacetic acid	2
Epinephrine	2
Histidine	2
5-Hydroxyindole	1

[a] Activating peak 385 mμ. Fluorescent peak 490 mμ. Compounds that give no measurable fluorescence: 6-hydroxytryptamine, 4-hydroxytryptamine, 5-methoxytryptamine, N,N-diethyltryptamine, tryptamine, indole, N,N-dimethyltryptamine, 6-methoxytryptamine, 6-methoxyindole, 5-methoxyindole, 5-hydroxy-6-methoxytryptamine, 6-hydroxy-5-methoxytryptamine, melatonin, norepinephrine, proline, cysteine, alanine, leucine, methionine, tyrosine, histamine, glutamic acid, tryptophan, N-acetylserotonin. All compounds tested at 3×10^{-6} M concentrations.

520 mμ. However, none of the amino acids studied is extracted to any appreciable extent.

2. Estimation of Serotonin in Tissues

The development of a sensitive method for serotonin makes it possible to measure this biogenic amine in tissues, such as heart and adrenal gland, in which it could not be detected by chemical methods previously used. Measurable amounts of serotonin are found in the adrenal glands and hearts of rats (Table VI). In all tissues, the activation and fluorescent spectra are the same as that of authentic serotonin. This amine has also been assayed in the rat pineal gland, large intestine, spleen, lung and brain by the ninhydrin method and by the method of Bogdanski et al. (1956). Close agreement in the serotonin concentration is obtained by both methods.

IV. SENSITIVE AND SPECIFIC ENZYMIC– ISOTOPIC ASSAY FOR TISSUE HISTAMINE

Tissue concentrations of histamine are usually measured by the ability of histamine to contract smooth muscle or by fluorescence after reaction with O-phthalaldehyde (Green, 1970). Bioassay procedures are relatively laborious and sometimes nonspecific. While the fluorometric assay for tissue histamine described by Shore et al. (1959) is sensitive and specific for most tissues, it gives falsely high values in the brain due to interference by brain sperimidine which also reacts with O-phthalaldehyde. Modifications of this procedure in which spermidine is separated from histamine prior to fluorescent assay have enhanced specificity, making it possible to measure brain histamine fluorometrically but have also greatly increased the time and effort needed

Table VI.   Serotonin Content of Several Tissues[a]

| | Serotonin content (μg/g) | |
	Method of Bogdanski et al.	Ninhydrin method
Tissue		
Rat pineal gland	62.2±6.5	64.07±.1
Rat adrenal gland	0.00	0.45±0.05
Cat superior cervical ganglion	0.00	0.00
Rat large intestine	1.75±0.20	1.78±0.2ᵃ
Rat spleen	3.09±0.30	3.05±0.22
Rat heart	0.00	0.19±0.02
Rat brain	0.44±0.06	0.45±0.06
Rat lung	1.01±0.20	1.10±0.14

[a] Groups of 3 to 6 rats were used for each tissue. Data are presented as means ± S.E.M.

to complete assay procedures (Anton and Sayre, 1969; Green and Erickson, 1964; Kremzner and Pfeiffer, 1965; Medina and Shore, 1966; Michaelson and Coffman 1969).

The method described here depends on the enzymic transfer of the methyl-^{14}C of S-adenosylmethionine-^{14}C (AMe-^{14}C) to tissue histamine to form methylhistamine-^{14}C. A tracer amount of histamine-^{3}H is added to correct for the efficiency of the reaction so that the final product formed is methylhistamine-^{14}C-^{3}H (Fig. 1). Endogenous AMe is destroyed by heating so that there is no dilution of the added AMe-^{14}C, while the histamine-^{3}H is diluted with endogenous histamine (Snyder *et al.*, 1966). The enzyme histamine methyltransferase used for the reaction is highly specific for histamine (Brawn *et al.*, 1959). The only tissue component that is methylated in the reaction is histamine. Thus the ratio ^{14}C/^{3}H is linearly related to the tissue content of histamine.

A. Materials

1. Reagents

Histamine-^{3}H generally labeled (9.6 Ci/mmole); S-adenosylmethionine-^{14}C (40 mCi/mmole).

Histamine methyltransferase is partially purified by a modification of the method of Brown *et al.* (1959). The brains of 6 adult male guinea pigs are homogenized in 10 volumes of 0.25 M sucrose and centrifuged at 78,000 g for 30 min. To 180 ml of the supernatant fluid, 50 g of ammonium sulfate are added (45% saturation), followed by centrifugation at 10,000 g for 20 min. To the decanted supernatant fraction 33 g of ammonium sulfate are added (70% saturation). The final precipitate obtained by centrifugation at 10,000 g for 10 min is dissolved in 25 ml of 0.01 M sodium phosphate buffer (pH 7.4). The specific activity of the final preparation is about 6 times greater than that of the original soluble supernatant fraction. The partially purified enzyme is stable for at least 3 months at $-15°$.

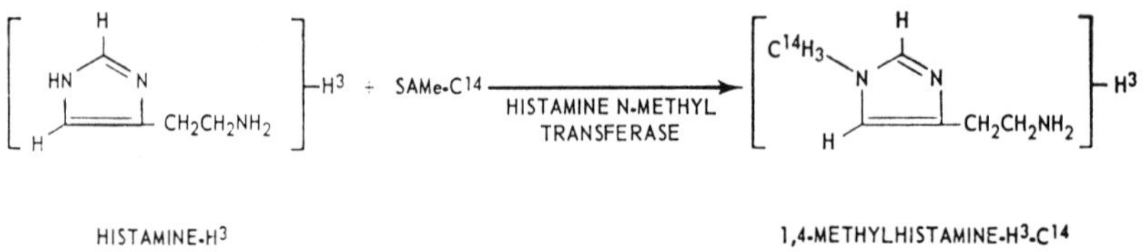

HISTAMINE-H^3 1,4-METHYLHISTAMINE-H^3-C^{14}

Fig. 1. Enzymic formation of methylhistamine-C^{14}-H^3.

B. Procedure

Step 1. Preparation of tissue extracts: Tissues are homogenized in 2–10 volumes of 0.05 M sodium phosphate buffer (pH 7.9). The homogenates are transferred to centrifuge tubes and heated for 10 min in boiling water to destroy tissue AMe and to free bound histamine. The resulting preparation is then centrifuged at 10,000 g for 20 min.

Step 2. Incubation: Aliquots (20–500 μl) of the supernatant fraction from step 1 containing 2–500 mμg of histamine are mixed in a 15-ml glass-stoppered centrifuge tube with 16 mμCi of histamine-[3]H (0.2 mμg). This is followed by the addition of 40 mμCi (1 mμmole) of AMe-^{14}C and 50 μl of the histamine methyltransferase preparation containing 15 units of activity (Brown *et al.*, 1959) and 0.05 M sodium phosphate buffer to make a total volume of 0.5 ml. The mixture is incubated for 1 hr at 37°C.

Step 3. Extraction and measurement of methylhistamine-[14]C-[3]H: The reaction is stopped by the addition of 2 ml of 1 N NaOH, the solution is saturated with sodium chloride, and the methylhistamine formed is extracted into 6 ml of chloroform. The aqueous phase is removed by aspiration, and the organic phase is washed with 2 ml of 1 N NaOH. Three milliliter of the organic phase are transferred to a counting vial and evaporated to dryness in a stream of hot air. One milliliter of absolute ethanol and 10 ml of toluene phosphor [0.4% 2,4-diphenyloxazole and 0.01% β-bis-(2-phenyloxazole)-benzene in toluene] are added to the vials and the radioactivity of ^{14}C and ^{3}H is measured in a scientillation spectrometer.

With each assay are included standard determinations of two concentrations of authentic histamine as well as histamine added to tissue homogenates before heating. Histamine added to tissues is recovered to the extent of 90–100%. The mean difference between duplicate determinations is 2.3% $\pm$ 0.2% of the values. An example of the data from a typical assay appears in Table VII.

The ^{14}C/^{3}H ratio in the methylhistamine formed is proportional to histamine concentration from 0.002 to 1.00 μg. Only about 3% of histamine-^{3}H and negligible amounts of AMe-^{14}C are extracted into chloroform under the experimental conditions.

In assays of brain tissue with the above procedure, extracts of brain tissue have appeared to contain substances which interfered with the activity of histamine methyltransferase. This difficulty, combined with the low endogenous levels of histamine in the brain, prompted the development of a semimicro procedure similar to that above but using smaller volumes and a higher concentration of AMe-[14]C. Tissue homogenates are prepared in the same way as described above. Small aliquots (50–100 μl) of the supernatant of tissue homogenates, containing 0.2–10 mμg of histamine, are mixed in a

Table VII. Typical Assay of Tissue Histamine by the Enzymic-Isotopic Method[a]

Sample	^{3}H (cpm)	^{14}C (cpm)	29% of ^{14}C[b] (cpm)	^{3}H corrected (cpm)	C^{14}/^{3}H (cpm)	Histamine in sample (ng)
Histamine (50 ng)	10,590	5,220	1,513	9,077	0.574	50
	11,340	5,960	1,730	9,612	0.620	50
Histamine (100 ng)	8,270	7,280	2,112	6,159	1.185	100
	7,625	6,870	1,984	5,668	1.213	100
No histamine	8,830	380	110	8,720	0.044	0
	9,540	484	140	9,402	0.051	0
Heart (200 μl)	4,504	1,934	560	3,944	0.489	40.7
	4,561	1,930	559	4,002	0.482	40.3
Stomach (25 μl)	7,149	3,186	924	6,225	0.512	42.6
	10,560	4,802	1,395	9,169	0.526	43.8
Stomach (25 μl) and 30 ng histamine	10,820	7,230	2,100	8,724	0.829	69.0
	12,140	8,550	2,480	9,657	0.885	73.6

[a] Tissues are homogenized in 10 volumes of 0.01 M phosphate buffer (pH 7.4), heated and centrifuged. Aliquots are assayed for histamine as described in the text. Histamine standard is added to a portion of the stomach homogenate prior to boiling.
[b] Under the experimental conditions, the scintillation spectrometer measures 29% of ^{14}C as ^{3}H, but only 2% of ^{3}H as ^{14}C.

15–ml glass-stoppered centrifuge tube with 16 mμCi of histamine-^{3}H (0.2 mμg/25 μl). This is followed by the addition of 200 mμCi (5 mμmole/25 μl) of AMe-^{14}C, 25 μl of the methyltransferase preparation, and 0.05 M sodium phosphate buffer to make a total reaction volume of 0.2 ml. The incubation, extraction, and liquid scintillation counting are carried out as described above for the macroassay. By these few modifications the sensitivity for the estimation of histamine is enhanced 10-fold so that in pure solution as little as 0.2 mμg of histamine gives a value twice blank readings. Histamine levels in the brain can be assayed with no preliminary concentrations of brain homogenates.

1. Specificity

Chloroform extracts from numerous tissues assayed by this method for histamine and chromatographed on paper with ethyl acetate–butanol–acetic acid–water (1:1:1:1) or ethanol–0.1 N HCl (19:1) show only a single peak of radioactivity which corresponds in R_f to authentic methylhistamine.

2. Tissue Concentrations of Histamine

The following rat tissues give the same values for histamine concentration when assayed by the present method or by the fluorometric technique of Shore et al. (1959): skin, stomach, heart, spleen. The histamine concentration of whole rat brain, determined by the present method, is 0.06 μg/g

(1966). In assays on the same samples, the unmodified method of Shore et al. (1959) gives histamine concentrations for whole rat brain of 0.31 μg/g (Snyder et al., 1966) and the fluorescent peak differs from that for authentic histamine. Careful bioassay of whole rat brain extracts gives histamine concentrations of 0.06 μg/g (Carlini and Green 1963a, b). Kremzner and Pfeiffer (1965) identified spermidine as a fluorescent contaminant in the fluorometric method for histamine. After spermidine is removed from extracts of whole rat brain by ion-exchange chromatography (Green and Erickson, 1964; Kremzner and Pfeiffer, 1965; Medina and Shore, 1966; Michaelson and Coffman, 1969) or appropriate organic solvents (Anton and Sayre, 1969), the fluorometric method also gives values for histamine of 0.06 μg/g.

Using semimicro modification, brain histamine can be assayed in small amounts of tissue (about 10 mg) so that it is possible to study the regional localization of histamine in rat brain (Table VIII). (Taylor and Snyder 1971b, 1972a). Highest concentrations of histamine occur in the hypothalamus, as has been reported previously by several investigators (Adam, 1961; Green, 1970).

V. MICROASSAY FOR HISTAMINE

Recently we have developed a single or double isotopic micromodification of the histamine assay permitting the determination of as little as 10 pg brain histamine. (Taylor and Snyder 1972b; Snyder and Taylor, 1972).

Tissues are homogenized in 5–20 volumes of ice-cold 0.01 M sodium phosphate buffer, pH 7.9, containing 0.1 % Triton X-100 and centrifuged at 50,000 g for 10 min. Aliquots of the supernatant fluid are heated in a boiling water bath for 10 min, cooled, and centrifuged at 50,000 g for 10 min.

Table VIII. Histamine Concentrations in Various Regions of the Rat Brain Determined by the Enzymic-Isotopic Procedure[a]

Region	Weight (mg)	Histamine (mμg/g)
Brainstem	228 ± 5	24 ± 3
Cerebellum	264 ± 4	22 ± 3
Midbrain	218 ± 12	57 ± 6
Hippocampus	152 ± 5	38 ± 4
Hypothalamus	68 ± 4	177 ± 9
Thalamus	66 ± 4	106 ± 8
Corpus striatum	148 ± 8	59 ± 4
Cerebral cortex	709 ± 10	57 ± 5

[a] Sprague-Dawley female rats (180–200 g) were used. Each value is the mean ± S.E.M. of 10 determinations.

Aliquots (1–20 μl) of the supernatant fluid are transferred to microfuge tubes for histamine assay, and made up to 20 μl with 0.05 M sodium phosphate buffer, pH 7.9, containing 0.1 % Triton X-100. This is followed by the addition of 10 μl of the histamine methyltransferase reactant solution. This solution is prepared at 4 °C immediately before addition and consists of 1 part AMe-^{14}C (5 μCi/ml), 1 part histamine-^{3}H (0.64 μCi/ml) and 2 parts of the guinea pig histamine methyltransferase preparation (3.8 mg protein/ml). Ten microliters of this solution contain 1.6 nCi (0.22 pmoles) histamine-^{3}H and 12.5 nCi (0.28 nmoles) AMe-^{14}C. The total reaction volume is 30 μl. Final concentrations of histamine-^{3}H and AMe-^{14}C are 7.35 nM and 9.35 μM, respectively.

The mixture is incubated for 1 hr at 37°C. The reaction is stopped by the addition of 5 μl of 1 M NaOH, the solution is saturated with NaCl, and the methylhistamine formed in the reaction is extracted into 250 μl chloroform by applying a vortex to the capped microfuge tubes for 30 sec using a Lab-line Supermixer (A. Thomas Co., Philadelphia, Pa.).

The aqueous phase is removed by aspiration and the organic phase washed with 100 μl 1 M NaOH by applying a vortex using the Lab-line for 10 sec. The aqueous phase is carefully removed by aspiration and the organic phase is transferred to a glass vial and evaporated to dryness in a stream of air. Then 1 ml ethanol and 10 ml of toluene phosphor (0.4 % 2.4-diphenyloxazole benzene in toluene) are added and the radioactivity of ^{14}C and ^{3}H is measured in a Packard Tri-carb liquid scintillation spectrometer for a counting period of 10–30 min. The efficiency of counting both ^{3}H and ^{14}C has been found to be constant. Each assay is performed on triplicate samples.

^{3}H and ^{14}C are counted at an efficiency of 24 % and 61 %, respectively. There is a 9 % overlap of ^{14}C into the tritium channel but no overlap of ^{3}H into the ^{14}C channel. This overlap is allowed for in the calculation of the ratio of ^{14}C/^{3}H.

With each assay are included standard determinations of two concentrations of authentic histamine as well as histamine added to tissue homogenates before heating. Histamine added to tissues is recovered to the extent of 93 to 98 %. There is a linear relationship between the amount of unlabeled histamine and the ^{14}C/^{3}H ratio in methylhistamine formed enzymically (Fig. 2). The ^{14}C/^{3}H ratio in methylhistamine is proportional to histamine concentration over the range of 0.02–5 ng. In pure solution and in tissue samples as little as 0.02 ng of histamine gives a value twice blank readings.

To demonstrate the presence of a single radioactive product, the chloroform extracts are evaporated to a small volume and chromatographed on Whatman No. 1 paper with ethyl acetate–butanol–glacial acetic acid–

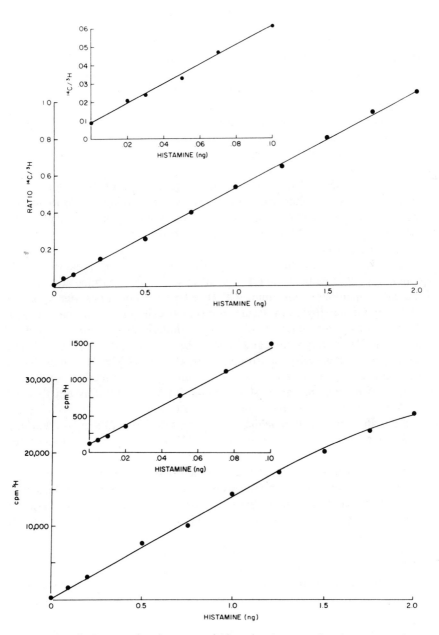

Fig. 2. Standard curves for the assay of histamine by enzymic microassays using double label (top) or single label (bottom) techniques.

water (1:1:1:1) or with ethanol–0.1 N HCl (9:1). In every brain region examined there is a single peak of radioactivity which corresponds in R_f to authentic methylhistamine. The amount of methylhistamine-^{14}C, histamine-^{3}H and AMe-^{14}C extracted into chloroform under conditions of the present assay are 84%, 4%, and 0%, respectively. These extractibility values do not vary with the amount of tissue in the homogenate sample. Therefore, the reagent blank containing no histamine is used as a tissue blank. Aliquots (5–20 μl) of a rat brain tissue extract are assayed for histamine. A linear plot of radioactive methylhistamine formed by the increasing volumes of tissue extract is obtained which passes through the point given by the reagent blank.

The enhanced sensitivity has been brought about by reducing the reaction volume and increasing the concentration of AMe-^{14}C so that more than 85% of the histamine in samples is methylated. Further increases in the concentration of AMe-^{14}C increase the blank value.

In experiments to measure the sensitivity of the reaction, 0.02 ng HA yields 5 cpm of methylhistamine-^{14}C after subtracting a blank value of 3 cpm in the ^{14}C channel (Table IX). In assays of brain histamine and internal standards of authentic histamine with the above method it has been apparent that histamine methylation occurs to a similar extent in all samples. Thus a double isotope technique involving the addition of a tracer amount of histamine-^{3}H to every sample ought not to be necessary. Accordingly we have developed a single enzymic-isotopic method using AMe-^{3}H, which has a specific activity 80 times that of the ^{14}C analog, as the methyl donor. The method is exactly the same as the double isotopic method except that the histamine methyltransferase solution consists of 1 part AMe-^{3}H (62.5 μCi/ml) and 1 part histamine methyltransferase solution (3.8 mg protein/ml). Ten microliters of this solution contain 312.5 nCi (0.78 nmoles) AMe-^{3}H. The final concentration of AMe-^{3}H in the 30-μl reaction volume is 26.1 μM. With each assay are included standard determinations of two concentrations of authentic histamine as well as two concentrations of histamine added to tissue homogenates before heating. Histamine added to tissues is recovered to the extent of 92–96%. There is a linear relationship between the amount of unlabeled histamine and methylhistamine-^{3}H formed enzymically over the range of 0.01–2.0 ng. In pure solutions and tissue samples as little as 0.01 ng of histamine gives a value twice blank readings.

Both the single and double isotope methods provide reliable estimates of tissue histamine under our experimental conditions (Table IX). The single isotope method is linear over a smaller range of histamine concentrntions than the double isotope technique. This is presumably attributable to the smaller proportion of histamine methylated at higher concentrations which, in the double isotope procedure, would be corrected by the isotopic

Table IX. Typical Assay of Histamine in Selected Regions of the Rat Brain by the Enzymic-Isotopic Method[a]

Sample	Double isotope method			Single isotope method		
	Ratio $^{14}C{:}^{3}H$	Internal standard sample	Histamine conc. (ng/g)	^{3}H cpm	Internal standard sample	Histamine conc. (ng/g)
Pure solution	0.009			61		
+ 0.1 ng histamine	0.57	0.048		1447	1386	
+ 0.2 ng histamine	0.118	0.109		2755	2694	
Hypothalamus (59 mg)	0.139		195	3471		206
+ 0.1 ng histamine	0.198	0.059		4810	1349	
+ 0.2 ng histamine	0.252	0.113		6101	2630	
Corpus striatum (115 mg)	0.066		46	1361		43
+ 0.1 ng histamine	0.121	0.055		2636	1275	
+ 0.2 ng histamine	0.172	0.106		3931	2570	
Cerebral cortex (166 mg)	0.083		40	1911		43
+ 0.1 ng histamine	0.135	0.052		3201	1290	
+ 0.2 ng histamine	0.191	0.108		4438	2527	

[a] Tissues were homogenized in 1 ml of 0.01 M phosphate buffer, pH 7.9, containing 0.1% Triton X-100, heated and centrifuged. Aliquots (20 μl) were assayed for histamine as described in the text. Histamine standards were added to aliquots of supernatant fluid prior to estimation for histamine.

ratio but which would decrease linearity in the single isotopic technique. Because of this limitation of the single isotope procedure, in all single isotope assays, internal standards of histamine are included. Assays are assumed to be valid only if the two concentrations of added internal standard histamine solutions and the reagent blank are related linearly (Table IX). In all experiments with the single isotope assay, the amount of internal standard of histamine added corresponds approximately to the amount of histamine in the tissue sample. Assays in which there is a marked discrepancy between these values are rejected.

To determine the optimal concentration of AMe in the two assays for histamine, varying amounts of ^{14}C or AMe-^3H have been employed with a range of histamine concentrations (Table X). With both single and double isotope techniques, the ratio of radioactivity in methylhistamine to blank values decreases at AMe concentrations in excess of 0.3–0.4 nmoles per 30 μl, presumably because maximal methylation of histamine occurs at this concentration, and at higher levels only blank values are increased. With lower concentrations of AMe the extent of methylation appears to decrease so that the reaction is not linear with increasing amounts of histamine.

Adding Triton X-100 to tissues prior to homogenization increases histamine values in all brain regions about 20–30%, suggesting that Triton enhances the extraction of histamine from tissue. Accordingly, histamine levels obtained without added Triton may be spuriously low. We also have observed that adding Triton to the tissues prior to the homogenization

Table X.   The Effect of the Concentration of AMe-^{14}C and AMe–^3H on the Enzymic-Isotopic Determination of two Concentrations of Histamine

Amount of AMe added in reaction	Histamine								
	0			0.2 ng			0.5 ng		
	^{14}C	^3H	$^{14}C/^3H$	^{14}C	^3H	$^{14}C/^3H$	^{14}C	^3H	$^{14}C/^3H$
AMe-^{14}C									
6.3 nCi	35	386	0.008	33	411	0.081	85	479	0.178
12.5 nCi	4	428	0.009	48	428	0.112	125	462	0.271
25 nCi	19	410	0.046	61	420	0.145	146	489	0.299
50 nCi	38	412	0.092	81	417	0.195	176	501	0.351
AMe-^3H									
78 nCi		116			2516			6118	
156 nCi		118			2918			7216	
312 nCi		132			2982			7015	
625 nCi		189			2778			6221	
1250 nCi		284			2043			4810	

increases the recovery of added histamine-^{3}H. Previously we reported that a certain amount of added histamine-^{3}H was bound to particulate tissue fractions, and could provide an erroneous indication of the amine's subcellular localization (Kuhar *et. al.* 1971). Homogenization in the presence of Triton appears to decrease this binding.

VI. SENSITIVE FLUOROMETRIC AND RADIOMETRIC ASSAYS FOR MONOAMINE OXIDASE AND DIAMINE OXIDASE

The enzymic oxidation of amines is associated with oxygen uptake, the production of ammonia, hydrogen peroxide, and the corresponding oxidation products of the amine. All of these parameters as well as the disappearance of substrate can be used as a basis for assaying oxidative deamination. The greatest sensitivity has been obtained by radiometric estimation of amine oxidation products (Okuyama and Kobayashi, 1961; Otsuka and Kobayashi, 1964; Wurtman and Axelrod, 1963). In a recently developed procedure (Snyder and Hendley, 1968; Tipton, 1969) a fluorescent product is formed from hydrogen peroxide released during oxidative deamination of substrate and homovanillic acid. This procedure is similar in sensitivity to the radiometric assays, and permits the use of multiple substrates and continuous monitoring. In this section, assays of monoamine and diamine oxidase activities by the fluorometric method of Snyder and Hendley (1968) and the radiometric assays of Otsuka and Kobayashi (1964) and Okuyama and Kobayashi (1961) will be described and compared.

A. Fluorometric Assay

1. Principle

The method depends on the finding of Guilbeault *et al.* (1967) that hydrogen peroxide formed in oxidase reactions can be measured by coupling it to the formation of a fluorophore with homovanillic acid in the presence of peroxidase. Accordingly, tissue preparations are incubated with amine substrate, homovanillic acid, and horseradish peroxidase, and the hydrogen peroxide evolved is measured fluorometrically (Snyder and Hendley, 1968). This permits the use of a number of substrates and continuous monitoring of the enzyme reaction. The method is comparable in sensitivity to the radiometric methods for amine oxidases and is relatively simple to perform so that as many as 50 assays can be completed in 2 hr.

2. Reagents

Horseradish peroxidase (Calbiochem)
Homovanillic acid
Hydrogen peroxide

3. Preparation of Tissues

Tissues are homogenized in 5–20 volumes of ice-cold 0.1 M Na-K phosphate buffer in a motor-driven glass homogenizer. Aliquots of whole homogenate are taken for monoamine oxidase assay whereas supernatant preparations are assayed for diamine oxidase activity. The latter are obtained after centrifuging the homogenates in the cold for 20 min at 12,000 g.

4. Procedure

Duplicate samples for incubation are made up to contain in a final volume of 3 ml: 0.1 M Na-K phosphate buffer, pH 7.8; 0.04 mg horseradish peroxidase; 1–2 units of tissue enzyme preparation; 0.25 mg homovanillic acid; and appropriate amine substrate. Before the addition of homovanillic acid and substrate, the tubes are preincubated for 10 min with shaking at 37 °C in a metabolic incubator (Dubnoff) to remove substrates of H_2O producing enzymes. This procedure lowers the tissue blanks between 15 and 45%. After preincubation, homovanillic acid and substrate are added and the tubes incubated for 1 hr at 36 °C with shaking. The reaction is stopped by chilling the tubes to 4 °C and the fluorescent intensity measured in a spectrophotofluorometer (Aminco-Bowman) at an activation wavelength of 315 mμ, and fluorescent wavelength of 425 mμ. When whole homogenates of tissues are used for assay, the tubes are centrifuged in the cold for 20 min at 12,000 g, after which fluorescence measurements are made on the supernatant fraction. Diamine oxidase activity has been examined in supernatant preparations from rat small intestine (0.2–10 mg of tissue) using concentrations of putrescine, cadaverine, histamine, and 1,4-methylhistamine [1-methyl-(β-aminoethyl)-imidazole] ranging from 10^{-6} M to 10^{-3} M. Monoamine oxidase activity has been measured in homogenates of rat liver (0.1–2.0 mg of tissue) and rat brain (0.4–10.0 mg) using tyramine, tryptamine, benzylamine, octopamine, normetanephrine, metanephrine, and 1,4-methylhistamine as substrates at 10^{-4} M concentration. With these tissues and substrates enzyme activity is linear for 90 min.

Blanks containing tissue enzyme but no added substrate are subtracted for calculation of enzyme activity. A calibration curve is determined in each experiment by adding increasing amounts of freshly prepared standard hydrogen peroxide solution, 1 mμmole per μl, to the cuvette containing in 3 ml: 0.1 M Na-K phosphate buffer, pH 7.8; horseradish peroxidase, 0.02 mg; and homovanillic acid, 0.25 mg. The exact molarity of the stock H_2O_2

solution is determined by titration with $KMnO_4$. The resultant fluorescence readings are used to calculate equivalent $m\mu$moles of substrate oxidized per hour. Fluorescence readings twice the blank reading are obtained with 1 $m\mu$mole hydrogen peroxide.

One unit of monoamine oxidase activity is defined as that amount which transforms 0.6 $m\mu$moles of tyramine at 10^{-4} M concentration per minute at 37 °C. One unit of diamine oxidase activity is defined as that amount which transforms 0.6 $m\mu$moles of putrescine at 10^{-4} M concentration per minute at 37 °C.

Under the standard assay condition, addition of 10 $m\mu$moles of authentic hydrogen peroxide to reaction mixture gives the same fluorescence as hydrogen peroxide reacted in pure solution with homovanillic acid.

5. Comparison of Radiometric and Fluorometric Techniques for Amine Oxidase Assay

The fluorometric method described here has been compared with radiometric assays for monoamine oxidase and diamine oxidase which will be described below. Putrescine has been used as substrate for rat small intestinal diamine oxidase and tyramine as substrate for brain monoamine oxidase. Incubation conditions for the simultaneous radiometric and fluorometric assays have been identical with respect to total volume, enzyme, and substrate concentrations, and incubation times except that radiometric assay mixtures do not contain homovanillic acid and horseradish peroxidase. Tyramine consumption by brain homogenates and putrescine consumption by small intestinal preparations is the same with fluorometric and radiometric techniques. In the radiometric assays of diamine oxidase and monoamine oxidase, the deaminated products are measured, while hydrogen peroxide production is assayed in the fluorometric method. Since these methods give the same results, the enzymic formation of detectable hydrogen peroxide would appear to be stoichiometric with the formation of deaminated products.

6. Substrates of Rat Brain and Liver Monoamine Oxidase

Of all the substrates examined (Table XI), the greatest activity has been observed using tyramine and tryptamine both in brain and liver. Benzylamine, octopamine, metanephrine, and normetanephrine are also active in both these tissues: The relative activity toward these substrates is the same in brain and liver. 1,4-Methylhistamine, an active substrate for liver, is not utilized by brain, although under these conditions the production of as little as 1.0 $m\mu$mole of hydrogen peroxide can be detected.

When norepinephrine, epinephrine, and serotonin are added to phosphate buffer containing horseradish peroxidase, homovanillic acid, and

Table XI. Substrates for Rat Liver and Brain Monoamine Oxidase

Amine[a]	mμmoles hydrogen peroxide produced in 1 hr[b]	
	Brain, 5 mg	Liver, 1.25 mg
Tyramine	36	52
Tryptamine	30	52
Benzylamine	14	41
dl-Octopamine	7	15
dl-Normetanephrine	2	5
dl-Metanephrine	2	4
1,4-Methyl histamine	0	4

[a] All at final concentration of 10^{-14} M.
[b] Values are obtained from a calibration curve using authentic hydrogen peroxide.

hydrogen peroxide, there is complete inhibition of the production of fluorescent product between homovanillic acid and hydrogen peroxide. When examined as possible substrates with brain and liver homogenates, no activity toward these catecholamines and serotonin can be detected. These results suggest that the catechol and 5-hydroxy groupings may interfere with the ability of homovanillic acid to react with hydrogen peroxide themselves.

B. Radiometric Assays for Monoamine Oxidase and Diamine Oxidase

1. Principle

In the assay for monoamine oxidase, tyramine-^{14}C is incubated with tissue extracts. After incubation, the reaction mixture is acidified, the deaminated products formed are extracted into a mixture of anisole and PPO (2,5-diphenyloxazole) and the radioactivity measured in a liquid scintillation spectrometer (Otsuka and Kobayashi, 1964). The assay for diamine oxidase activity is similar except that putrescine-^{14}C or cadaverine-^{14}C are used as substrates, the reaction is terminated with NaHCO$_3$, and the deaminated products extracted into a mixture of toluene and PPO (Okuyama and Kobayashi, 1961).

C. Monoamine Oxidase Assay

1. Reagents

Tyramine-^{14}C (4.6 mCi/mmole) is diluted with nonradioactive tyramine to give about 50,000 dpm/0.3 μmoles.

Anisole (reagent grade) containing 0.6% PPO.

2. Preparation of Tissues

Tissues are homogenized in 10 volumes of ice-cold 0.1 M Na-K phosphate buffer, pH 7.8.

3. Procedure

The incubation mixtures contain 0.3 μmoles of tyramine-^{14}C, 1–2 units of enzyme preparation, and 0.1 M Na-K phosphate buffer, pH 7.8 in a final volume of 3 ml. Incubation is performed in a screw-cap culture tube (10 × 1.5 cm) at 37 °C in air with shaking for 60 min. At the end of the incubation period 0.5 ml of 2 M citric acid is added to the culture tube followed by 10 ml of the anisole-PPO solution. The mixture is then shaken vigorously for 5 min, centrifuged at 900 g for 5 min and allowed to stand at −20 °C until the lower aqueous phase is frozen. The upper layer is then poured into a counting vial and the radioactivity measured in a liquid scintillation spectrometer. Values are corrected for a small heated enzyme blank (30–50 cpm) which presumably represents extraction of a very small amount of tyramine-^{14}C into the organic phase under these conditions. The deaminated products are extracted into the organic phase to the extent of 80–85%. The counting efficiency of the anisole-PPO mixture under these conditions is 75% in a Nuclear-Chicago Unilux I liquid scintillation spectrometer. Enzyme activity rate in preparations from rat brain and rat liver is linear for 90 min.

The formation of ^{14}C-deaminated products is stoichiometric with the formation of hydrogen peroxide (Snyder and Hendley, 1968) and the consumption of oxygen (Otsuka and Kobayashi, 1964).

D. Diamine Oxidase Assay

1. Reagents

Putrescine-[14]C (9 mCi/mmole) and cadaverine-[14]C (4 mCi/mmole) are diluted with nonisotopic putrescine and cadaverine respectively to give about 50,000 dpm/0.3 μmoles.

Toluene (reagent grade) containing 0.35% PPO.

2. Preparations of Tissues

Tissues are homogenized in 10 volumes of ice-cold 0.1 M Na-K phosphate buffer, pH 7.8. Since diamine oxidase is a soluble enzyme in most tissues, homogenates are centrifuged at 12,000 g in the cold for 20 min. The enzyme assay can also be used with crude homogenates.

3. Procedure

The incubation mixtures contain 0.3 μmoles of putrescine-^{14}C or cadaverine-^{14}C, 1–2 units of enzyme preparation and 0.1 M Na-K phosphate buffer, pH 7.8 in a final volume of 3 ml. Incubations are performed in a screw-cap culture tube (10×1.5 cm) at 37 °C in air with shaking, for 30 min. At the end of the incubation period, 1 g of solid NaHCO₃ is added to the culture tube followed by 10 ml of the toluene-PPO solution. The mixture is shaken vigorously for 5 min, centrifuged at 900 g for 5 min and allowed to stand at -20 °C until the lower aqueous phase is frozen. The upper layer is then poured into a counting vial and the radioactivity measured in a liquid scintillation spectrometer. Values are corrected for a small heated enzyme blank (40–60 cpm) which presumably represents the extraction of small amounts of putrescine-^{14}C or cadaverine-[14]C. The deaminated products are extracted into the organic phase to the extent of 65–70% with both putrescine and cadaverine (Okuyama and Kobayashi, 1961). The counting efficiency of the toluene-PPO mixture under these conditions is 70% in a Nuclear Chicago Unilux I liquid scintillation spectrometer. The rate of enzyme activity in supernatant preparations from the rat small intestine is linear for 90 min.

Other sensitive techniques for the measurement of monoamine oxidase in crude tissue extracts include a radiometric method in which tryptamine-^{14}C is the substrate and the indoleacetaldehyde-^{14}C or indoleacetic acid-^{14}C formed is measured by liquid scintillation spectrometry (Wurtman and Axelrod). A microradiometric method uses tyramine-^{14}C or serotonin-^{14}C with the extraction of the deaminated products into organic solvents (McCaman et al., 1965). In the technique of Lovenberg et al. (1962), tryptamine is used as substrate and indoleacetaldehyde formed is converted to indoleacetic acid by the addition of aldehyde dehydrogenase. The indoleacetic acid is then measured spectrophotofluorometrically.

REFERENCES

Adam, H. M. (1961) in *Regional Neurochemistry* (S. S., Kety and J. Elkes, eds.), Pergamon Press, London, p. 293.

Anton, A. H., and Sayre, D. F. (1964) *J. Pharmacol. Exp. Ther.* **145,** 326.

Anton, A. H., and Sayre, D. F. (1969) *J. Pharmacol. Exp. Ther.* **166,** 285.

Bogdanski, D. F., Pletscher, A., Brodie, B. B., and Udenfriend, S. (1956) *J. Pharm. Exp. Ther.* **117,** 82.

Brown, D. D., Tomchick, R., and Axelrod, J. (1959) *J. Biol. Chem.* **234,** 2948.

Carlini, E. A., and Green, J. P. (1963a) *Brit. J. Pharmacol.* **20,** 264.

Carlini, E. A., and Green, J. P. (1963b) *Biochem. Pharmacol.* **12,** 1448.

Carlsson, A., and Lindquist, M. (1962) *Acta Physiol. Scnad.* **54,** 83.

Carlsson, A., and Waldeck, B. (1958) *Acta Physiol. Scand.* **44,** 293.

Carlsson, A., and Waldeck, B. (1964) *Scand. J. Clin. Lab. Invest.* **16,** 133.

Engelman, K., Portnoy, B., and Lovenberg, W. (1968) *Am. J. Med. Sci.* **255,** 259.

Euler, U. S. von (1959) *Pharmacol. Rev.* **11,** 262.

Euler, U. S. von (1961) in *Hormones in Blood* (C. H. Gray, ed.), Academic Press, New, York p. 515.

Green, H., and Erickson, R. W. (1964) *Int. J. Neuropharmacol.* **3,** 315.

Green, J. P. (1970) *Handbook of Neurochemistry*, Vol. 4 (A. Lajtha, ed.), Plenum Press, New York, p. 221.

Guilbeault, G. G., Kramer, D. N., and Hackley, E. (1967) *Analyl. Chem.* **39,** 271.

Häggendal, J. (1966) *Pharmacol. Rev.* **18,** 325.

Jepson, J. B., and Stevens, B. J. (1953) *Nature,* **172,** 772.

Juorio, A. V., Sharman, D. F., and Trajkov, T. (1966) *Brit. J. Pharmacol.* **26,** 385.

Kremzner, L. T., and Pfeiffer, C. C. (1965) *Biochem. Pharmacol.* **14,** 1189.

Kuhar, M. J., Taylor, K. M., and Snyder, S. H. (1971) *J. Neurochem.* **18,** 1515.

Laverty, R., and Taylor, K. M. (1968) *Analyt. Biochem.* **22,** 269.

Lovenberg, W., Levine, R. J., and Sjoerdsma, A. (1962) *J. Pharm. Exp. Ther.* **135,** 7.

McCaman, R. E., McCaman, M. W., Hunt, J. M., and Smith, M. S. (1965) *J. Neurochem.* **12,** 15.

Medina, M., and Shore, P. A. (1966) *Biochem. Pharmacol.* **15,** 1627.

Michaelson, I. A., and Coffman, P. Z. (1969) *Analyt. Biochem.* **27,** 257.

Okuyama, T., and Kobayashi, Y. (1961) *Arch. Biochem. Biophys.* **95,** 242.

Otsuka, S., and Kobayashi, Y. (1964) *Biochem. Pharmacol.* **13,** 995.

Saelens, J. K., Schoen, M. S., and Kovacsics, G. B. (1967) *Biochem. Pharmacol.* **16,** 1043.

Shore, P. A., and Olin, J. S. (1958) *J. Pharmacol. Exp. Ther.* **122,** 295.

Shore, P. A., Burkhalter, A., and Cohn, V. H. (1959) *J. Pharmacol. Exp. Ther.* **127,** 182.

Snyder, S. H., Baldessarini, R. J., and Axelrod, J. (1966) *J. Pharmacol. Exp. Ther.* **153,** 544.

Snyder, S. H., and Hendley, E. D. (1968) *J. Pharmacol. Exp. Ther.* **163,** 386.

Snyder, S. H., Axelrod, J., and Zweig, M. (1965) *Biochem. Pharmacol.* **14,** 831.

Snyder, S. H., and Taylor, K. M. (1972) in *Perspectives in Neuropharmacology* (S. H. Snyder, ed.), Oxford University Press, New York (in press).

Taylor, K. M., and Laverty, R. (1969) *J. Neurochem.* **16,** 1361.

Taylor, K. M., and Snyder, S. H. (1971*a*) *Science* **172,** 1037.

Taylor, K. M., and Snyder, S. H. (1971*b*) *J. Pharm. Exp. Ther.* **179,** 619.

Taylor, K. M., and Snyder, S. H. (1972*a*) *J. Neurochem.* **19,** 341.

Taylor, K. M., and Snyder S. H. (1972*b*) *J. Neurochem.* (in press).

Tipton, K. F. (1969) *Analyt. Biochem.* **28,** 318.

Vanable, J. W. (1963) *Analyt. Biochem.* **6,** 393.

Wurtman, R. J., and Axelrod, J. (1963) *Biochem. Pharmacol.* **12,** 1439.

Chapter 13

Enzymes Involved in the Catalysis of Catecholamine Biosynthesis

M. Goldstein*

Department of Psychiatry
Neurochemistry Laboratories
New York University Medical Center
New York, New York

I. INTRODUCTION

The postulated biosynthetic pathway (Blaschko, 1939) for the formation of the adrenergic transmitters (Fig. 1) was the subject of several studies and was confirmed with the use of radioactive labeled precursors. Three enzymes are involved in the catalysis of norepinephrine biosynthesis: tyrosine hydroxylase (TH), dopa decarboxylase (DDC), and dopamine-β-hydroxylase (DβH; a fourth enzyme, namely, phenylethanolamine-N-methyltransferase (PNMT) catalyzes the biosynthesis of epinephrine from norepinephrine. Two enzymes, namely, TH and DβH, can be classified as mixed-function oxidase (Mason, 1957) or monooxygenase (Hayaishi, 1964). The general reaction catalyzed by monooxygenases is shown in Reaction (1) where RH stands for the substrate to be hydroxylated, ROH for the hydroxylated product, and XH_2 for the electron donor.

$$RH + O_2 + XH_2 \longrightarrow ROH + H_2O + X \qquad (1)$$

Two different electron donors function as coreactants in the NE biosynthetic pathway. A tetrahydropteridine (DMPH$_4$) is the coenzyme in the systems that hydroxylate phenylalanine (Kaufman, 1958) and tyrosine

* Research Scientist Awardee of USPHS, NIH Grant MH-14918.

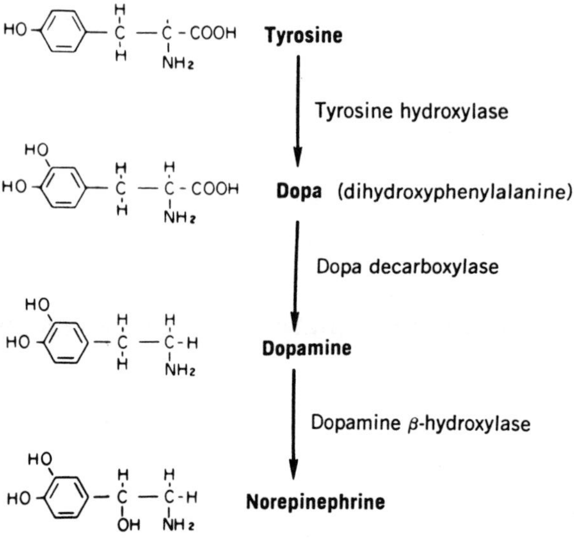

Fig. 1. Biosynthetic pathway for catecholamines.

(Nagatsu *et al.*, 1964a), and ascorbate is the coenzyme for DβH (Levin *et al.*, 1960) (The oxygen in the hydroxylated products comes from the atmosphere and not from water and therefore the rate of NE formation might depend on the oxygen concentration in the atmosphere.

This review will describe methods for purification of enzymes involved in catecholamine biosynthesis as well as methods for determination of their activities. The characteristics of the catecholamine biosynthetic enzymes and the mechanisms of the enzymic reactions will be briefly discussed.

II. PROPERTIES AND PURIFICATION OF INDIVIDUAL ENZYMES

A. Tyrosine Hydroxylase

L-Tyrosine, tetrahydropteridine; oxygen oxidoreductase (3-hydroxylating)

Tyrosine hydroxylase is a monooxygenase which catalyzes the first step in norepinephrine biosynthesis (Nagatsu *et al.*, 1964a) The tetrahydropteridine-dependent enzymic hydroxylation reaction is formulated in Reaction 2.

$$\text{Tyrosine} + O_2 + DMPH_4 \longrightarrow \text{dopa} + H_2O + DMPH_4 \qquad (2)$$

1. Purification of Tyrosine Hydroxylase

The enzyme was first partially purified from the supernatant fractions of adrenal homogenates by $(NH_4)_2SO_4$ fractionation (Nagatsu et al., 1964). In the same study it was shown that various regions of the brain as well as different sympathetic innervated tissues contain tyrosine hydroxylase activity. Subsequently TH was partially purified from the particulate fractions of bovine adrenal medulla. The particulate enzyme was solubilized with trypsin and further purified by $(NH_4)_2SO_4$ fractionation (Petrack et al., 1968). Some additional purifications were obtained by adsorption on hydroxylapatite (Nagatsu et al., 1970) or calcium phosphate gel (Goldstein and Joh, unpublished data). However, the enzyme became unstable following these purification procedures.

More recently, the particulate tyrosine hydroxylase was further purified (Shiman et al., 1971). The stoichiometry of the reaction catalyzed by the enzyme, as well as its regulatory properties, have been found to vary with different pterin cofactors. In addition to tyrosine, tyrosine hydroxylase accepts phenylalanine as a substrate (Ikeda et al., 1965). In presence of tetrahydrobiopterin the rate of hydroxylation of phenylalanine is even greater than the rate of tyrosine hydroxylation (Shiman et al., 1971). In striatal slices dopamine can be formed from phenylalanine or from tyrosine without the addition of any external cofactor (Frenkel et al., 1971). Tyrosine seems to have a slightly higher affinity for the hydroxylating enzyme than phenylalanine in the striatal slices.

Catalase and peroxidase protect tyrosine hydroxylase activity in crude tissue homogenates (M. Goldstein, unpublished data; Sedvall and Kopin, 1967) and more recently it was shown that the purified enzyme has to be protected by catalase, peroxidase, or Fe^{2+} from H_2O_2-mediated inactivation (Shiman et al., 1971).

2. Assays of Enzyme Activity

Two isotopic procedures are generally employed for the determination of tyrosine hydroxylase activity. In the first procedure the conversion of tyrosine-^{14}C to dopa-^{14}C is measured (Nagatsu et al., 1964a) The enzymically formed dopa-^{14}C is adsorbed on alumina and subsequently eluted with acid. The principle of the second procedure is based on the release of ^{3}H from 3,5-tyrosine-^{3}H into the water during the enzymic conversion of tyrosine to dopa (Nagatsu et al., 1964b). The rate of tritium released as water is directly proportional to the rate of the enzymic hydroxylation. The tritiated water is separated from tyrosine-^{3}H by passage through an ionexchange column. Both procedures require purification from contaminant catechols which are present in the commercially available ^{14}C or ^{3}H-labeled tyrosine preparations. The second procedure is simpler and has a higher sensitivity than the first procedure. This procedure is very useful for the determination of the activities in purified enzyme preparations while in crude homogenates the first procedure might be preferable.

The enzyme purified from the supernatant as well as from the particulate fractions of bovine adrenal medulla has similar characteristics. Both preparations require tetrahydropteridine as a cofactor. The activities from both preparations are stimulated by addition of Fe^{2+} and are inhibited by sulf-hydryl reagents, tyrosine analogs, and catechol derivatives.

The results of the gel filtration experiments suggest that TH might appear in different molecular forms (Wurzburger *et al.*, 1970), but definite molecular weight data cannot be calculated until the enzyme is isolated in a pure form. For maximal stimulation the guinea pig brain enzyme requires a 10 times higher concentration of $DMPH_4$ than the adrenal enzyme (Petrack *et al.*, 1970). These findings, in conjunction with the reported different molecular forms, may indicate that TH exists in different forms with different catalytic and regulatory activities.

3. Kinetic Studies

The kinetic properties of TH obtained from the supernatant preparations and from the particulate preparations were investigated. The initial velocity patterns obtained from the supernatant enzyme preparations indicate a "ping-pong" mechanism (Ikeda *et al.*, 1966) in which the enzyme is reduced by $DMPH_4$ followed by dissociation of the oxidized pteridine with the subsequent addition of O_2 and tyrosine to the reduced form of the enzyme producing dopa and reoxidation of the enzyme.

The initial velocity pattern obtained with the partially purified particulate enzyme preparation points to a sequential mechanism in which all three substrates, namely, O_2, tyrosine, and $DMPH_4$ add to the enzyme before a product is released (Joh *et al.*, 1969a; Joh *et al.*, 1969b). The pattern is very distinctive and indicates the obligatory addition of O_2 prior to $DMPH_4$ with the addition of these molecules being at thermodynamic equilibrium (Fig. 2). The rate equation reproduces the kinetic pattern under the assumption

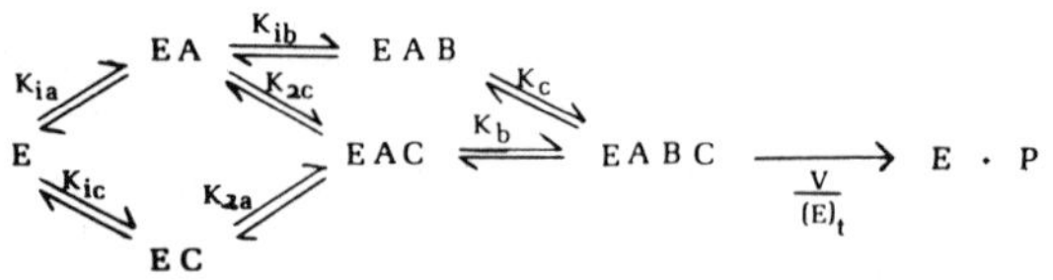

Fig. 2. Kinetic mechanism of the enzymic tyrosine hydroxyla-tion. A = O_2; B = $DMPH_4$; C = tyrosine; E = enzyme; p = products.

that equilibrium is rapid and that molecule B cannot combine until after molecule A does (see Fig. 2). The product inhibition patterns and inhibition by α-methyl-*p*-tyrosine are consistent with this mechanism if both dopa and DMPH$_4$ combine at the DMPH$_4$ site and if α-methyl-*p*-tyrosine combines at the tyrosine site.

The discrepancy between the kinetic results obtained with the supernatant and particulate preparation is most likely due to differences in the experimental conditions, such as differences in the range of the substrate concentrations and differences in incubation periods, and not as might be assumed, to the different enzyme preparations.

B. Dihydropteridine Reductase

Dihydropteridine reductase was partially purified from bovine adrenal medulla (Musacchio, 1969). Although this enzyme is not directly involved in the catecholamine biosynthesis, it might indirectly influence the rate of catecholamine biosynthesis by catalyzing the regeneration of the pteridine cofactor which is required for the TH activity.

C. Aromatic L-Amino Acid Decarboxylase
(Dopa Decarboxylase)

The enzyme which catalyzes the decarboxylation of dopa to dopamine (DA) also catalyzes the decarboxylation of all the naturally occuring aromatic L–amino acids and therefore, according to the suggestion of Lovenberg *et al.* (1962), the enzyme was referred to as "aromatic L-amino acid decarboxylase" (AADC). The enzyme requires pyridoxal phosphate as a cofactor.

The properties and purification procedures for AADC were recently reviewed (Sourkes, 1966; Aures *et al.,* 1970). Recently, AADC was extensively purified from bovine adrenal glands (Ceasar *et al.,* 1970) and from bovine kidneys (Christenson *et al.,* 1970). The purification procedure of AADC from bovine adrenal glands as described by Ceasar *et al.* (1970) is summarized in Table I. During the purification procedure it became apparent that we were dealing with a rather labile enzyme and that tne addition of dithiothreitol resulted in a significant stabilization of the enzyme activity.

In the standard polyacrylamide gel electrophoresis system, the enzyme activity is associated with two major protein bands (Fig. 3). Studies are in progress to determine the nature of the two protein bands.

1. Methods for the Assay of AADC Activity

AADC activity can be estimated with specific biological assays (Holtz

Table I. Purification of Supernatant Dopa Decarboxylase from
Bovine Adrenal Medulla

Purification step	Total protein (mg)	Specific activity (units/mg protein)[a]	Purification (-fold)
$(NH_4)_2SO_4$, 80% ppt.[b]	4948	44.7	—
		(28.8)	
$(NH_4)_2SO_4$, 35–40% ppt.	541	179.5	4.0
		(133.7)	(4.6)
Sephadex G-100[c]	59.6	1014.7	22.6
		(1000.4)	(34.4)
DEAE-cellulose	5.7	2353.0	52.4

[a] One unit is expressed as $m\mu$moles of substrate decarboxylated per mg protein per hour. Values in parentheses, 5-HTP decarboxylase activity.
[b] $(NH_4)_2SO_4$ ppt. of 100,000 g supernatant.
[c] Additional purification (approx. 4-fold) of the enzyme has been achieved by passage of the Sephadex G-100 enzyme preparation through a hydroxylapatite (Hypatite C) column, prior to chromatography on the DEAE cellulose column.

et al., 1942) or with biochemical procedures. The principle for the biochemical decarboxylase assays is shown in the following reaction.

$$\text{Aromatic L-amino acid} \longrightarrow \text{Amine} + CO_2 \qquad (3)$$

It is evident from reaction (3) that the determination of either one of the two enzymically formed products will reflect the enzymic activity.

The liberated CO_2 can be estimated by manometry or when carboxyl-labeled amino acids are used as substrate the radioactivity of labeled CO_2 can be measured. The enzymically formed amines separate from the substrate by ion-exchange chromatography. The amines are then determined fluorometrically or when radioactive amino acids are used as substrates the amount of radiolabeled amine can be measured.

An isotopic procedure for the determination of AADC activity in tissues was described (Hakanson and Owman, 1965) and with some modification was used in our laboratory for the determination of AADC activities in various tissues and in purified enzyme preparations.

2. Substrate Specificity

Although aromatic L-amino acid decarboxylase is usually regarded as a single enzyme, this is not yet a universally accepted fact. In the course of our studies we have been able to shed some light on the problem, with particular emphasis on dopa decarboxylase and 5-HTP decarboxylase activity.

AADC was purified from bovine adrenal glands and the purified enzyme was submitted to disc-gel electrophoresis. From the results presented in Fig. 4 it is evident that following elution of the protein bands after disc-gel elec-

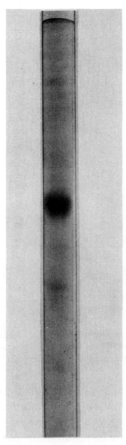

Fig. 3. Photograph of poly-acrylamide gel electrophoresis of purified AADC preparation.

trophoresis the pattern of enzyme activity was similar, whether dopa or 5-HTP was used as substrate.

The problem of whether the same enzyme catalyzes the decarboxylation of dopa and 5-HTP was studied by another experimental approach. The reagent 6-hydroxydopamine causes a specific degeneration of adrenergic nerve terminals both centrally and peripherally. Thus, 6-hydroxydopamine was injected intraventricularly into rats and some 8–10 days later decarboxylase activity was assayed in the striatum of 6-hydroxydopamine-treated and untreated animals. The results of this experiment have shown that treatment with 6-hydroxydopamine reduced decarboxylase activity to the same extent whether dopa or 5-HTP was used as enzyme substrate. Thus, the degeneration of the adrenergic nerve terminals affected the decarboxylation of dopa as well as of 5-HTP.

In another experiment we determined decarboxylase activity in monkeys

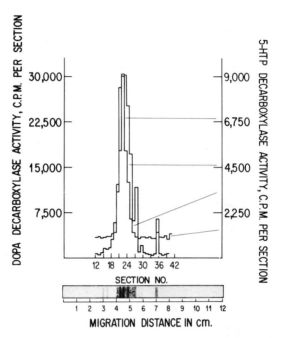

Fig. 4. The distribution of dopa and 5-HTP activity after polyacrylamide gel electrophoresis. (This enzymic preparation was not purified on hydroxylapatite column.)

with nigral lesions. These monkeys exhibited tremor and showed decreased levels of dopamine and 5-hydroxytryptamine in the striatum on the lesion side. The results of this experiment have shown that decarboxylase activity is reduced on the lesion side of the striatum when both dopa and 5-HTP were tested as substrates. These results suggest that most likely the same enzyme is responsible for the decarboxylation of dopa and 5-HTP in the striatum (Goldstein *et al.,* 1969; Goldstein *et al.,* 1970). However, it is conceivable that in specific regions of the brain a separate enzyme catalyzes the decarboxylation of dopa and of 5-HTP. The purification of AADC from the brain is now in progress and the substrate specificity of brain AADC will be investigated.

In the past few years there has been a lot of interest in L-dopa therapy in parkinsonism. The effectiveness of L-dopa therapy in parkinsonian patients may depend on the activity of dopa decarboxylase in the brain. Since it was reported that DDC cannot be detected in human postmortem brains (Vogel *et al.,* 1970) and that DDC activity was not present in the basal ganglia of parkinsonian patients, it became somewhat questionable whether the therapeutic effectiveness of L-dopa is due to the alleviation of the dopamine deficiency. We have therefore investigated dopa decarboxylase activity in the basal ganglia obtained from a postmortem parkinsonian patient who was treated with L-dopa for a long period of time prior to death. We found that dopa decarboxylase activity is present in the basal ganglia of the post-mortem parkinsonian patient. Although the activity is extremely low, it might be sufficient for replacement of the missing dopamine. This finding supports the view that the effectiveness of L-dopa therapy is due to substitution of the missing in the basal ganglia.

D. Dopamine-β-Hydroxylase

[3,4-dihydroxyphenylethylamine, ascorbate: oxygen oxidoreductase (hydroxylating) E.C. 1.14.21]

The enzyme DβH is a monooxygenase which catalyzes the terminal step in the biosynthesis of norepinephrine. The conversion of DA to norepinephrine has been demonstrated *in vitro* with the use of adrenal slices (Hagan, 1956), homogenates (Goodal and Kirschner, 1957), and aqueous extracts of acetone powders (Neri *et al.*, 1956). The enzymic dopamine-β-hydroxylation is coupled to a stoichiometrically equivalent oxidation of ascorbic acid according to Reaction (4) (Levin *et al.*, 1960).

$$DA + Ascorbate + O_2 \longrightarrow 1\text{-}NE + Dehydroascorbate + H_2O \qquad (4)$$

Fumarate and related decarboxylic acids stimulate the enzymic reaction (Levin *et al.*, 1960). The enzyme is nonspecific and accepts a variety of sympathomimetic amines structurally related to dopamine as substrates (Goldstein and Contrera, 1961; Levin and Kaufman, 1961; Pisano *et al.*, 1960; Creveling *et al.*, 1962).

DβH is a copper enzyme (Goldstein *et al.*, 1965; Blumberg *et al.*, 1965; Friedman and Kaufman, 1965) and various chelating agents effectively inhibit the enzymic activity *in vivo* and *in vitro* (Goldstein *et al.*, 1964). Electron paramagnetic resonance (EPR) and chemical studies have shown that the copper of the enzyme undergoes reduction and oxidation during the enzymic hydroxylation reaction (Friedman and Kaufman, 1965; Blumberg *et al.*, 1965). The mechanism of the enzymic dopamine-β-hydroxylation was further investigated with kinetic studies (Goldstein *et al.*, 1968). The kinetic data as well as the EPR studies support the mechanism which is outlined in the scheme presented in Fig. 5. In this scheme the first product, dehydroascorbate, leaves the enzyme before the addition of the subsequent substrates (ping-pong). The subsequent substrates (dopamine or tyramine and oxygen) add to the reduced enzyme intermediate before either product is released. The interconversion of the central ternary complexes seems to be the rate-limiting step in the overall β-hydroxylation reaction. The kinetic pattern also indicates

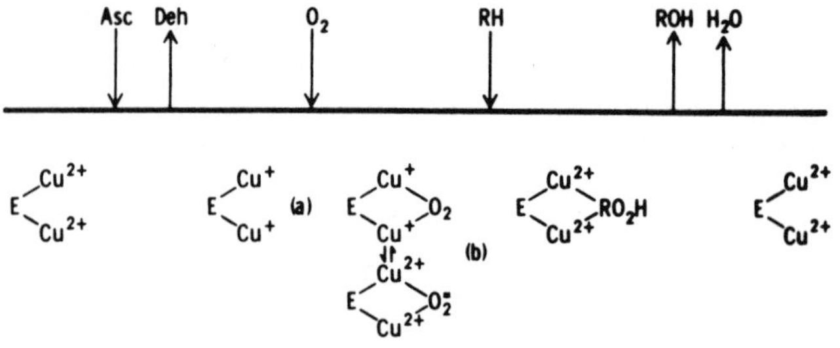

RH = tyramine or dopamine
ROH = product (octopamine or norepinephrine)
Asc = ascorbate
Deh = dehydroascorbic

Fig. 5. Schematic presentation of the enzymic dopamine-β-hydroxylation. RH = dopamine or tyramine, ROH = product (norepinephrine or octopamine), ASC = ascorbate, Deh = dehydroascorbic.

the obligatory addition of oxygen prior to the addition of dopamine. Fumarate and oxygen stimulate the enzymic activity at low substrate (RH) concentrations and both change the K_m of the substrate but not the V_{max}. Fumarate facilitates the interaction of the reduced enzyme intermediate with oxygen and most likely induces a conformational change of the enzyme (Goldstein *et al.*, 1968).

1. Purification of Dopamine-β-Hydroxylase

The extraction and purification of DβH from bovine adrenal medulla was described (Levin *et al.*, 1960). An essentially pure form of the enzyme was obtained and a molecular weight of approximately 290,000 was estimated (Friedman and Kaufman, 1965). Another shorter procedure yielded higher recoveries but the enzymic specific activity was lower (Goldstein *et al.*, 1965). More recently, the procedure for the purification of DβH was modified (Goldstein and Joh, unpublished data) and a highly purified enzyme preparation was obtained. The purification steps of this modified procedure are summarized in Table II. The enzyme obtained by this procedure shows one major single band and one very minor band following acrylamide disc gel electrophoresis. The major band (approximately 90% of the total protein) is associated with DβH activity.

2. Methods for the Assay of Dopamine-β-Hydroxylase Activity

The composition of the incubation mixture which is required for maximal DβH activity was described (Levin *et al.*, 1960). A standard incubation mixture contains the following components: ascorbic acid, 6 μmoles;

Table II. The Purification of Dopamine-β-Hydroxylase

Fraction	Protein (mg)	Total activity units[a]	Specific activity (units/mg protein)	Purification (-fold)
80% (NH$_4$)$_2$SO$_4$	520	1,872	3.6	0
25-35%	49	882	18.0	5
DEAE Sephadex A-50	7.2	684	95.0	26.4
Sephadex G-200	6.0	840	140.0	38.9

[a] The activity is expressed as μmoles of product formed per milligram protein per 20 min of incubation time.

fumaric acid, 10 μmoles; catalase, 100 units, and dopamine, 2 μmoles (or any other phenylethylamine which is a substrate for the enzyme). After the addition of the enzyme preparation, the reaction mixture is incubated at 37°C for 30 min. The reaction is stopped by the addition of 3% trichloroacetic acid.

The procedure employed for measuring the enzymic activity will depend on the substrate used in the incubation mixture. When dopamine is used as a substrate, the enzymic activity can be measured by assaying the enzymically formed NE fluorometrically (von Euler and Flooding, 1955). When tyramine is used as a substrate, the enzyme activity can be assayed by the spectrophotometric procedure of Pisano et al. (1960) .The procedure of Pisano can also be employed when other radioactive labeled phenylethylamines are used as substrates. For example, when DA labeled with ^{14}C in the terminal position was used as a substrate, the enzymically formed 1-NE-^{14}C was treated with periodate to liberate formaldehyde which was then trapped and counted (Levin et al., 1960). When uniformly labeled tyramine was used as a substrate, the enzymically formed octopamine was treated with periodate which resulted in the formation of uniformly labeled p-hydroxybenzaldehyde. The labeled p-hydroxybenzaldehyde was extracted into toluene and the radioactivity was subsequently determined (Fischer et al., 1964). The DβH activity can also be measured by separation of the substrate from the enzymically formed product with the use of paper chromatography. A procedure was developed in which the amines are acetylated and subsequently separated by paper chromatography in the "C" solvent system of Bush (Goldstein et al., 1959). Although this procedure is more elaborate, it is especially suitable for the determination of enzymic activity when nonradioactive phenylethylamines are used as substrates for the enzyme.

3. Dopamine-β-Hydroxylase Assay in Tissues

Although DβH activity was demonstrated in vivo in various sympathetic innervated tissues, the enzyme activity could not be measured in homogenates obtained from these tissues. Evidence has been presented that endogenous inhibitors interfere with the assays of DβH activity *in vitro* (Nagatsu *et al.*, 1967; Duch *et al.*, 1968).

Recently a sensitive and specific enzymic assay for DβH was developed and the activity of this enzyme measured in various tissues and in the serum (Bonnay *et al.*, 1970; Molinoff *et al.*, 1970).

The principle of the assay is outlined in reaction (5).

$$RCH_2CH_2NH_2 + O_2 + XH_2 \xrightarrow{DBH} RCHOHCH_2NH_2 + H_2O + X$$

$$RCHOHCH_2NH_2 + {}^{14}CH_3\text{-}S\text{-}AM \xrightarrow{PNMT} RCHOHCH_2NHC^{14}H_3 + SAHCys \qquad (5)$$

XH_2 = ascorbate; X = dehydroascorbate; ${}^{14}CH_3\text{-}S\text{-}AM$ = S-adenosylmethionine; $S\text{-}AHCys$ = S-adenosylhomocysteine

It can be seen from reaction (5) that the assay depends on two enzymic reactions. In the first reaction tyramine is added to the homogenate and is converted by DβH to octopamine. In the subsequent second reaction the enzymically formed octopamine is further converted by the added PNMT to N-methyl octopamine. ${}^{14}CH_3\text{-}S\text{-}AM$ serves as a methyl donor and the amount of -N-methyl octopamine-${}^{14}C$ is proportional to DβH activity.

4. Determination of Dopamine-β-Hydroxylase Activity in the Serum

The following procedure was developed in our laboratory for the determination of DβH activity in the serum (Goldstein, *et al.*, 1971). Serum obtained from humans was diluted 50–100-fold and used for enzyme activity assay. The incubations were carried out in two separate steps.

Step 1. To an aliquot of diluted serum (0.05 ml–0.1 ml) 10 μmoles of acetate buffer pH 5.5 and 0.1 μmole of N-ethylmaleimide (NEM) were added in a volume of 0.2 ml. The mixture was preincubated at room temperature for 10 min and then the following components in a total volume of 0.3 ml were added (in mμmoles): fumarate, 10; ascorbate, 6; pargyline, 0.7; tyramine, 0.4; and 1000 units of catalase (Sigma). The mixture was incubated for 20 min at 37°C.

Step 2. At the end of the incubation 0.1 μmole of dithiothreitol (Cleland's reagent) (DTT) in 0.1 ml was added and after 5 min the following components were added; tris buffer, pH 7.5, 100 μmoles; ${}^{14}CH_3\text{-}S\text{-}AM$, 2 m$\mu$moles and 0.1 ml of purified PNMT. (A PNMT preparation purified by chromatography on Sephadex G-100 column was used: see Section V,E.). The reaction mixture was incubated for 30 min at 37°C. The incubation was stopped by the addition of borate buffer, pH 10.5 (500 μmoles). The ${}^{14}C\text{-}N$-methylated octopamine was extracted into a mixture of toluene–isoamyl alcohol (3:2) as previously described (Axelrod, 1962). An aliquot of the organic phase was transferred into a counting vial and the radioactivity was determined. A sample of boiled enzyme preparation served as blank.

5. Determination of Dopamine-β-Hydroxylase Activity in Tissues

The same procedure as described for serum was used for the determination of DβH activity in tissues. Tissues were homogenized in 30 volumes of 0.05 M tris buffer, pH 6.8, containing 0.1% Triton X-100. The homogenate was centrifuged at 27,000 g for 20 min at 0°C. Aliquots of the supernatant were used for enzyme activity and for protein determination. When the DβH activity in the homogenates of some tissues was too low, the enzyme in the supernatant was concentrated by precipitation with 80% $(NH_4)_2$ SO_4. The precipitant was collected on Millipore filter and dissolved in a minimum volume of 0.05 M tris buffer, pH 6.8 (20–30 mg of protein per milliliter). The dissolved protein was dialyzed against 0.15 M acetate buffer, pH 5.5, and the volume adjusted to contain 20 gm of protein per milliliter. Aliquots of these preparations were used for determination of enzyme activity and protein as described in the previous section.

E. Phenylethanolamine N-Methyltransferase

(S-Adenosyl methionine: phenylethanolamine N-methyltransferase)

The enzyme phenylethanolamine N-methyltransferase (PNMT) catalyzes the last step in the catecholamine biosynthesis, namely, the Nmethylation of norepinephrine to epinephrine. The enzyme is present mainly in the adrenal glands but the presence of enzymic activity in the brain was also reported (Axelrod, 1962; Pohorecky et al., 1969).

The N-methylation of norepinephrine to epinephrine was first described by Bulbring (1949) in incubations of adrenal glands with ATP. Kishner and and Goodal (1957) have shown that the reaction occurs in the soluble fraction of homogenates obtained from adrenal glands and requires S-adenosylmethionine as a methyl donor. The enzyme was partially purified from adrenal glands of monkeys and its distribution as well as the substrate specificity was studied (Axelrod, 1962). It was reported that the enzyme shows an absolute specificity toward phenylethanolamine derivatives, but recent studies have shown that phenylethylamines can also serve as substrates for the enzyme (Goldstein and Joh, unpublished data). The reactions catalyzed by the enzyme are formulated in Reaction (6).

$$RCHR'CH_2NH_2 \longrightarrow RCHR'CH_2NHCH_3 \rightleftharpoons RCHR'CH_2N(CH_3)_2 \quad (6)$$

$$R' = OH \text{ or } H$$

The enzyme catalyzes the N-methylation of secondary phenylethanolamines (Axelrod, 1960; Goldstein and Joh, 1971). The secondary phenyl-ethanolamines have a low affinity for the enzyme (high K_m) and the pH optimum of the enzymic reaction differs when phenylethylamines, primary or secondary phenylethanolamines are used as substrates (Goldstein and Joh, 1971).

1. Purification of PNMT

The enzyme was partially purified from adrenal glands by $(NH_4)_2$ SO_4 fractionation and calcium gel adsorption (Axelrod, 1962). More recently the enzyme was obtained in almost pure form following purification by similar procedures used independently in two laboratories (Connet and Kirshner, 1970; Goldstein and Joh, 1970). The purification procedure as described by Goldstein and Joh (1970) is summarized in Table III. During the purification procedure it became apparent that the enzyme was unstable and that the addition of dithiothreitol resulted in a stabilization of enzyme activity.

2. Methods for Assay of PNMT Activity

The most common assay depends on the transfer of the methyl group from $^{14}CH_3$-S-AM to the nitrogen of a phenylethanolamine derivative to form a ^{14}C-N-methylated product (Axelrod, 1962). The enzymically formed product is then separated from unreacted $^{14}CH_3$-S-AM by extraction into an organic solvent. When normetanephrine or other phenylethanolamine derivatives were used as substrates, the ^{14}C-N-methylated products were

Table III.   Purification of Supernatant PNMT from Bovine Adrenal Medulla[a]

Purification step	Total protein (mg)	Total activity (units × 10)	Specific activity (units/mg protein × 10)	Purification (-fold)
$(NH_4)_2$ SO_4, 80%	2,980	13,500	4.5	0
$(NH_4)_2$ SO_4, 35–55%	450	7,880	17.5	3.9
Sephadex G-100				
Fraction 1	270	5,400	20.0	4.4
Fraction 2	76	3,200	42.3	9.4
pH 5.5 Supernatant	60.5	3,500	58.0	12.9
CM-Cellulose				
Fraction 1	26.4	2,196	83.2	18.5
Fraction 2	6.0	900	151.5	33.7
DEAE-Sephadex A-50	7.3	2,392	327.7	81.7

[a] The enzyme activities were tested in incubation mixtures at pH 7.9 using phenylethanolamine as substrate. The reaction mixtures were incubated for 15 min. A unit of enzyme activity is defined as mμmole of product formed per hour.

extracted into a mixture of toluene–isoamyl alcohol at pH 10, and the radioactivity in the solvent was measured after the addition of phosphor. When catechols were used as substrates (e.g., norepinephrine), the *N*-methylated products were extracted into *n*-butanol from NaCl-saturated solution which was acidified with HCl (Axelrod, 1962).

Another procedure for determination of PNMT activity is based on the precipitation of $^{14}CH_3$-*S*-AM with reineckate solution. The ^{14}C-*N*-methylated enzymic formed product is then measured in the supernatant (Fuller and Hunt, 1966). This procedure appears to be sensitive and specific for determining PNMT activity with norepinephrine as a substrate.

3. Properties of the Purified Enzyme

The molecular weight of purified PNMT was determined by the sucrose gradient density centrifugation method as described by Martin and Ames (1961) and a value of 38,000 was obtained (Connet and Kirshner, 1970). the sedimentation coefficient from the purified PNMT was found to be 3.9 S and a molecular weight of 38,000–40,000 was obtained by the Yphantis (1964) meniscus depletion method (Goldstein and Joh, 1971). Electrophoresis of the enzyme on a sodium dodecyl sulfate polyacrylamide gel gave one major protein band which represents 90% of the total protein. The molecular weight was also determined by disc gel electrophoresis in the presence of sodium dodecyl sulfate and a value of 38,000–40,000 was calculated (Goldstein and Joh, unpublished data).

In the standard polyacrylamide gel electrophoresis system the PNMT activity is associated with two major bands and with several minor bands (Fig. 6). The electrophoretic pattern suggests that the different PNMT bands represent conformational isozymes (Market and Whitt, 1968). Evidence has been presented that a glucocorticoid inducible form of PNMT is present in adrenal glands of mammals while an uninducible form of the enzyme is present in the frog (Wurtman *et al.,* 1968). It is conceivable that both forms might be present in the same species and studies are now in progress to determine whether some of the protein bands separated on the electrophoresis represent the two different forms of the enzyme.

III. CELLULAR LOCALIZATION OF ENZYMES INVOLVED IN CATECHOLAMINE BIOSYNTHESIS

The studies with hisotchemical fluorescence method for the determination of catecholamines and 5-HT in central nervous system have not only contributed to the mapping out of new specific neuronal systems but also markedly increased our knowledge on specific CNS functions. Further

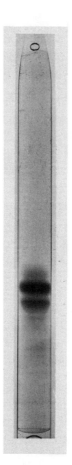

Fig. 6. Photograph of polyacrylamide gel electrophoresis of purified PNMT.

mapping of specific neuronal systems and better understanding of neurotran-
smitter functions might be achieved by immunohistochemical localization
of enzymes involved in catecholamine biosynthesis. Cellular localization
of the synthetic enzymes involved in catecholamine biosynthesis can provide
some new information which may not be obtainable by direct staining of
catecholamines in the tissues (Hillarp *et al.*, 1966). Antibodies to DβH were
prepared by Gibb *et al.* (1967) and subsequently the subcellular localization
of DβH in various tissues was reported with the use of immunohistochemical procedures (Geffen *et al.*, 1969; Udenfriend *et. al.* 1970; Fuxe
et al., 1970). More recently, antibodies toward PNMT and dopa decarboxylase were prepared (Goldstein and Joh, unpublished data; Goldstein and
Ceasar, unpublished data).

A. Cellular Localization of Dopamine-β-Hydroxylase

1. Preparation of Antibody

The enzyme DβH was purified as described in the previous section. As a final step in purification, the enzyme was subjected to disc gel electrophoresis and the segments containing pure enzyme were combined from several tubes and homogenized in 2 ml of saline and 2 ml of complete Freund's adjuvant (Hartman and Udenfriend, 1970). Aliquots of the homogenate were then injected subcutaneously and each rabbit received 0.4 mg of protein. The dose was repeated every 2 weeks for 6–8 weeks. Immunoglobulin was precipitated from the serum at 50% saturation with $(NH_4)_2SO_4$ and further purified on DEAE cellulose (Fahey, 1962; Kochwa et al., 1961). Immunoelectrophoresis of the DβH antibody showed only one line against the purified enzyme (Fig. 7).

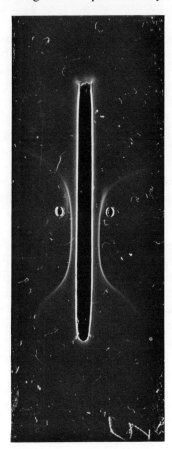

Fig. 7. Immunoelectrophoretic pattern between DβH and antiserum.

2. Histochemical Localization of DβH in Various Tissues

Since the antibody to bovine DβH cross reacts with the enzyme derived from the adrenals of other species (Gibb *et al.,* 1967), it was possible to use the antibody for fluorescent studies in tissues of other species. The immuno-fluorescent procedure has been described (Geffen *et. al.,* 1969; Hartman and Udenfriend, 1970; Fuxe *et al.,* 1970). It was demonstrated with immuno-histochemical techniques that DβH is present in peripheral adrenergic nerve cells and in adrenal medullary cells. The localization of DβH in various tissues was studied by Fuxe *et al.* (1970) and the preliminary results obtained by these authors are summarized as follows:

a. Rat Adrenal Gland. Most of the adrenal medullary cells showed a relatively weak green fluorescence and a few exhibited no specific fluore-scence at all. Several islands of adrenal medullary cells (10–20% of total population) exhibited a strong specific green fluorescence (Fig. 8). In view of these results, the adrenal medullary cells are probably heterogeneous with regard to their content of DβH. It may be that the strongly fluorescent cells represent the norepinephrine cells which are present in small numbers and also are found in islands of similar morphology (Hillarp and Hökfelt, 1953, 1955; Eränkö, 1951).

No specific fluorescence was found in the cells of the adrenal cortex.

b. Rat Superior Cervical Ganglion. The cytoplasm of the vast majority of the norepinephrine ganglion cells contained specific green immuno-fluorescence (Fig. 9). The brightness of fluorescence varied from weak to strong, and the fluorescence was localized diffusely throughout the cyto-plasm. No specific fluorescence was found in axon terminals or nonterminal axons, nor in the primitive catecholamine storing system of these ganglia which consists of small cells containing large concentrations of catechola-mines (Norberg *et al.,* 1966).

These results indicate that the DβH contents of norepinephrine ganglion cells vary considerably, which is true also for their contents of norepine-phrine (Norberg and Hamberger, 1964). However, the norepinephrine is mainly localized to the periphery of the norepinephrine cells whereas the DβH is evenly distributed throughout the cytoplasm. It is possible that some norepinephrine storage granules do not contain DβH which has been shown to be localized in amine storage particles.

In view of the probable lack of DβH in the primitive catecholamine cells, these cells probably store dopamine and not norepinephrine.

c. Rat Sciatic Nerve. Nerve fibers containing specific immunofluore-scence could only be identified following ligation of the nerve. Twenty four hours following operation, a strong immunofluorescence was observed immediately cranial to the ligation in nerve fibers with the same distribution

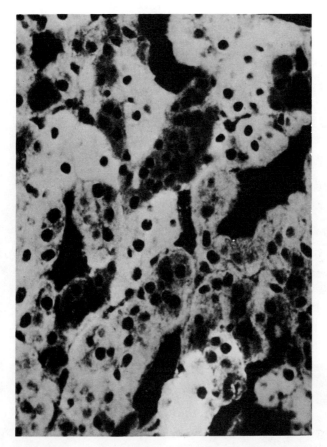

Fig. 8. DβH immunofluorescence of rat adrenal medulla (×200).

and appearance as norepinephrine fibers have following such ligations (Dahlström and Fuxe, 1964a; Dahlström, 1965). Increased reaction to antisera against DβH has also been found by Geffen et al. (1969) cranial to a ligation and increased DβH activity has been measured biochemically above a ligation by Laduron and Belpaire (1968). All these results are in accordance with the view that DβH may mainly be localized in the large granular vesicles, since high amounts of such vesicles are found in transected adrenergic fibers (Kapeller and Mayor, 1967; Geffen and Ostberg, 1969; Hökfelt and Dahlström, 1970). The accumulation of norepinephrine and DβH above a transection is therefore probably the result of interruption of the axonal flow of large granular amine vesicles which are synthesized in the cell bodies and transported down to the terminals.

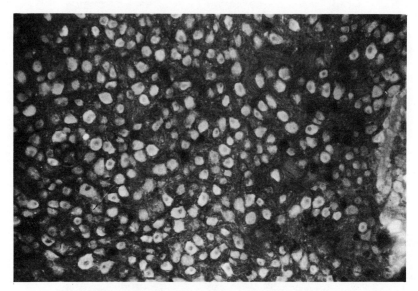

Fig. 9. DβH immunofluorescence of rat superior cervical ganglion.

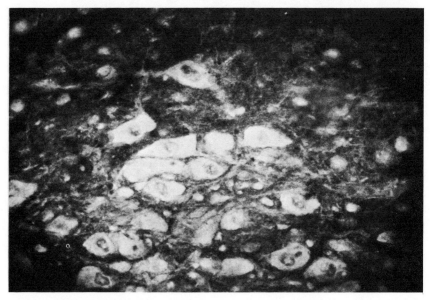

Fig. 10. DβH immunofluorescence in the nerve cells of the locus coeruleus.

d. Rat Central Nervous System. Specific immunofluorescence was only found in the catecholamine-containing cell bodies of the pons and medulla oblongata (Fig.10). These catecholamine cell bodies consititue the catecholamine cell groups A1-A2 and A4-A7 of Dahlström and Fuxe (1964b). They are localized mainly to the reticular formation and A6 is practically identical with locus coeruleus. These results show that the norepinephrine cell bodies are exclusively located in the pons and the medulla oblongata.

No specific fluorescence was observed in the dopamine cell bodies of the mesencephalon and hypothalamus and in the 5-HT cell bodies.

No specific immunofluorescence was observed in the norepinephrine pathways unless stereotaxic lesions had been made. When the lesion was placed in the ascending catecholamine bundles from the pons and the medulla oblongata on the border between pons and mesencephalon, strong specific immunofluorescence was observed in the catecholamine fibers close to the lesion on the cell body side. These results demonstrate that the ascending catecholamine bundles from the pons and the medulla oblongata are norepinephrine bundles. After a corresponding lesion of the nigroneostriatal dopamine pathway, no specific immunofluorescence was observed in the dopamine fibers on the cell body side of the lesion. However, it is known that

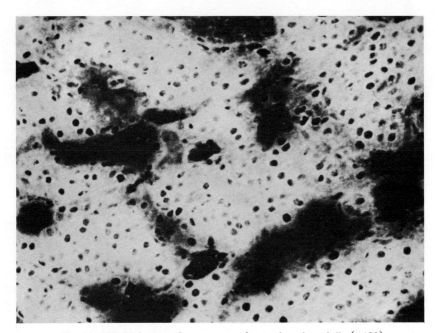

Fig. 11. PNMT immunofluorescence of rat adrenal medulla ($\times 120$).

dopamine does accumulate in these fibers (Anden *et. al.,* 1964, 1965). Thus the negative results indicate the absence of DβH in these fibers.

3. Histochemical Localization of PNMT and AADC in Various Tissues

PNMT and AADC were purified as described in the previous sections, and the antibodies were produced in a similar manner as described for DβH.

Figure 11 shows the immunofluorescence of PNMT in the rat adrenal gland. In contrast to the DβH reaction in which the fluorescent islands were sharply defined, the immunofluorescence developed in the cells in the PNMT reaction showed indistinct borders and the cell islands appeared indistinct. PNMT is a cytoplasmic enzyme (Axelrod, 1962) and perhaps therefore the cell islands appear indistinct, while DβH is a particulate enzyme and the immunofluorescence appears distinct in cell islands.

AADC was localized in the catecholamine-containing cells of the adrenal glands. In the rat kidneys AADC is localized in the proximal and distal tubuli. Figure 12 shows AADC immunofluorescence in the substantia nigra of rats. The fluorescence is localized in the cytoplasm of the cell bodies and no fluorescence is visible in the nuclei. The localization of these immunofluorescent cell bodies corresponds to the catecholamine-containing cells.

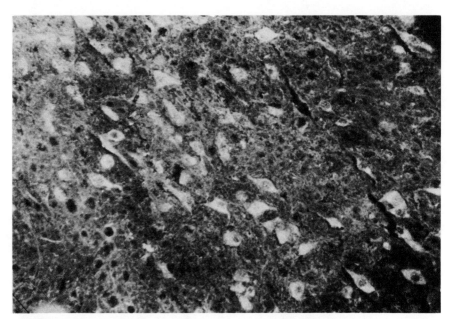

Fig. 12. AADC immunofluorescence in the cell bodies of the substantia nigra obtained from a rat (× 400)·

Studies on the localization of PNMT and AADC in different tissues are now in progress (Fuxe *et al.*, unpublished data).

REFERENCES

Anden, N.-E., Carlsson, A., Dahlström, A., Fuxe, K., Hillarp, N.-A., and Larsson, K. (1964) *Life Sci.* 3, 523.
Anden, N.-E., Dahlström, A., Fuxe, K., and Larsson, K. (1965) *Amer. J. Anat.* 116, 329.
Aures, D., Hakanson, R., and Clark, W. G. (1970) in *Handbook of Neurochemistry,* Vol. 4 (Abel Lajtha, ed.), New York, Plenum Press, pp. 165–196.
Axelrod, J. (1960) *Biochim. Biophys. Acta* 45, 614.
Axelrod, J. (1962) *J. Biol. Chem.* 237, No. 5, 1657.
Blaschko, H. (1939) *J. Physiol.* 96, 50 P.
Blumberg, W. E., Goldstein, M., Lauber, E., and Peisach, J. (1965) *Biochim. Biophys. Acta* 99, 188.
Bonnay, M., Troll, W., and Goldstein, M. (1970) *Fed. Proc.* 29, No. 2, 278.
Bulbring, E. (1949) *Brit. J. Pharmacol.* 4, 234.
Ceasar, P. M., Anagnoste, B. F., and Goldstein, M. (1970) 160th National Meeting American Chemical Society, Abstract No. 102.
Christenson, J. G., Dairman, W. M., and Udenfriend, S. (1970) *Fed. Proc.* 29, No. 2, 867.
Connett, R. J., and Kirshner, N. (1970) *J. Biol. Chem.* 245, No. 2, 329.
Creveling, C. R., Daly, J. W., Witkop, B., and Udenfriend, S. (1962) *Biochim. Biophys. Acta* 64, 125.
Dahlström, A. (1965) *J. Anat.* 99, 677.
Dahlström, A., and Fuxe, K. (1964a) *Z. Zellforsch.* 63, 602.
Dahlström, A., and Fuxe, K. (1964b) *Acta Physiol. Scand.* 62, Suppl. 232, 1.
Duch, D. S., Viveros, O. H., and Kirshner, N. (1968) *Biochem. Pharmacol.* 17, 255.
Eränkö, O. (1951) *Acta Physiol. Scand.* 25, Suppl. 89, 22.
Fahey, J. L. (1962) *J. Biol. Chem.* 237, 440.
Fischer, J. E., Musacchio, J. M., Kopin, I. J., and Axelrod, J. (1964) *Life Sci.* 3, 413.
Frenkel, R., Backstrom, T., Anagnoste, B., and Goldstein, M. (1971) *Pharmacologist* 13, No. 2, 253.
Friedman, S., and Kaufman, S. (1965) *J. Biol. Chem.* 240, 552.
Fuller, R. W., and Hunt, J. M. (1966) *Analyt. Biochem.* 16, No. 2, 349.
Fuxe, K., Goldstein, M., Hökfelt, T., and Joh, T. H. (1971) in *Progress in Brain Research* (O. Eranko, ed.), Vol. 34, Elsevier Publishing Company, Amsterdam, pp. 127–138.
Geffen, L. B., Livett, B. G., and Rush, R. A. (1969) *J. Physiol.*, 204, 593.
Geffen, L. B., and Ostberg, A. (1969) *J. Physiol.* 204, 583.
Gibb, J. W., Spector, S., and Udenfriend, S. (1967) *Mol. Pharmacol.* 3, 473.
Goldstein, M., Anagnoste, B., Battista, A. F., Owen, W. S., and Nakatani, S. (1969) *J. Neurochem.* 16, 645.
Goldstein, M., Anagnoste, B., Ceasar, P. M., Battista, A. F., Nakatani, S., and Ogawa, M. (1972) in *Association for Research in Nervous and Mental Disease* (I. J. Kopin, ed.), Vol. 50, Chapter 21, The Williams and Wilkins Co., Baltimore.
Goldstein, M., Anagnoste, B., Lauber, E., and McKereghan, M. R. (1964) *Life Sci.* 3, 763.
Goldstein, M., and Contrera, J. F. (1961) *J. Biol. Chem.* 237, 1898.
Goldstein, M., Friedhoff, A. J., and Simmons, C. (1959) *Experientia,* XV/2, 80.
Goldstein, M., Freedman, L. S., and Bonnay, M. (1971) *Experientia* 27, 632.
Goldstein, M., and Joh, T. H. (1970) *Fed. Proc.* 29, No. 2, 278.
Goldstein, M. and Joh, T. H., (1971) to be published.
Goldstein, M., Joh, T. H., and Garvey, III, T. Q. (1968) *Biochemistry* 7, 2724.
Goldstein, M., Lauber, E., and McKereghan, M. R. (1965) *J. Biol. Chem.* 240, 2066.

Goodall, McC., and Kirshner, N. (1957) *J. Biol. Chem.* **226**, 213.
Hagen, P. (1956) *J. Pharmacol.* **116**, 26.
Hakanson, R., and Owman, C. (1965) *J. Neurochem.* **12**, 417.
Hartman, B. K., and Udenfriend, S. (1970) *Mol. Pharmacol.* **6**, 85.
Hayaishi, O. (1964) in *Oxygenases,* Sixth International Congress of Biochemistry, Proc. Plenary Sessions, New York, pp. 31–43.
Hillarp, N. -A, Fuxe, K., and Dahlström, A. (1966) *Phramacol. Rev.* **18**, (1), 727.
Hillarp, N. -A, and Hökfelt, B. (1953) *Acta Physiol. Scand.* **30**, 55.
Hillarp, N. -A, and Hökfelt, B. (1955) *J. Histochem. Cytochem.* **3**, 1.
Hökfelt, T., and Dahlström, A. (1970) *Z. Zellforsch.* in press.
Holtz, P., Credner, K., and Koepp, W. (1942) *Arch. Exp. Path. Pharmak.* **200**, 356.
Ikeda, M., Levitt, M., and Udenfriend, S. (1957) *J. Lab. Clin. Med.* **50**, 733.
Ikeda, M., Fahien, L.A., and Udenfriend, S. (1966) *J. Biol. Chem* **241**, 4452.
Joh, T. H., and Goldstein, M. (1969) *American Chemical Society,* Article No. 231.
Joh, T. H., Kapit, R., and Goldstein, M. (1969) *Biochim. Biophys. Acta.* **171**, 378.
Kapeller, K., and Mayor, D. (1967) *Proc. Royal Soc. B.* **167**, 282.
Kaufman, S. (1958) *Biochim. Biophys. Acta.* **27**, 428.
Kirshner, N., and Goodall, McC. (1957) *Biochim. Biophys. Acta.* **24**, 658.
Kochwa, S., Rosenfield, R. E., Talal, L., and Wasserman, L. R. (1961) *J. Clin. Invest.* **40**, 874.
Laduron, P., and Belpaire, F. (1968) *Biochem. Pharmacol.* **17**, 1127.
Levin, E. Y., and Kaufman, S. (1961) *J. Biol. Chem.* **236**, 2043.
Levin, E. Y., Levenberg, B., and Kaufman, S. (1960) *J. Biol. Chem.* **235**, 2080.
Lovenberg, W., Weissbach, H., and Udenfriend, S. (1962) *J. Biol. Chem.* **237**, 89.
Markert, C. L., and Whitt, C. S. (1968) *Experientia* **24**, 977.
Martin, R. G., and Ames, B. N. (1961) *J. Biol. Chem.* **236**, 1372.
Mason, H. S. (1957) in *Advances in Enzymology,* Vol. 19 (F. F. Nord, ed.), New York, Interscience Publishers, Inc., pp. 79–233.
Molinoff, P. B., Weinshilboum, R., and Axelrod, J. (1970) *Fed. Proc.* **29**, No. 2, 278.
Musacchio, J. M. (1969) *Biochim. Biophys. Acta* **191**, 485.
Nagatsu, T., Kuzuya, H., and Hidaka, H. (1967) *Biochim. Biophys. Acta* **139**, 319.
Nagatsu, T., Levitt, M., and Udenfriend, S. (1964a) *J. Biol. Chem.* **239**, 2910.
Nagatsu, T., Levitt, M., and Udenfriend, S. (1964b) *Analyt. Biochem.* **9**, 122.
Nagatsu, T., Yamamoto, T., and Nagatsu, I. (1970) *Biochim. Biophys. Acta* **198**, 210.
Neri, R., Hagan, M., Stone, D., Dorfman, R. I., and Elmadjian, F. (1956) *Arch. Biochem.* **60**, 297.
Norberg, K.-A., Ritzen, M., and Ungerstedt, U. (1966) *Acta Physiol. Scand.* **67**, 260.
Petrack, B., Fetzer, V., Sheppy, F., and Manning, T. (1970) *Fed. Proc.* **29**, No. 2, 277.
Petrack, B., Sheppy, F., and Fetzer, V. (1968) *J. Biol. Chem.* **243**, 743.
Pisano, J. J., Creveling, C. R., and Udenfriend, S. (1960) *Biochim. Biophys. Acta* **43**, 566.
Pohoreckey, L. A., Zigmond, M. J., Heimer, L., and Wurtman, R. J. (1969) *Fed. Proc.* **28**, No. 2, 295.
Sedvall, G. C., and Kopin, I. J. (1967) *Biochem. Pharmacol.* **16**, 39.
Shiman, R., Akino, M., and Kaufmann, S. (1971) *J. Biol. Chem.* **246**, 1330.
Sourkes, T. L. (1966) *Pharmacol. Rev.* **18**, No. 1, 53.
Vogel, W. H., McFarland, H., and Prince, L. N. (1970) *Biochem. Pharmacol.* **19**, 618.
Von Euler, U. S., and Flooding, I. (1955) *Acta Physiol. Scand.* **33**, 45.
Wurzburger, R. J., D'Angelo, G. L., and Musacchio, J. M. (1970) *Fed. Proc.* **29**, No. 2, 277.
Yphantis, D. A. (1964) *Biochemistry* **3**, 297.

Chapter 14

Detection and Quantitative Analysis of Some Noncatecholic Primary Aromatic Amines

Alan A. Boulton

Psychiatric Research Unit, University Hospital
Saskatoon, Saskatchewan, Canada

and John R. Majer

Department of Chemistry, University of Birmingham
Edgbaston, Birmingham, England

I. INTRODUCTION

The extensive literature on the catecholamines and 5-hydroxytryptamine has arisen not just because of their physiological importance but also, to some extent, because of the availability of adequate methods for their detection. As a result of this and continuing efforts to improve the specificity, accuracy, and reproducibility of the available methods, we now possess considerable data on the presence and distribution of these monoamines in the brain and other organs and tissues of a wide variety of species. It is known that they are not uniformly distributed within the brain but are concentrated in certain regions; furthermore, we know that within the neuron they are to be found in varicosities present in the cell processes in both the bound and unbound forms. The elegant fluorimetric histological studies of the Swedish groups have allowed a precise mapping within the brain of certain of the noradrenergic, dopaminergic, and serotoninergic fibers.

Despite many indications that other non-catecholic primary aromatic amines (such as *p*-tyramine, octopamine, phenylethylamine, tryptamine) are of interest in certain psychiatric and neurological disease states (Boulton, 1967; Boulton and Milward, 1971; Boulton, Pollitt, and Majer, 1967;

Fisher, 1968; Oates *et al.,* 1963; Pscheidt *et al.,* 1966), in behavior (see Faubye, 1968) and in aspects of physiology, no extensive knowledge of their location or distribution exists. The reason for this is essentially because these particular amines have not been considered to be as important as the catecholamines and adequate methodology, at the sensitivity levels required, did not exist.

Such studies as there have been on the identification and quantitation of these amines to date have not been very revealing. In many cases the procedures used lacked the specificity required for claims of identification to be substantiated. Spector *et al.* (1963) using the fluorophore produced in solution from 1-nitroso-2-naphthol claimed that *p*-tyramine existed in rat brain at a concentration level of about 2 μg/g. Boulton and Quan (1969) and Quan (1970) were unable to confirm this using the same fluorophore by a more specific procedure based on chromatographic separations. Gunne and Jonsson (1965) were unable to find any *p*-tyramine in a cat brain using an ion-exchange procedure; they concluded that if *p*-tyramine was present at all it must be at a concentration level of less than 10 ng/g. Kakimoto and Armstrong (1962a, b) demonstrated, in a variety of chromatographic solvent systems, a spot isographic with *p*-tyramine in tissue extracts obtained from animals that had been treated with a monoamine oxidase inhibitor. Asatoor (1968) found labeled *p*-tyramine after a subcutaneous injection of ^{14}C-labeled tyrosine in rats. In a repeat of this experiment using tritiated tyrosine, Hempel and Männl (1966) could not find any labeled tyramine. Such studies can therefore only be interpreted as being perhaps indicative of the presence of tyramine in mammalian tissues. Following an intraventricular injection of labeled *p*-tyramine, Goldstein's group (1967, 1970) showed that the *p*-tyramine was distributed with the highest concentration in the hypothalamus and the caudate nucleus respectively. This group also demonstrated, by chromatographic means, the conversion of the *p*-tyramine to octopamine and *p*-hydroxyphenylacetic acid.

Kakimoto and Armstrong (1962b) have identified octopamine in urine and tissue extracts. Many groups have shown that *p*-tyramine may be hydroxylated *in vivo* in the side chain in a fashion analogous to dopamine $\longrightarrow$ noradrenaline. Molinoff and Axelrod (1969) have recently described an enzymological assay based on the transfer of the methyl group of ^{14}C-labeled S-adenosyl methionine to the nitrogen of octopamine. They estimated the level of octopamine in rat brain to be 2.4 ng/g.

Phenylethylamine does not appear to have been studied much at all. It has been identified in urine (Oates *et al.,* 1963) and is claimed to be increased in phenylketonuria and either reduced or nonexistent in urine taken from patients suffering with depression (Boulton and Milward, 1971; Fisher, 1968).

More is known of tryptamine but until recently most of the quantitative work was based on the measurement of natural or a derived fluorescence as present after organic solvent extraction (Udenfriend, 1962). Although it has been known for some time that tryptamine will condense with formaldehyde and other similar aldehydes (Bell and Somerville, 1966; Boulton, 1968; Procházka, 1958; Seiler and Weichmann, 1964; Seiler *et al.*, 1963), producing intense fluorophores, the technique has not been widely used. In our own experience, using urine extracts, we observed that there are numerous substances that are capable of forming these fluorophores; the separation and quantitation of the tryptamine fluorophore produced by formaldehyde was not possible. Björklund and Falck (1969) using fluorophore condensation *in situ* have recently demonstrated the histochemical localization of a tryptaminelike substance in the mammalian adenohypophysis.

II. CHROMATOGRAPHIC TECHNIQUES

In order to have confidence in the detection and quantitative determination of a particular metabolite suspected to be present in minute quantities in a tissue or biological fluid extract, by chromatographic means alone, it is necessary first to produce a chromogen or fluorogen (preferably exhibiting some specificity) which exists and can be quantitated at concentrations below those at which the metabolite in question is suspected to exist. Next it is necessary to demonstrate isographic behavior between a synthetic sample of the suspected metabolite and the substance in question in many different solvent systems. Metabolites existing in the brain are usually present in such small quantities that only by using their natural fluorescence or by converting to fluorescent derivatives will the required sensitivity be achieved. For those substances possessing a reactive hydroxyl, phenolic, amino, or sulfydryl group it is possible to use the DNS reagent* first introduced by Weber (1952) but elegantly exploited by Gray and Hartley (1963) (see also recent reviews by Boulton, 1968, 1969; Seiler, 1970; Seiler and Wiechman, 1970.

In our experience it has proved difficult to obtain satisfactory results with substances possessing multireactive groups (such as the catecholamines) or from the dansylation of complex extracts without some further fractionation or purification. Isolation of a group of substances by organic solvent extraction and ion exchange or absorption column chromatography followed by separation of the specific metabolite of interets on paper or thin layer chromatograms before dansylation is to be preferred. Even in these cases numerous fluorescent derivatives are formed which must arise from impurities

---

* DNS = Dansyl = 1-Dimethylaminoaphthalene-5-sulfonyl derivative.

in the chromatographic medium and/or from contaminants in the solvents used (see Figs. 1 and 2).

Crowshaw *et al.* (1967) used the dansyl reagent to investigate the amino acids present in a superfusate of the cat cerebral cortex; they located 21 different amino acids and attempted a semiquantitative assessment of the amounts present. Because of nonreproducible losses occurring during the dansylation of certain amino acids when they are present in a mixture (Boulton, 1971; Neadle and Pollitt, 1965) it is unlikely that this technique can be made quantitative. Simple amines are much superior to the ampholytes in this respect and reproducible data may be obtained.

We describe below a detailed procedure for the analysis of *p*-tyramine in rat brain. Preliminary details have been published (Boulton and Majer, 1970; Boulton and Quan, 1969; Majer and Boulton, 1970). Slight modifications of this procedure, obtained on the basis of trial and error, will allow the analysis of other suitably reactive metabolites.

A. Materials, Methods, and Results

The DNS reagent and *ortho* and *para* tyramine are available from Calbiochem, Los Angeles, California. In our work crystalline bis-DNS *para*-tyramine was donated by Dr. Nikolaus Seiler (Frankfurt); *meta* tyramine was kindly provided by Dr. J. B. Jepson (London) and Dr. P. Smith (Farmborough). Pen-bred male Wistar rats as supplied by the Medical Research Annex of the University of Saskatchewan were used as the source of brain tissue.

Rats are stunned, decapitated, and the heads chilled in an ice-salt freezing mixture. Whole brains or certain dissected areas are washed in ice-cold saline solution, blotted, weighed and homogenized (motor-driven Teflon-glass homogenizer; clearance, 0.10–0.15 mm on the radius) in 10 ml of 0.4 N HClO$_4$ solution. In order to determine the recovery of amine through the overall procedure, *p*-tyramine free base (usually 1 μg) is added at this stage. The homogenate, maintained at 4 °C, is centrifuged at 10,000 g for 20 min. After centrifugation the supernatant is adjusted to pH 5–6 with 1 M-NaOH and the phenolicamine fraction (Kakimoto and Armstrong, 1962a) isolated by percolating the extract through a column (1 × 2.5 cm) of Biorad AG50W-X2 resin (H$^+$ form) and washing sequentially with 5 ml of distilled water, 10 ml of 0.1 M sodium acetate and 5 ml of water. The phenolicamines are then eluted with 5 ml 1 M NH$_4$OH in 65 % ethanol into a 50-ml round-bottomed flask, evaporated to dryness under reduced pressure in a rotary evaporator, dissolved in 500 μl of 70 % ethanol, transferred to a 5-ml conical flask, re-evaporated to dryness and then triturated in 100 μl of 70 % ethanol. This whole extract is then quantitatively transferred to a strip of Whatman No. 2

paper and developed by the descending technique overnight (14 hr), in the solvent system, *n*-butanol–acetic acid–water, 4:1:1 (v/v). Synthetic *para* tyramine (5 μg) is spotted on two additional strips and run on either side of the brain extract or series of extracts in the same tank. The *p*-tyramine zones on the brain extract chromatograms are located by comparison with the two marker chromatograms following visualization of these two chromatograms with ninhydrin reagent according to the procedure described by Smith (1969). The *p*-tyramine zones are then excised from the stips, cut into small pieces, and shaken in stoppered tubes with 5 ml of 90% methanol for 30 min at room temperature. After centrifugation the methanol supernatants are removed and rotary evaporated to dryness. A control extract is obtained by subjecting a blank chromatogram to the whole process. The extracted paper residues are then reextracted by shaking for 5 min with 90% methanol and the extract and washings, in 25-ml round-bottomed flasks, evaporated to dryness on the rotary evaporator. These dried methanolic eluates are then transferred to 5-ml tubes with 100 μl of 0.1 M-NaHCO$_3$; 100 μl dansyl reagent, 1 mg DNS chloride in 1 ml acetone, added, shaken, stoppered, and left overnight at room temperature. Next morning 0.8 ml of acetone is added and after shaking, the precipitated NHCO$_3$ removed by centrifugation. The supernatants are placed into 5-ml round-bottomed flasks, evaporated to dryness and dissolved in 100 μl of benzene–glacial acetic acid, 99:1 (v/v).

These DNS reaction products from whole brain and/or brain areas, sometimes supplemented with *para* tyramine, and the control are then streaked (about 5 cm) onto a layer of silica gel (Eastman 6061). DNS *para* tyramine obtained by dansylating a *para* tyramine eluate from a paper chromatogram is run alongside as marker. Development is in chloroform–*n*-butyl acetate, 5:1 (v/v) for 1.5 hr at room temperature. On removal from the system the plates are allowed to dry in air until the excess solvent has evaporated (30–60 sec) and then sprayed with triethanolamine–isopropanol, 1:4 (v/v) to stabilize the fluorescence (Seiler and Wiechmann, 1966). The thin layer sheets are dried in air for 1 hr and then inspected in ultraviolet light (365 nm) and the fluorescent zones delineated in pencil. The zones corresponding to the maximum fluorophore from the DNS *para* tyramine marker are scraped off the plate, the gel placed in stoppered tubes and eluted during 15 min at room temperature, with 2 ml of benzene–acetic acid, 99:1 (v/v). After centrifugation the supernatant is transferred to a 5-ml conical flask, rotary evaporated to dryness, and then dissolved in 100 μl of benzene–acetic acid, 99:1 (v/v). This DNS *p*-tyramine zone extract is then reapplied as a streak (about 5 cm) to a further silica gel thin-layer chromatogram (Eastman 6061) and developed in the solvent system-ethyl acetate–cyclohexane, 2:3 (v/v). After initial air drying the plates are sprayed with triethanolamine–isopropanol, 1:4 (v/v), dried completely and the DNS *para* tyramine zone (as assessed by comparing with

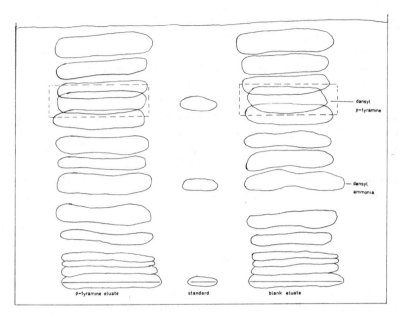

Fig. 1. Chromatographic separation of the dansyl reaction products in the solvent system chloroform–butyl acetate, 5:1 (v/v).

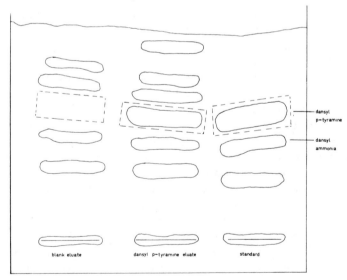

Fig. 2. Chromatographic separation of the dansyl *p*-tyramine zone eluate in the solvent system ethylacetate–cyclohexane, 2:3 (v/v).

the eluted qualitative DNS *para* tyramine marker run alongside, eluted with 2 ml of benzene–acetic acid, 99:1 (v/v). The amount of fluorescence in this final extract is measured in the Aminco Bowman spectrophoto-fluorimeter (activation 340 nm, emmission 510 nm).

Figures 1 and 2 illustrate the qualitative pattern of spots obtained following separation of the DNS reaction products obtained from the paper chromatogram eluate and the eluted DNS *p*-tyramine zone from the first thin-layer separation respectively. It can be seen that there are numerous fluorescent zones and that the paper chromatogram blank contributes most of them. The final DNS *p*-tyramine (Fig. 2) separation, however, appears to be complete and the brain DNS *p*-tyramine separated in this way is completely isographic with crystalline DNS *para* tyramine. As compared with crystalline DNS *p*-tyramine, the amount of fluorescence in the zone selected in these experiments represents a 70% conversion (see Fig. 3). A calibration curve for DNS *p*-tyramine is shown in Fig. 4. The minimum detectable quantity is approximately 5 ng but more than this is required for a satisfactory quantitative evaluation. The useful working range is 10^{-8} to 2×10^{-6} g with an error of $\pm 10.2\%$ (95% fiducial limits). The overall recovery of *p*-tyramine through the entire procedure is $56.1 \pm 8.1\%$ (mean $\pm$ mean deivation, $n = 4$). The total laboratory working time involves 3 days.

The values obtained for the amount of *p*-tyramine present in whole rat brain are given in Table I and the range of values for certain regions of the rat brain in Table II.

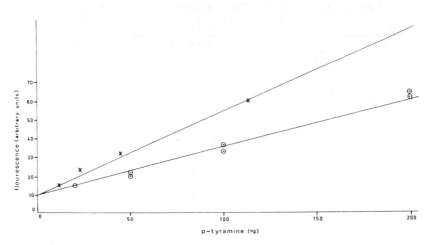

Fig. 3. Efficiency of the dansylation of *p*-tyramine. DNS *p*-tyramine zone eluted from thin-layer chromatogram in 90% methanol and the amount of fluorescence measured (activation 340 nm, emission 510 nm). ×, crystalline DNS *p*-tyramine; ⊙, DNS *p*-tyramine prepared from synthetic amine.

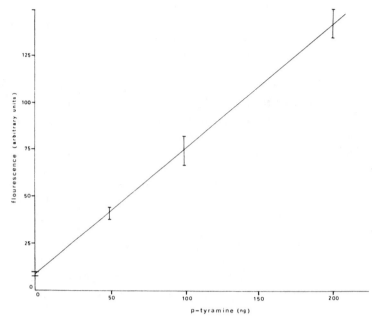

Fig. 4. Calibration curve for DNS *p*-tyramine.

Table I.   Concentration of *p*-Tyramine in Whole Rat Brain by the
DNS and I.I.C. Techniques[a]

	p-Tyramine (ng)	*p*-Tyramine (ng/g tissue)
DNS Technique (*n*=7)	365±35	192±24
I.I.C. Technique (*n*=9)	373±62.5	189±33

[a] Results are expressed as mean ± standard deviation.

Table II.   Regional Distribution of *p*-Tyramine in Rat Brain
DNS Technique

Brain region[a]	Weight (g)[b]	Total *p*-tyramine (ng)[c]	ng *p*-Tyramine/g issue[c]
Hypothalamus	0.072±0.010	104–282	1410–4270
Caudate	0.196±0.034	74–210	441–890
Cerebellum	0.554±0.054	95–204	203–368
Stem	0.553±0.056	20–275	38–456
"Rest"	2.51 ±0.090	92–260	39–104

[a] Regions from two rat brains pooled.
[b] Mean ± standard deviation.
[c] These values represent the range of results obtained in seven different experiments.

B. Comments

As mentioned in the introduction, it is very difficult positively to identify a substance by chromatographic means alone. The procedure described above for the analysis of *para* tyramine is time consuming and complicated. Although the results obtained seem quite good, at least with respect to the whole brain, an unambiguous identification is not achieved and it is a fact that the *meta* isomer of tyramine (Boulton and Quan, 1971), subjected to this procedure is eluted along with the *para* isomer. It is desirable and necessary, therefore, to utilize in addition to chromatography some other physicochemical method of identification. With a total yield of 206 ng (56 % of 365 ng; see Table I) for a single rat brain, this is not possible by conventional techniques (ultraviolet, visible, or infrared spectroscopy). This amount is, however, quite sufficient for a mass spectrometric analysis. Since the processes involved in the isolation of the DNS *p*-tyramine are based on several different chromatographic separations, it may be assumed that the final DNS *p*-tyramine eluate is not going to be contaminated by more than one or two alternatives. Because of this a qualitative mass spectrum as produced by a relatively small mass spectrometer would suffice to confirm the identity and in addition give an indication of the extent of contamination. Clearly, many different substances in brain and other tissues are amenable to analysis in this way and in fact the DNS methodology has already been used to separate and quantitate γ-amino butyric acid (Seiler and Weichman, 1968, 1969) and spermine and spermidine (Seiler and Weichmann, 1967). It could also be used to measure histamine. Under development in our laboratory at this time are procedures for the isolation and quantitative analysis of octopamine, tryptamine, and phenylethylamine. Although in the next section we describe a new technique of analysis based completely on the mass spectrometer, it is essential to have chromatographic and other techniques of analysis available since it is now desirable to investigate the metabolism of these noncatecholic amines using radioactive tracer techniques.

A possibility not yet explored but potentially of considerable significance in metabolic studies is the use of stable isotopes instead of radioactive ones. In such cases the mass spectrometer would give not only an unambiguous and quantitative assessment of the natural metabolite but data on the distribution, metabolism, and kinetics of the metabolic processes involving the metabolite of interest.

III. MASS SPECTROMETRY

Until recently most mass spectrometric analyses of metabolites of biological interest have been of a qualitative nature. Frequently the substance of interest has been separated by gas-liquid chromatography and the identity established by a fast scan in a single focusing mass spectrometer. More recently substances have been identified following their elution from chromatograms (Creveling, Kondo, and Daly, 1968; Knoche *et al.,* 1969; Seiler, 1971). A new method of considerable promise is the so-called "integrated ion current technique" (Boulton and Majer, 1970; Jenkins and Majer, 1967; Majer and Boulton, 1970). It has proved possible to identify a suspected metabolite in an extract by precise mass analysis using the molecule ion or one or more of the fragment ions and then to quantitate this ion by measuring the ion current during evaporation from the probe. The advantages accruing from such an analytical procedure are not just the unambiguity of analysis and the extreme sensitivity, but the fact that identification and quantitation may be achieved in a highly complex and/or contaminated extract. So far four different aromatic primary amines have been positively identified in a simple benzene extract of a rat brain homogenate and the quantitative distribution of *p*-tyramine has been established. The technique is not limited to any particular class of metabolites however, and it has been used positively to identify in brain or urine extracts the following substances: *p*-tyramine (Boulton and Majer, 1970; Majer and Boulton, 1970); phenylethylamine, tryptamine, octopamine (Boulton *et al.,* 1970), bufotenin, *p*-hydroxyphenylacetic acid (Boulton and Majer, 1971a) and kryptopyrrole (Irvine *et al.,* 1969).

In the conventional use of a mass spectrometer, a large reservoir of sample vapor is usually maintained at a constant low pressure while a very small fraction flows into the instrument through a constriction. The ion currents recorded during ionization of the sample are proportional to the partial pressures of the respective components of the mixture in the reservoir; the ratio between the partial pressure and the ion current at any particular m/e value may be regarded as being constant during the period of the recording. This does not apply for small amounts (nanogram quantities) of materials present in mixtures obtained from biological sources, since these materials usually possess low vapor pressures. In these cases an alternate procedure is to record the ion current at a significant m/e value as the sample in the solid state is evaporated from the probe which is inserted into the vacuum system and close to the ionizing beam. In this situation it is possible to relate the integrated ion current at the selected m/e value to the weight of pure material evaporated, and so calibrate the machine.

A. Materials, Methods, and Results

The MS-9 (Associated Electrical Industries Ltd., Manchester, U.K.) mass spectrometer was used in all the work reported here. The source of chemicals and the preparative procedures up to the supernatant obtained from the brain homogenates are the same as described in the previous section, except that the hypothalamus, caudate, cerebellum and stem, as dissected from the whole rat brain, were homogenized in 5-ml samples of 0.4 N HClO$_4$ in a smaller (5-ml) Teflon-glass homogenizer. The further treatment of the supernatant is related to the particular amine to be analyzed. In the case of p-tyramine, isolation of the phenolic amine fraction is as previously described except that 3 drops of 3 N HCl are added to the alcoholic solution at the time of transfer to the 5-ml round-bottomed flask. This treatment results in the formation of the hydrochloride salt which is useful for purposes of storage and transport. Organic solvent extraction may be used for the analysis of the other amines.

Prior to analysis the residue is described in 100 μl elthanol: ammonium hydroxide (28–30% NH$_3$) and 5μl samples of this solution are introduced into the tip of the direct insertion probe with the aid of a calibrated microsyringe. The probe tip consists of a Pyrex glass tube (length 27 mm, diameter 1 mm, internal dimensions); it is used in any series of measurements and then discarded. The probe is inserted through the vacuum lock into the vacuum system of the mass spectrometer so that the probe tip is in the cool part of the ion source region. During this stage the ethanolic ammonia evaporates, leaving the pure amine standard (now free base) or the constituents of the brain extracts (also as free amine) in the solid state on the probe tip. A measured pressure of heptacosa-fluoro-tri-n-butylamine (this acts as an internal standard with constant partial pressure and as a mass scale marker) is admitted to the gasinlet system. The reference peak is selected and displayed on the oscilloscope. The decadic resistance is then set to a value corresponding to the ratio of the ions responsible for the reference and characteristic mass peaks (for which an unambiguous atomic constitution has been assigned by precise mass analysis where necessary), and the peak switching system so adjusted that the oscilloscope gives an alternate display of the reference and characteristic peaks. At this stage in the analysis the characteristic peak does not appear. The galvanometer recorder is then set in operation so as to record only the one peak pair displayed on the oscilloscope. The probe tip is now lowered into the heated region of the ion source to allow evaporation of the sample. When evaporation beings the characteristic peak appears on the oscilloscope and is recorded. Evaporation is complete in 10–20 sec, depending upon the sample size and then the characteristic peak disappears from the oscilloscope and the recorder trace. The amount of sample evaporated is proportional to the integrated ion current at the characteristic peak, and therefore to the area enclosed under the envelope from the characteristic peak on the recorder trace. The most suitable ion to select as the characteristic peak is the molecule ion itself. For those molecules that do not exhibit a satisfactory mass peak at their molecular weight, an intense alternate peak at a high m/e value must be used. If two substances coevaporate and possess closely similar peaks, then the recorded ion current is additive; the possibility that two compounds will evaporate at the same temperature and provide almost identical ions is a slight one. In the event that coevaporation of two or more ions differing by only a few parts per million in their mass occurs, the high resolution mass spectrometer can record the ion currents produced as two separate peaks. Such an effect was observed for the molecule ion peak (m/e 137) and the base peak (m/e 108) of *para* tyramine in rat brain. If two or more ions cannot be separated even after searching among the fragmentation peaks then a suitable derivative could be prepared for one of them. This is, of course, likely to be necessary only on rare occasions.

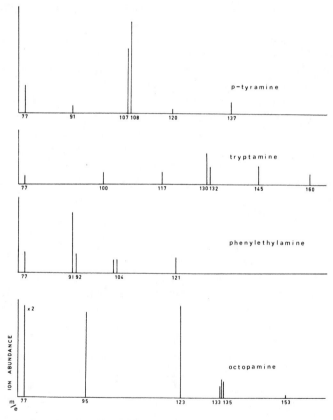

Fig. 5. Simplified monoisotopic mass spectra of *p*-tyramine, octopamine, phenylethylamine, and tryptamine.

Simplified monoisotopic mass spectra for p-tyramine, octopamine, tryptamine, and phenylethylamine are shown in Fig. 5. The following peaks are recommended for quantitative procedures: p-tyramine m/e 108 and 137; octopamine m/e 123; phenylethylamine m/e 121; tryptamine m/e 160. A record of the ion current m/e 137 during evaporation at 220°C of 1 ng of p-tyramine is shown in Fig. 6. This record is typical of the results obtained for all the amines analyzed.

Typical calibration curves for p-tyramine, octopamine, phenylethylamine, and tryptamine are shown in Fig. 7. The working range in our hands is 10^{-12} to 10^{-5} g with an error of $\pm$ 5.0% (95% fiducial limits). A complete analysis takes approximately 2 hr.

When brain extracts are analyzed for p-tyramine at both m/e 137 and m/e 108, the ion current record is as shown in Fig. 8. It is clear that this record is of two ions which overlap; they were shown by precise mass analysis to be, at m/e 137 $C_8H_{11}ON^+$ 137.0841 from p-tyramine and a hydrocarbon contaminant $C_{10}H_{17}^+$ 137.1330, at m/e 108 the ions were $C_7H_8O^+$ 108.0575 from p-tyramine and $C_8H_{12}^+$ 108.0939 from the hydrocarbon (Boulton and Majer, 1970, 1971b; Majer and Boulton, 1970). Quantitation of the p-tyramine portion of the curve provided the data listed in Tables I and III. As can be seen, there is agreement between the I.I.C. figures and values obtained using the DNS methodology.

B. Comment

It seems likely that mass spectrometric techniques (precise mass analysis and the I.I.C. procedure) are capable of development to provide unambiguous and sensitive analyses of most metabolites as these exist in complex tissue

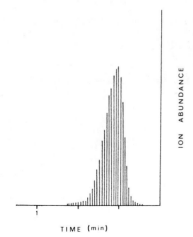

TIME (min)

Fig. 6. Record of the ion current at m/e 137 during evaporation at 220 °C of 1 ng of p-tyramine.

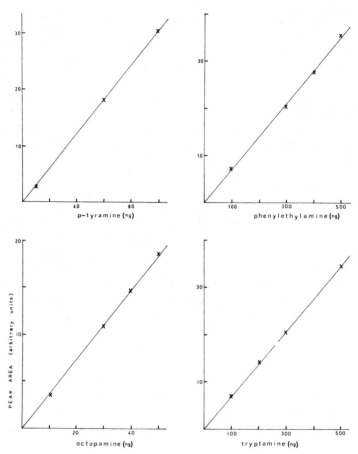

Fig. 7. Typical calibration curves, as obtained by I.I.C. analysis, for *p*-tyramine, octopamine, phenylethylamine, and tryptamine.

Table III.   Regional Distribution of *p*-Tyramine in Rat Brain I.I.C. Technique

Brain Region	Weight (g)[a]	*p*-Tyramine (ng/g tissue)[b]
Hypothalamus	0.044 ± 0.007	1940 ± 224
Caudate	0.076 ± 0.008	892 ± 256
Cerebellum	0.269 ± 0.010	316 ± 49
Stem	0.228 ± 0.011	198 ± 21
"Rest"	1.307 ± 0.035	53 ± 3

[a] Mean $\pm$ standard deviation ($n = 6$).
[b] Mean $\pm$ mean deviation ($n = 5$).

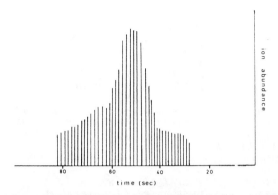

Fig. 8. Record of the ion current at m/e 137 during evaporation at 220 °C of a rat brain phenolic amine extract.

and body fluid extracts. In addition to straightforward analysis as is the case when only a single ion exists at any selected m/e value, it is often possible in addition to make use of the ability of identical ions (isomers) and/or ions with very similar masses to evaporate differentially from the probe and so separate and quantitate each constituent (Boulton and Majer, 1971b, c).

ACKNOWLEDGMENT

We thank Miss M.J.A. Reade for the mass spectrometric determinations and Miss L. Quan for certain of the chromatographic data and for help in obtaining the various rat brain fractions. One of us (AAB) thanks the Psychiatric Services Branch of the Province of Saskatchewan and the Candaian Medical Research Council for continuing support.

REFERENCES

Anagnoste, B., and Goldstein, M. (1967) *Life Sci.* **6**, 1535.
Asatoor, A. M. (1968) *Clin. Chim. Acta* **22**, 223.
Bell, L. E., and Somerville, A. R. (1966) *Biochem. J.* **98**, 16.
Björklund, A., and Falck, B. (1969) *Acta Physiol. Scand.* **77**, 475.
Boulton, A. A. (1967) *Prog. Neurogenetics* **1**, 437.
Boulton, A. A. (1968) *Meth. Biochem. Anal.* **16**, 327.
Boulton, A. A. (1969) in *Chromatographic and Electrophoretic Techniques,* Vol. I (I. Smith, ed.) Heinemann Medical Books Ltd., London, p. 887.
Boulton, A. A. (1971) Unpublished observations.
Boulton, A. A., and Majer, J. R. (1970) *J. Chromatog.* **48**, 322.
Boulton, A. A., and Majer, J. R. (1971a) Unpublished observations.

Boulton, A. A., and Majer, J. R. (1971b) *Meth. Biochem. Anal.* **21** (in press).
Boulton, A. A., and Majer, J. R. (1971c) *Can. J. Biochem.* **49**, 993.
Boulton, A. A., and Milward, L. (1971) *J. Chromatog.* **57**, 287.
Boulton, A. A., Pollitt, R. J., and Majer, J. R. (1967) *Nature.* **215**, 132.
Boulton, A. A., and Quan, Lillian, (1969) 2nd Int. Meeting Int. Soc. Neurochem., Milan.
Boulton, A. A., and Quan, Lillian (1971) Unpublished observations.
Boulton, A. A., Quan, Lillian, and Majer, J. R. (1970) Communication No. 82, 13th Annual Meeting Can. Fed. Biol. Soc., Montreal.
Creveling, C. R., Kondo, K., and Daly, J. W. (1968) *Clin. Chem.* **14**, 302.
Crowshaw, K., Jessup, S. J., and Ramwell, P. W. (1967) *J. Biochem.* **103**, 79.
Faurbye, A. (1968) *Comp. Psychiat.* **9**, 155.
Fischer, E. (1968) *Arz. Forsch.* **18**, 1486.
Goldstein, M., Anagnoste, B., Yamamoto, A., and Felch, W. C. (1970) *J. Pharmac. Exp. Therap.* **171**, 196.
Gray, W. B., and Hartley, B. S. (1963) *J. Biochem.* **89**, 59p.
Gunne, L. M., and Jonsson, J. (1965) *Acta Physiol. Scand.* **64**, 434.
Hempel, K., and Männl, H. F. K. (1966) *N. S. Arch. Pharmak. Exp. Path.* **254**, 448.
Irvine, D., Bayne, W., Miyushita, H., and Majer, J. R. (1969) *Nature* **224**, 811.
Jenkins, A. E., and Majer, J. R. (1967) *Talanta* **14**, 777.
Kakimoto, Y., and Armstrong, M. D. (1962a) *J. Biol. Chem.* **137**, 208.
Kakimoto, Y., and Armstrong, M. D. (1962b) *J. Biol. Chem.* **237**, 422.
Knoche, H., Alfes, H., Mollman, H., and Reisch, J. (1969) *Experientia* **25**, 315.
Majer, J. R., and Boulton, A. A. (1970) *Nature* **225**, 658.
Molinoff, P., and Axelrod, J. (1969) *Science* **164**, 428.
Neadle, D. J., and Pollitt, R. J. (1965) *J. Biochem.* **97**, 607.
Oates, J. A., Nirenberg, P. F., Jepson, J. B., Sjoerdsma, A., and Udenfriend, S. (1963) *Proc. Soc. Exp. Biol. Med.* **112**, 1078.
Procházka, Z. (1958) in *Handbuch der Papier Chromatographie* (I. M. Hais and K. Macek, eds.), Fischer-Verlag, Jena.
Pscheidt, G. R., Berlet, H. H., Spaide, J., and Himwich, H. E. (1966) *Clin. Chim. Acta* **13**, 218.
Seiler, N. (1970) *Meth. Biochem. Anal.* **18**, 259.
Seiler, N. (1971) Personal communication.
Seiler, N., and Wiechman, M. (1964) *Hoppe-Seyler's Z. Physiol. Chem.* **337**, 229.
Seiler, N., and Wiechman, M. (1966) *Zeit. Anal. Chemie.* **220**, 109.
Seiler, N., and Wiechman, M. (1967) *Hoppe-Seyler's Z. Physiol. Chem.* **348**, 1285.
Seiler, N., and Wiechman, M. (1968) *Hoppe-Seyler's Z. Physiol. Chem.* **349**, 588.
Seiler, N., and Wiechman, M. (1969) *Hoppe-Seyler's Z. Physiol. Chem.* **350**, 1493.
Seiler, N., and Wiechman, M. (1970) in *Progress in Thin Layer Chromatography and Related Methods.* Vol. I (A. Niederwieser and H. Pataki, eds.), Ann Arbor-Humphrey, Ann Arbor.
Seiler, N., Werner, G., and Wiechman, M. (1963) *Naturwissenschaften.*
Udenfriend, S. (1962) *Fluorescence Assay in Biology and Medicine,* Academic Press, New York.
Smith, I. (1969) in *Chromatographic and Electrophoretic Techniques,* Vol. I, Heineman Medical Books, London, 104.
Smith, I., and Kellow, A. H. (1969) *Nature* **221**, 1261.
Spector, S., Melmon, K., Lovenberg, W., and Sjoerdsma, A. (1963) *J. Pharm. Exp. Therap.* **140**, 229.
Quan, Lillian (1970) M. Sc. Thesis, University of Saskatchewan.
Weber, G. (1952) *J. Biochem.* **51**, 157.

Index